CELL SHOCK

Our starving cells
The biological energy crisis of our time

AF823982

Dr Rodney Lopez

MBBS (Sydney) Grad.Cert.Nutri.Med (RMIT) FASLM

Bulk Ordering Information: Special discounts are available on quantity purchases by corporations, associations, and others. Contact the "Special Sales Department" at this email address: **admin@a8h.com.au**

Connect with the author and keep up to date with the latest research:

www.a8h.com.au

Cell Shock/Dr Rodney Lopez. —1st ed
ISBN: 978-1-7636667-6-4

Disclaimer

This book is intended to provide general information only about nutrition, dietary supplements, and health.

The author and publisher have made every effort to ensure the accuracy and completeness of the information contained within. However, we do not guarantee the accuracy of the information, and it may be subject to change over time. The views are those of the author and not of any reviewer mentioned as a contributor. The author and publisher expressly disclaim responsibility for any adverse effects arising from the use or application of the information contained herein.

While this book does discuss health, nutrition, and medical topics, it is not meant to replace professional medical advice. Always seek the advice of your physician or other qualified health provider with any questions you may have regarding a medical condition. Never disregard professional medical advice or delay in seeking it because of something you have read in this book. However, it is also important for you to know that it is your inalienable right to pursue health solutions beyond orthodoxy, which you know to be the correct path but to do so with detailed knowledge from various professionals and from your research into the concepts presented.

Suppose you choose to use any supplements or follow any nutritional advice within this book. In that case, you do so of your own accord and accept any risk and adverse outcome that may occur. Adverse reactions may apply to any pharmaceutical, supplement or herbal preparation. The author and publisher are not responsible for any harm or injury that may result. It is always recommended to consult with a healthcare provider before starting any new diet, exercise program, or dietary and supplement regimen.

Contents

Introduction: Our Cellular Energy Crisis 9
A medical war we have already lost 114
"Prediabetes": A huge missed opportunity 178
Creating a starving cell is very easy in the 21st-century! 233
Fiendish Fructose: Swift ATP depletion, insulin resistance, fatty liver 295
That's no way to treat a metabolic biomarker 325
Revolution Time 381
Nutritional Ketosis (NK) 409
Appendix-1: Fructose Metabolism 480
Appendix-2: AMPK Function 481
Appendix-3: The Randle Cycle 482
Appendix-4: Excess Glucose & Intracellular Fat Cells 483
Appendix-5: Statins, Heme-A, CoQ10 Impacts 484
Appendix-6: How Does Epigenetics Work? 485
Appendix-7: Krebs Citric Acid Cycle B-Group, Minerals & Vitamins 486
Appendix-8: High and Low Fructose Foods 487
Appendix-9: High Energy Triglycerides 488
Appendix-10: Lipoproteins 489
Appendix-11: NAD^+ 490
Appendix-12: Citrulline, Nitric Oxide & Erectile Dysfunction 491
Appendix-13 Insulin Resistance 492
Appendix-14: Insulin Resistance & Diabetes 493
Appendix-15: The 3 Stages of ATP Production 494
Appendix-16: OXPHOS 495
Appendix-17: Electron Transport Chain (ETC) Components 496
Appendix-18: Postprandial (After-Eating) Effects 497
Appendix-19: Choline and the GABA Switch 498
Appendix-20: The Critical Nature of Magnesium in Vitamin D Activation 499
Appendix-21: Vegetable & Fruit Nutrients 500

Appendix-22: Activ8Health Resources 501
Appendix-23: Omega-3, Omega-6 Pathways 502
Appendix-24: Hidden Hunger. The Myth of an Optimal Diet 503
Appendix-25: Drug vs Supplement Risk Bar Chart 504
Appendix-26: Drugs vs Supplement Risk Bubble Chart 505
Appendix-27: NAD^+ Sirtuins and Protein Activation 506
Appendix-28: NAD^+ vs NADH 507
Appendix-29: Krebs Cycle NADH & FADH2 508
Appendix-30: Long-term trends in diabetes. CDC Graph 509
Appendix-31: Early IR Markers 510
Appendix-32: AETT, Toxic Wounds, Perfume & Fragrance Toxicity 511
Appendix-33: Lessons From The Laron Syndrome 512
Appendix-34: Brain Impacts 513
Appendix-35: Adverse Drug Reactions (ADRs) 514
Appendix-36: Multivitamin Components 515
Appendix-37: The Activ8Health Antioxidant Plate (One variation) 516
Appendix-38: The Food Pyramid 1992 – 2005 517
Appendix-39: The DASH Diet: Recommendations & Flaws 518
Appendix-40: Exercise 519
Appendix-41: Vitamin-C, Scurvy Haptogobin (HP-2-2) Genetic Variant 520
Bibliography 521

Lisa Pearson (King) Dietitian (APD)

This book is the health wake-up call everyone needs. It is a passionate, interesting, and well-researched read that highlights the importance of preventative health and why current medical and nutrition interventions are failing us. This book helps to point us in the right direction with useful insights into how we can improve our health. After reading this, you'll be convinced of the need for change in health prevention, diagnosis, treatment, and public health recommendations.

Accredited Practising Dietitian (APD)

Accredited Nutritionist (AN)

BNutrDiet (Hons), Dip Nut, Cert III/IV Fitness

Olwen Chell Dietitian (APD)

After graduating in 2004 and having worked in South Africa, New Zealand and Australia, it has been a privilege to work with Dr Rodney Lopez for the past few years. His book "Cell Shock" contains fascinating insights into cellular and metabolic processes. The book sheds light on nutritional choices and eating patterns and how changes in dietary inputs can improve health and energy levels and significantly reduce the risk of chronic disease. He provides a compelling case that much of the nutritional advice that is given today is based on outdated information and needs to be updated to take into account the latest research. Thank you, Dr Lopez, for your very informative book and insights.

Accredited Practising Dietitian (APD)

BSc Diet Postgrad Dipl Diet

Diabetes Educator

Master Trainer in the Stanford Model of Care

Postgraduate paper on Eating Disorders

I dedicate this book to my clever daughters, Courtney and Caitlin; my bright son, Jamison; my wonderful son-in-law, Andrew; and my amazing grandsons, Luca (5), Tyler (3); and our newborn, Noah.

"A new scientific truth does not triumph by convincing its opponents and making them see the light, but rather because its opponents eventually die, and a new generation grows up that is familiar with it."... **Max Planck**

*"You never change things by fighting the existing reality. To change something, build a new model that makes the existing model obsolete."...***Buckminster Fuller**

Our Cellular Energy Crisis

Insulin Resistance (IR), Metabolic Dysfunction, Prediabetes, Metabolic Syndrome (MetS), Many Cancers, Mental Health Disorders, Obesity, Diabetes, Heart & Vascular Disease and an Explosion of Chronic Metabolic Diseases: ***All wicked problems, all linked, and all an inconvenient truth***

"Medical science has made such tremendous progress that there is hardly a healthy human left."

---Aldous Huxley---

"***In this world, nothing can be said to be certain, except death and taxes***". This quote is attributed to Benjamin Franklin, but we can now add another to this list of certainties in 21st-century life:

ACQUIRED CHRONIC METABOLIC DISEASES.

Chronic illnesses are wicked diseases with wicked outcomes.

Thomas Hobbes, one of history's most famous cynics, stated that life is '***nasty, brutish, and short.***' Yet, there is nothing cynical about these terms when we view them through the lens of anyone suffering from debilitating chronic illnesses.

None of us can escape chronic metabolic diseases in our lifetime, at least not if we continue to adopt the current undeniably failed medical and dietary models. In life, we bide our time and wait for those telltale signs of a chronic illness to strike and hope a lethal and preventable cancer, heart attack or stroke doesn't take us out quickly. Mental health problems are a part of this abnormal metabolic process, as we will discuss. We will inevitably all witness loved ones suffer slowly and die from many highly preventable chronic diseases. In them, we will see our future and realise that similar fates await all of us one day. We can thus appreciate Hobbes' aphorism that life is indeed ***nasty***, ***brutish***, and, in many instances, way too ***short.***

Frightening prevalence statistics have emerged in recent decades for chronic metabolic diseases, which make up, by far, the majority of diseases threatening all of us. These are the same diseases flooding every doctor's appointment scheduler and are the very same diseases filling beds in hospitals that are crushing our healthcare systems globally. Even more frightening are the prevalence statistics that are yet to come in the next two to three decades. An article in the American Heart Association's publication ***Circulation*** has warned of the coming ***tsunamis*** of chronic diseases with cardiovascular (heart and blood vessel) diseases at the crest of this tsunami of death and destruction, merely one to two decades ahead (Califf 2021). A massive surge of killer diseases is coming our way.

Every human on this planet will face a chronic disease sooner or later. Often, it's sooner rather than later, and frequently, multiple diseases will emerge in your lifetime, threatening to destroy your life prematurely. Please don't hold your breath waiting for governments or public health bodies to come to your rescue anytime soon. It's up to you, the fleet-footed individual, to make changes and a difference in your own life. You don't need sweeping societal changes to protect your health. By making deeply personal choices, you can avoid preventable medical disasters and thrive in the prime of your life, full of health and vitality, rather than being riddled with sickness.

The sad fact is that on that large population scale, we can correct this whole mess of a problem through doable changes in food and other harmful 21st-century inputs. So why are we all facing destructive and deadly diseases in our lifetimes, and why are we putting populations and nations at great risk rather than changing highly modifiable inputs? This question is not hard to answer and is, in fact, very easy to answer if we consider that money and economic imperatives matter more than lives. Money and greed are the ugly (nasty) side of human nature. So it is no wonder that we are all facing metabolic disease armageddon in our own lives and within populations, causing nations to struggle unnecessarily.

This book aims to unpack how and why this monstrous chronic disease pandemic has been "set on fire" as a result of overt, covert or naïve policies that have enabled self-interest and vested interests to call the shots. I will also discuss how governments are major players in this metabolic disease crisis, and politicians need to know their huge and undeniable role in propelling this healthcare nightmare into the stratosphere.

What is never done in this metabolic disease story is putting the pieces together where dots are joined, thus shedding light on all the synergistic inputs and blunders in medical (and dietary) thinking that have allowed humanity to reach a crisis point that is yet another existential threat. Using my extensive medical experience and postgraduate studies, I will unpack this story and join the dots for you. Without this educational background and deep nutritional insights, it would be unbelievably difficult for anyone to make sense of this disaster. Otherwise, it becomes very easy for the medical profession, Pharma, agricultural and food corporations to hoodwink politicians or the lay public through complexity and gaslighting.

After you see a clear picture emerge and how we have lost opportunities to reverse this healthcare disaster, you may be angered by what you learn. I am sure you will wonder why we have allowed such neglect to take hold that has allowed highly modifiable and reversible diseases to reach dizzying heights in populations and are now set to threaten humanity. Far-fetched, you may be thinking? I will prove it to you page by page.

It's important to remember that we are talking about highly preventable diseases that we as a society allow to run rampant in populations due to poor leadership in governments and weak, ineffective medical and dietary professions. If we take into consideration the horrendous health-damaging toll on individuals (all of us eventually) and then the massive death toll globally due to chronic metabolic diseases, it is then unforgivable for governments and the medical and dietetic professions to stay passive in the face of this healthcare disaster, and yet they do.

The top of the list of chronic metabolic diseases we see ending our lives includes "diabetes", a heart attack (highly likely), a stroke (also very likely), dementia (more and more likely) or a preventable cancer of one kind or another. Once these diseases manifest in our lives, then life changes drastically. Mortality comes knocking on your door. Throughout this book, I will be greatly challenging your ideas about what causes chronic disease and what constitutes "healthy food". I do take a swipe at both the medical and dietetic professions, but with good reason. These are noble fields that have been hijacked and undermined by self-interest and vested interests. It is time for integrity and honour to reemerge. It is time for governments to understand how they are helping to fan the flames of this devastating pandemic of chronic illness, including mental health disorders. The way we treat chronic metabolic diseases and mental health issues (also metabolic problems) is unbelievably primitive.

My wish for my medical profession and for that of dietetics is that they must take up the challenge to strip themselves of all commercial interests that do not meet the criteria for individual and population health. As I will discuss, both the medical and dietetic professions are facing unprecedented enormous challenges in the 21st-century. However, they continue to rely on outdated models that are woefully inadequate for addressing the chronic metabolic diseases prevalent today. ***We know this as we have already lost this war.***

From Pharma to agriculture and food production, manufacturing and distribution, political interests are present at all points in this chain, poised to siphon duties or taxes and quid pro quo agreements at every turn in the food-related money-making process. Governments wield coercive force over dietary recommendations, bending the will of those to suit their agenda. From food pyramids to government-backed food guidelines, what hope does an individual have when food inputs are the greatest threat to our health in our lifetimes and where financial imperatives distort these food inputs?

Governments need to rally teams of ***polymaths*** in every food-related department to change the very nature of food and strip away the harmful impacts of foods and food components that damage us meal-by-meal and snack-by-snack. We will look at the huge harm that after-eating (postprandial) impacts have on our health.

Later on, I will describe a proposed department under a Future Generations Healthcare Commissioner (FGHC), a brilliant concept that began in Wales (UK) whose focus is entirely on the health of current and future generations. I propose a health department full of highly intelligent polymaths who are experts in multiple areas and called "***Renaissance men or women***". No medical or dietetic guru would dare try to pull the wool over the eyes of these polymaths with mumbo jumbo facts for fear of looking downright foolish in the eyes of a polymath. More on this much-needed FGHC department is in the chapter ***Revolution Time***.

Many laws are designed to protect people from themselves, and yet the greatest personal danger to an individual is made up of ignored food inputs. Society eventually picks up the tab for the slack controls that are in place for food consumption, which ultimately leads to preventable diseases that will need to be dealt with through our increasingly failing healthcare systems. It is not about destroying agriculture or food interests. What we must do, however, is change the very nature of food. Otherwise, we will all go over the cliff soon, all because medicine and dietetics are failing to halt this juggernaut of chronic metabolic diseases. We must help change agricultural practices and alter food production and manufacturing processes. Is agriculture and food production so special that we exempt them from having to adapt and change in a world beset by change? We must force change upon these industries. It is a huge opportunity.

I will be discussing the many impacts of foods few people ever consider in the causation of diseases, along with other critical factors driving this never-ending, ever-increasing pandemic of debilitating and deadly chronic metabolic diseases. Medicine needs to admit fault in a *mea culpa* moment that acknowledges the many blunders made over decades now that are propelling this metabolic disease pandemic to ever greater heights. Let's look at these factors in-depth to understand why you are at huge risk. Let me now pull the rug from under our cherished ideas about common staple foods and introduce you to the concept of food-related biological damage.

The dark side of staple foods

I will put forward compelling evidence to show you how a large number of staple foods we regard as "healthy" are, in fact, a major player in causing and accelerating disease processes throughout our lives, pushing all of us towards nasty and brutish chronic illnesses that are seemingly inevitable in all humans. That food harms us all biologically with every meal and snack is not something that can be contested. The extensive existing research shows how food damages all of us from the cradle to the grave, and the weight of this research is overwhelming. That food causes biological damage is beyond any sane argument to the contrary, but this does not mean that food-related damage cannot be gaslighted by those with skin in the game where money is at stake to create doubt and confusion about food inputs in everyone. Medical and dietetic models are swamped with vested interests from every angle, and as the Americans say, we must drain the swamp if we are to have any chance to avoid the inevitable chronic disease armageddon ahead.

So, for governments to steer the food-related ship from paddock to plate, siphoning money along the whole way is a huge conflict of interest between financial imperatives and the health of their populations and nations. This conflict of interest is an ethical disgrace. Remember, we have ***tsunamis*** of chronic disease heading our way soon. Also, it is vital to consider that, as mentioned, we have already lost this war on chronic metabolic diseases in a big way.

Medical and dietary models must be updated to meet the urgent needs of our time, far beyond the silver bullet approaches that have been used to great effect, like antibiotics in the last century. However, the current 21st-century "silver bullets" used for chronic metabolic diseases simply bounce off these diseases, allowing the underlying progressive ***biological rot*** to continue untouched in the background. After-eating (postprandial) impacts are ignored as a powerful factor that drives ***biological rot*** throughout our lives. These well-documented, highly researched staple food impacts in our bloodstream after eating, if ignored, will ensure we have no hope of stopping this outrageous pandemic of chronic diseases.

Biological Rot

Biological rot is a term I have coined so you can conceptualise the biological damage caused to all our cells, tissues, large and small vascular networks, and organ systems, just like any other organic or inorganic material that is allowed to undergo progressive damage (rot) like iron rusting without intervention to halt this process. Biological rot occurs throughout our lifetimes and is driven by multiple factors, where dietary inputs lead the charge towards ongoing cumulative biological rot in all those cells and tissues.

Biological rot is ongoing "rust" that starts in the womb and accelerates to our tombs. This rot occurs every day in everyone. The terms biological rot and biological damage will be used interchangeably. Failing to target this biological rot seals our fates. Drugs never halt and reverse biological rot; hence, their abject failure to halt the march of chronic disease despite a bagful of drugs that are essentially useless in this war on highly preventable diseases.

We imagine that we have mythical creatures walking among us that are medically "normal" with pristine cells, tissues, and vascular and organ systems. Yet, "normal" doesn't exist. "Normal" is a fantasy. No one is left untouched by biological rot that accelerates from the womb to the tomb. Children are not untouched. We just don't have the ultra-sensitive tools to detect biological damage at extremely early points as yet. Yet this damage will undoubtedly be there unseen at an undetected biochemical and molecular level, just waiting to accelerate and destroy lives in the chronic phase of this process, which we will discuss soon. However, we do have very early biomarkers that I will discuss later, indicating abnormal metabolic processes are occurring far earlier in our lives than we would like. Ignoring these early warning signals also seals our fates.

Illness doesn't begin with a disastrous resounding medical alert; it has been brewing beneath the surface, often unnoticed, until it reaches a critical point. Chronic diseases are a lifelong enterprise. This ***biological rot*** is driven from the time a pregnant woman consumes volumes of high-energy, low-nutrient, low-fibre staples or ultra-processed foods to the time we inflict staple foods on our babies with nutrient-poor cereal purees or bland nutrient-deficient and carb-loaded gruels or when we expose these babies to a flood of dairy, animal flesh, sugar, fructose, etc. To think that these staple food exposures with those massive after-eating impacts will not affect the future health outcomes of those babies is indeed fantastical thinking. We trigger long-term biological rot in our babies.

Yet when we have "selfish" political hands that encourage such eating patterns to push their agricultural economic agendas, then what can we expect other than staple foods being presented by dietitians as the norm and where damaging staple foods become the only way to nourish our children and all of us as adults? You will be amazed at how each staple food type can inflict such enormous biological damage on all of us. From the time of the Neolithic Revolution around 12,000 years ago to the Green and Farming Revolutions of the 1960s and 70s, we have truly distorted staple foods to unrecognizable horror foods that inflict so much damage to us biologically, thus driving biological rot to our graves.

Regarding societal, governmental, and public health neglect, you have a choice: either become a victim of structural neglect or take a stand for yourself and your loved ones.

Cereal Grains: Our nemesis in many ways

I will touch upon the ignored risk of consuming grain-based foods, from micronutrient inadequacy to the surges in glucose and insulin/IgF-1 that occur in our bloodstream after consuming high-starch cereal grains. This rise in glucose in our bloodstream after eating can stay elevated for many hours after consumption. High glucose levels may never come down in someone with insulin resistance (most of us now). Grains make up a major part of food consumption in wealthy and developing countries. Grain micronutrient inadequacies and glucose-spiking effects can lead to heart disease, vascular disease, dementia and Alzheimer's. All these diseases make up the bulk of deaths worldwide. Is it any wonder?

As Professor Loren Cordain stated in his brilliant paper, ***Cereal Grains: Humanity's Double-Edged Sword***, it is unbelievable to think that out of 195,000 edible plants, we have chosen less than 0.1% of them, or around 300 species, as edible food. We are driven by the idea of grain yield and not nutrient density. We pay no attention to the potentially harmful after-eating effects or weak nutrient or fibre content of foods created from grains. I will expose the dark side of individual staple foods in the BIG-10 Womb-to-Tomb list at the end of the next chapter. Be prepared to be surprised by the effects of common foods you grew up with and no doubt love.

There are far healthier options than many staple foods. These staples include eggs, dairy, animal flesh, grains, cereals, legumes, high-starch root vegetables, fructose, sugar, fructose-rich fruits, fructose-rich fruit juices and vegetable oils, and yet, due to propaganda, people feel compelled to consume these foods out of fear their health will suffer. They fear their babies will become weak and sick and will not grow if they are not fed a high-staple food diet. I will put my case forward that it is because of these very staple foods that we are not seeing chronic diseases plummet and why they are at the heart of food-generated ***biological rot throughout our lifetimes,*** putting all of us at risk from poor food intake and poor food composition. We prime our babies for future poor health by the very staples inflicted on them. Chronic disease all starts in the womb and our baby stage. Chronic disease is driven from childhood onwards.

Staple foods (not all of them) are the reason people get sicker and why we program babies to fail health-wise long-term. It is no wonder that deadly health outcomes are occurring in younger and younger people. We do have horror processed staple foods, but it is not the processing that makes them bad; staple foods are ***intrinsically damaging*** to our bodies as all these foods have to be digested, and the digested components are then carried to cells in our bloodstream after eating a meal, and these digested components are glucose or fats (triglycerides), amino acids and a range of nutrients needed by our trillions of cells and organ systems to survive. But there is a price to pay for nourishing our bodies with digested food components, triggering all the frightening changes we see in the blood after we consume a meal, as summarised in Appendix-18.

What is stated above is the reason we have such conflicting research between processed, ultra-processed and whole foods all because we are convinced that whole foods can do absolutely no harm, and so we consume staples thinking we will be fine because, after all, governments, dietetic bodies and dietitians endorse staple foods as "healthy" and encourage us to consume them without fear.

We inflict this adverse health destiny in many dietary ways as we cling to agricultural economic imperatives. Professions playing dumb about these obvious drivers of disease keep disease creation ongoing. Food corporations understandably ignore the effects of their enterprises on disease causation, and then we have Pharma benefitting enormously from a world saturated with never-ending, ever-increasing disease prevalence. Pharma heaven, right?

Governments, farming groups or food boards don't want to hear about food-induced biological damage? And yet, we would all be crushed by the weight of scientific research that has documented the damaging effects of various staple foods in the after-eating (postprandial) period for decades now, leading to biological damage (biological rot). After-eating impacts are so easily modified but are ignored and are a wasted opportunity for good. The damaging effects of "healthy" staple foods are a very inconvenient truth.

When Titans Clash: Insulin Resistance Meets After-Eating Impacts Head-On

Making matters much worse is a ubiquitous scourge of a problem in insulin resistance and metabolic dysfunction globally that meets after-eating impacts head-on to produce a combined damaging juggernaut of lifelong biological damage. This clash of insulin resistance and metabolic dysfunction, along with these after-eating (postprandial) effects, merge to become the mega engine driving abnormal metabolic processes, leading to all our feared chronic illnesses. Dreadful food inputs can also spark the insulin resistance-metabolic dysfunction process in the first place, and I will show you how this happens due to various food-related after-eating effects and the many food-related strikes on energy-generating biochemical and metabolic pathways adversely impacting energy (ATP) production. As cell energy declines, entropy (chaos, decay, and deterioration) begins to dominate within our cells. We ignore cell bioenergetics to our peril and allow entropy to run rampant.

The time has come for the medical and dietetic professions to either adapt or perish, as disruptive technologies in both occupations are here now. From nutrigenomics (nutrition genetics) to complete gut microbiome analysis to functional laboratory tests, all of these are moving forward at a rapid, highly disruptive pace. We also have food technologies like 3D food printing and the monumental changes in the very nature of staple foods now happening. These health professions will need to jump on board or look downright foolish in the face of the lay public, who will be far more knowledgeable in terms of diet-related impacts than them.

We are reaching a dangerous point now in this pandemic of preventable diseases. The public can sense the deceit in the medical and dietetic management options being forced upon them. There is a huge and justifiable distrust of pharmaceuticals and a great distrust of the medical and dietary models that see all of humanity destined for ongoing biological damage and chronic diseases despite any treatment being offered. Dietary advice just fans the flames.

The staggering changes in supermarket food options over the past decade, from plant-based protein sources to dairy-free and egg-free alternatives, have nothing to do with the medical or dietetic professions. These professions are too entrenched in their self-interested bubbles to recognise the food revolution being driven by the public and their demands. The medical and dietetic professions are peripheral to this revolution instead of driving it.

Like feral animals cornered, vested interests will fight back during this time of upheaval that challenges their interests. But this challenge will only accelerate. Crunch time looms over the horizon, and gaslighting by vested interests will take on a steroid-driven frenzy. The day of reckoning is very near, but who will pay for this healthcare disaster that has taken 100s of millions of lives over 60 years? Who will be tarred and feathered? Will all the gurus of medicine and dietetics in the pockets of vested interests that have helped drive this healthcare disaster scurry up their Ivy League towers and vanish, or will they be held to account? Time will tell.

Our failed medical and dietetic models will crash and burn, but out of the ashes, hopefully, wonderful models will emerge with health at the heart of everything they do.

Let my challenge to the medical and dietetic models begin

One of the challenges I will start with is something extremely important and has to do with the very flimsy framework we have created around metabolic disease biomarkers and our focus on certain glucose cut-off points. Most of this framework is now totally outdated and belongs to a bygone era. This shaky metabolic diagnostic and management framework is now adding to the explosive prevalence of acquired chronic metabolic diseases globally. This construct of biomarker cut-offs must disappear.

Each year, millions undergo tests for blood biomarkers, the critical indicators that signal metabolic dysfunction – which is our cellular processes going off course. These biomarkers will normally include glucose or lipid fractions such as cholesterol, LDL or triglycerides, to name a few. "Diabetes" will be diagnosed on the basis of a high fasting blood glucose level or through a 2-hour Glucose Tolerance Test (GTT) as the main tests used for diagnosis.

You may have noticed I have written "diabetes" in inverted commas, indicating this disease is not what it seems to be. Yet 100s of millions of people are diagnosed with it and will suffer the deadly consequences of this problem globally. The medical implications of this "disease" are horrendous and include heart disease, strokes, dementia, mental health problems, kidney failure, gangrene, and blindness, to name a few. More diseases are listed on the back cover.

Yet, these blood glucose levels are just a snapshot frozen in time along a continuum of change that, more likely than not, will accelerate towards the devastating chronic diseases we will all face in our lifetimes. More on fake cut-offs and fake labels will come.

I will use the term "diabetes" synonymously with "Type-2 Diabetes Mellitus (T2DM)". T2DM is an acquired form of diabetes and the most common by far. More than 95% of cases are T2DM, according to the WHO. Our obsessive focus on T2DM has been an unmitigated disaster for reasons that will unfold as you read on.

"Diabetes" is often referred to as the "***mother***" of chronic metabolic diseases with an early (acute) and late (chronic) phase (Bengmark 2004). Waiting for glaring biomarker signals like a high blood glucose level has been our absolute downfall. It has, in fact, been a complete tragedy that allows tremendous biological damage to occur ***long before*** and ***long after ANY*** biomarker signal. This flimsy biomarker cut-off framework has done nothing to stop the steamroller of metabolic diseases now crushing healthcare systems worldwide. We are fragmenting a process that should never be fragmented: ***One process, many "diseases", many outcomes.***

We wait and wait for biomarker signals to "shout" "look at us," but then what? As I will discuss, no drug has come anywhere near halting and reversing the damage done to our vascular and organ systems caused by unstoppable ***biological rot***, but that doesn't stop medical practitioners from making the diagnosis in the first place and then scratching their heads as if to say, "what do we do now"? We don't have even one curative drug that says "***you shall not pass***" beyond this biomarker point (cut-off) and then push this metabolic process back to a normal state. Not one drug will halt and reverse the relentless disease-generating process that is biological rot. This biological rot continues uninterrupted in the background of all of us towards vascular and multiple organ failure. Do you know of anyone immune to organ failure? So, no drug stops this rot. Why have we ignored this obvious and deadly process that ***CAN*** be halted and pushed back through nutrient-based interventions? Vested interests, do you think? Money and not life matter in corporate thinking.

As you will see, Metformin, the go-to drug, is pathetic and has an adverse effect on an Electron Transport Chain (ETC) component in the mitochondria, affecting energy production. Metformin is no saviour. Yet we write millions of scripts for Metformin just to do something. This gaslighting of drugs that does its best to squeeze out even remotely positive drug results has seen the rise and rise of chronic diseases worldwide. The slow creep towards multiorgan failure and polypharmacy (multiple drugs) is never held back, and so we walk a tightrope by adding more and more drugs. Why do we need to add other "drug buddies" if any drug alone is brilliant?

Relentless ***biological rot*** is the underlying reason we see more and more complicated presentations in our healthcare systems that require more and more drugs to deal with this or that complication. Our healthcare system is totally ill-prepared for these highly complex multiorgan failure presentations, and so this pandemic of ever-increasing medical complexity presentations marches on.

It is time to push for a definitive cure and not just the band-aid approaches that drugs offer. Metabolic disease is a vicious beast with a ferocious bite that you cannot tame with pharmaceuticals. It is no victory in the least that we simply hold back a catastrophic medical event with a drug— simply delaying a deadly condition in individuals is not curative or brilliant in the least. We have ignored established dietary interventions that have led to cures and decreased ***all-cause***

mortality all because we kneel at the altar of Pharma and failed drug-centric approaches.

Our true "mother" of chronic metabolic diseases

Once again, the term "mother" of chronic diseases as applied to "diabetes" is misplaced because the true "mother" of not only "diabetes" but all the other fake metabolic labels, such as "prediabetes" or "Metabolic Syndrome (MetS)" is discussed below and in chapters ahead. These labels are simply points on a ***continuum*** of glucose and metabolic changes leading to an increasing risk of multi-organ damage and failure being propelled from the cradle to the grave by multiple modifiable inputs.

Which organs fail will then define our fake disease labels, such as heart disease, kidney, Alzheimer's, etc. "Diabetes" is only a mere stop on the way to all these diseases. "Diabetes" is not a bona fide disease, as suggested in the literature, but is defined by an arbitrary glucose cut-off point on a continuum of glucose change. Renowned metabolic disease experts have fiercely challenged cut-off points.

The glucose cut-off for diabetes is an extremely high glucose level on this continuous (yet fixable) path towards horrendous (wicked) diseases with wicked outcomes. As we will discuss, this continuum of risk for disease occurs long ***before, between and long after*** cut-off points and even between our normal range goalposts (Kahn, Cooper et al. 2014). More on normal ranges and what I have coined "***quintile climbs***" later. Any result falling between two laboratory goalposts doesn't mean all is well and that you can relax, far from it.

How can any blip on the way to chronic disease along a continuum of increasing risk be considered a disease? However, I do get that a continuum of risk was never considered in the early stages of this disease emerging from the 1960s. Diabetes was as rare as hen's teeth before 1960. We have been left with a broken and distorted legacy of biomarker cut-offs and labels as having more significance and relevance than other points on this continuum of risk when ***ALL*** points on this continuum have the potential to reach the end of the line – our acquired chronic metabolic diseases.

As an individual reading this book, it is important to understand that you already have biological damage from birth, and the aim is to halt and reverse this rot as much as possible by knowing what drives it. Luckily, that information is found in this book.

Like many dead ends in medicine, cut-offs and fake labels are an embarrassing but understandable historical *faux pas*, and yet I am looking in hindsight with the clarity of knowledge we only now have, so I can't be too smug about this. Everything is absolutely clear in retrospect, as we all know. What I can be angry about is why these false medical constructs continue in the face of undeniable failure, as shown in horrendous chronic disease prevalence statistics—failure to act results in the loss of tens of millions of lives every year.

Advanced glucose cut-off points make the medical profession think they are doing something worthwhile in dividing a continuum of glucose change with "***GPS tags***" along a continuous track, but by doing so, they allow a tremendous amount of biological damage to occur irrespective of "GPS tags". How does a cut-off stop the rot?

Our concepts of "normal ranges" are now highly embarrassing and adding to chronic disease prevalence. They are not "normal" by any means but are simply a continuum of risk between laboratory goalposts that doctors are reassured by and, in turn, reassure their patients. In fact, risk starts even before the lower goalpost. An ignored "Quintile Climb" within a normal range warns of risk.

High blood pressure, high blood glucose, high uric acid levels

It is staggering that over 100 years ago, a Swede Eskil Kylin published an article in 1923 that suggested the existence of the "***hypertension-hyperglycemia-hyperuricemia***" syndrome, and if I put this in lay terms, this is the high blood pressure (hypertension), high blood glucose (hyperglycemia) and a high uric acid level (hyperuricemia) syndrome.

Many of those with gout or kidney stones will know about high uric acid level complications. 100s of millions of people now have this exact cluster of clinical problems, as described by Eskil Kylin, diagnosed in them. Vast numbers are clueless that they even have these problems. It took Gerald Reaven's 1988 Banting Lecture to cement what Eskil Kylin stated 65 years before him, and Reaven labelled this cluster of medical problems as "Syndrome-X", now termed "Metabolic Syndrome (MetS)" (Bengmark 2004).

MetS is exploding in prevalence worldwide, where an alarming 1 in 3 people in their mid-20s onwards have this problem diagnosed in them. This prevalence is in Australia and many other countries. It is incredibly shocking then that we condemn masses of 20-somethings to a life of cardiovascular disease and early death. Metabolic Syndrome (MetS), in fact, is not a clinical diagnosis by a long shot. It is only a jumble of clinical problems that, like "diabetes", occurs along this metabolic dysfunction continuum.

The components of MetS, like high blood pressure, large waist circumference, high glucose levels, etc., are all adaptations or branches that come off the one metabolic thread, which is our ***insulin resistance-metabolic dysfunction continuum.*** These adaptations, as I will explain, are not random events but can all be seen as survival mechanisms for cells in distress crying out for help.

Why, then, does the medical profession move at the pace of a snail on opioids? That someone over 100 years ago, long before Gerald Reaven had the brilliance to join the dots without all of the technology and data resources of today to see a connection (a thread) is a sad reflection on medical reductionism and vested interest distortion. I will expand on this scourge of medical reductionism under the ***Gordian Knot*** later in this chapter.

Scientific reductionism has been a disaster for humanity. Focusing on drug targets is a victory for a few genetic diseases. Yet drugs have failed for billions at risk of chronic diseases that have no killer genetic cause and no sledgehammer single factor. So, why do we adopt reductionism for diseases beyond reductionism? Many corporations, though, do thrive in a world riddled with diseases.

This cluster of problems mentioned by Kylin over a century ago became a nightmare from the 1960s on, as I will discuss. We sweat the small things where, in the end, all we need to do is modify the blatantly obvious inputs and, ultimately, as far as managing these metabolic diseases is concerned, only prevention and cure matters. Who cares about the biochemical or molecular mechanisms in-depth, as that may take centuries to completely unravel (if we even survive chronic disease armageddon) and indulge in research while we watch people drop off like flies from one disease after another that we could have prevented without such reductionism?

However, Pharma does care as they salivate at the thought that they can find the slightest chink in the biochemical or molecular armour and develop a drug that has even some remote impact on chronic metabolic disease, not to cure anything but only to manage disease states, gaslight effectiveness and make a ton of money. There is no altruism here, only the quest for pharmaceutical gold.

Both the medical and dietetic professions will be ripped apart with great disgrace as we all see the deep chasms emerging in healthcare. ***We have an abundance of drugs and yet no cure for even a single chronic metabolic disease.*** What a complete disgrace. As I will discuss in this chapter, the failure of drugs is highly predictable. We do nothing for the inputs, with diet being the most impactful, and we do nothing for the ongoing "***biological rot***" that takes all of us out. Thus, we face tsunamis of disease ahead.

Our medical and dietary assumptions are tremendously flawed, and I want to explain why. Suppose we don't target the drivers of biological rot. In that case, we have no chance at all as it is highly naïve of reductionism to think one biochemical or molecular drug target can overcome the wealth of cellular insults over a lifetime from the womb to the tomb that causes harm.

High blood pressure, high blood glucose, high blood uric acid, insulin resistance, "Prediabetes", "Type-2 Diabetes Mellitus (Diabetes)", and "Metabolic Syndrome (MetS)" are all undeniably a part of the insulin resistance–metabolic dysfunction continuum and yet how many doctors know this? Many doctors see these labels as ***standalone*** problems, which they are not. ***Metabolic dysfunction*** can be seen as cell metabolism behaving badly, causing multiple long-term conditions (Khunti, Chudasama et al. 2023).

Reaching the point of "diabetes" is a complete failure in my mind. This failure occurs when a continuum of glucose change and risk is not seen as a threat from even the earliest glimmer of **metabolic** change and is just left to run rampant with no drug to halt the underlying damage caused over time. We look into these disease "faces" (labels) and see and treat individual organs failing. By doing so, we miss the point completely, which is that ***one process drives multi-organ failure simultaneously.*** The skyrocketing prevalence of chronic metabolic diseases is due to this failure to see one path with many disease labels (disease "faces").

Multi-organ failure starts at the level of cells. It is our cells that make up organs and are thus the fundamental unit of an organ that needs to be protected at all costs. Cells becoming starved of energy (bioenergetic decline) and structurally damaged (increasing entropy) are all highly predictable problems. The brilliant ***Cell Starvation Model (CSM)*** will be our metabolic disease guide.

For far too long, we have used failed drug approaches and totally ignored the foundational cause of chronic disease, which is cellular bioenergetic (energy) decline, thus sealing the fate of billions of people worldwide. This failure of both the medical and dietetic professions to focus on cell bioenergetics has combined to drive the greatest healthcare disaster of all time in world history. Unless we challenge the very nature of the medical and dietetic models and challenge what we consider to be "healthy foods," then all is lost.

Peak bodies in medicine want to move from ***disease-care*** to ***health-care***, but how will this happen? Add more failed drug approaches? Invest in more failed scientific reductionism? Build more healthcare infrastructure? Hire more and more medical personnel? Buy more ambulances? Or do we create more quasi-wannabe doctors who never went to medical school and who have a fraction of the hard-earned knowledge and experience of a doctor and yet increasingly are given the licence to act as doctors? What could go wrong? However, doctors do need to change their game dramatically, as I will discuss later, to deal with 21st-century diseases. Medical training has only created drug-centric lunacy.

Our aimless goal is simply to keep on mopping up the increasing numbers that are getting sicker and sicker but never curing them. All we want to do is keep on absorbing the vast volumes of the walking wounded riddled with diseases that are never fixed.

As they say, talk is cheap, but action is priceless. When do we stop talking and take meaningful action?

Our mega-engine driving metabolic disease

Three gigantic parts to this metabolic mega-engine generate all our chronic metabolic diseases and demand to be addressed if we are to get anywhere. It is frightening to see that this insulin resistance-metabolic dysfunction process is a natural part of life as we age but is driven by the factors below:

1. Dietary inputs (A huge multi-factor food problem)
2. Epigenetic programming in pregnancy – is a monumental yet preventable problem that will lead to an exponential explosion of metabolic disease in the coming two decades. This programming unfairly affects future generations.
3. Environmental toxicities range from forever chemicals found everywhere to fragrances, perfumes and energy-robbing medications. There are 350,000 environmental toxins.

I will discuss what needs to be done as far as dietary inputs are concerned throughout this book. Point two above is also driven by dietary inputs, but this time in pregnancy. Obesity in pregnancy and Gestational Diabetes Mellitus (GDM) are rising rapidly. GDM is a driver of ***intergenerational and transgenerational diabetes*** and chronic illness. GDM will be a powerful, exponential force that will drive the coming tsunamis of "diabetes" in the decades to come and will destroy the lives of generations to come (Khan 2019).

A 2024 research paper in Australia published in the journal ***Psychiatry Research*** stated the following about obesity in pregnancy (Duko, Mengistu et al. 2024):

- Increases the risk of ADHD in children by 32%
- Doubles the risk of Autism Spectrum Disorder (ASD)

- Increases the risk of conduct (behavioural) disorders by 16%

With high rates of obesity in pregnancy, we are setting the scene for a worsening mental health disorder crisis in future generations. Together, GDM and dreadful dietary inputs are the major drivers of the expected tsunamis of metabolic disease that are coming our way. Unless we tackle these huge problems head-on, everything will be simply pointless and worthless talk. The medical profession seems lost as to what to do, and yet I have pointed out exactly what needs to be done above. Shuffling deck chairs on a sinking ship is downright loony, and yet the fear of change means nothing changes.

I will discuss the "tap" and "sponge" analogies later, explaining why our health systems are being crushed. We must turn off the causes of diseases pouring out of the "tap" rather than fiddle around with the "sponge", where the sponge is a metaphor I use for the healthcare system that must absorb diseases pouring out of the "tap". Building and maintaining a bigger and bigger "sponge" is a ridiculous notion that is highly expensive and a futile model of healthcare.

We must embrace all these metabolic diseases as a continuum of change and risk. Damage to biological systems occurs throughout this continuum from the earliest point to the furthest, where organs start to fail. Thus, early intervention using nutrition-based approaches is priceless. Any organ reaching failure is negligence in the extreme. Sadly, we allow deadly diseases to occur in our lives.

Every new textbook on medicine and endocrinology will state that we are dealing with continuums of metabolic change. Decrees from expert committees on metabolic diseases to a profusion of recent research articles on metabolism will only discuss metabolic dysfunction, glucose increases, vascular disease, high blood pressure, fatty liver, Alzheimer's, etc., as continuums of change and risk. All of this means that medicine and dietetics need to pull themselves out of that outdated, deep, dark hole they have dug themselves into. Anachronistic ideas have no role to play. ***Diabetes should never be our focus.*** Only a continuum of risk should command our attention.

It is this "mother" of metabolic dysfunction as a continuum of biological damage (rot) that drives us all towards chronic diseases. No one eventually escapes these miserable, wicked diseases with wicked medical outcomes due to ongoing biological rot. Should increasing metabolic damage be seen as a natural and irreversible process of ageing? Should most people suffer multiple organs crumbling before their genetic potential is reached? Should individuals suddenly die before they even age? Should people age rapidly and look like shrivelled and hunched prunes before they should? Reach 115 or 122 years of age, as some have? Not likely.

We just have to view the onslaught of statistics coming out of our healthcare watchdogs, such as the WHO, CDC and homegrown observers, to know that the failure of the medical and dietetic professions is no small problem but a monumental disaster worldwide that only increases and never plummets. Don't be fooled by mortality statistics showing we are doing anything worthwhile. Such rosy mortality figures are deceptive and all about preventing death short term, maybe for a few years, thus making statistics look good within a particular window of time. Yet all we have done is kick the can down the road to a future point that is not considered in these deceptive figures. Bad medicine, wanting to look good.

The *acute* and *chronic* phases of the "mother" of *biological rot* and chronic metabolic diseases

Towards the end of this chapter, I describe this whole area of chronic metabolic disease as a "dog's breakfast". It is shockingly messy and way too complex when it doesn't have to be. No one has bothered to see this whole process as being unified, with one thread linking all our cells, tissues, blood vessels and organs. One thread weaves its destructive force throughout our entire biological system. As indicated, it all starts at the level of cells. Ultimately, we have triggers that weaken cells bioenergetically, which in turn results in a cascade of increasing entropy (chaos, decay, degeneration) and increasing cellular structural decline.

This "mother" of chronic disease leading to ***biological rot*** and multiorgan failure is made up of two phases (Bengmark 2004). There has to be a beginning, and this beginning is made up of multiple ultra-common 21st-century insults that weaken vulnerable energy-producing systems in cells. This energy decline (bioenergetic decline), in turn, increases entropy. This sequence is not arguable and obeys the laws of physics and the universe. More on energy and entropy will be discussed later in this chapter.

Medicine conveniently ignores the laws of physics to continue with drug management that does nothing to ensure cell "batteries" are fully charged, enabling them to have the energy reserves (ATP) to drive back entropy. Entropy is constant and unrelenting. We have a never-ending battle between energy needs and entropy control.

1. ***An acute (early) phase (our beginning)***: If insulin resistance and the metabolic dysfunction continuum (the "mother") produce all our medical enemies in terms of blood biomarker changes like glucose, which we have declared war on unsuccessfully or produces hypertension, vascular disease, fatty liver or a range of other medical continuums, the question then that demands an answer is what is the focal point or beginning of these disastrous metabolic continuums that lead to chronic diseases? None of this happens out of thin air or happens overnight. It is all small, incremental and cumulative damage over a lifetime towards chronic illness.

   Initially, we have multiple insults or "shocks" on our vulnerable cells to kick-start energy and structural decline. It all starts in our mother's wombs and is then propelled along through ongoing cellular insults over our lifetimes. These shocks occur daily, and in the case of dietary shocks, multiple times a day. I will expand on these dietary impacts throughout this book. You will be surprised at how incredibly easy it is to pull the rug from under cell energy production.

   These shocks gradually lead to a cellular energy decline (bioenergetic decline), resulting in increasing entropy (chaos, decay), and structural decline then follows within cells, vascular systems and organs. Disastrous 21st-century cellular insults hammer our cells in many ways, which we will discuss in detail. It is a womb-to-tomb lifelong struggle of ongoing bioenergetic decline. There is no shortage of insults to our cells in the 21st-century that are "***energy bandits***".

There has been gross negligence in failing to halt cellular energy decline by ensuring that all our cells are fully "charged" through the supply of nutritional resources needed for ATP production and repair. We have been drug-dazed, which has produced a gold rush fever as we have focused on metabolic targets using pharmaceuticals, not nutrients.

Balance in cells will ***never occur*** without a significant investment of energy in those cells. Energy is king throughout the cosmos, and our biological universe is no different. Ignore energy levels, and we will suffer increasing entropy. Plain and simple. False prophets in medicine and dietetics have slammed effective dietary and nutrient management, which is the only game in town. Drugs are not nutrients and never will be. You cannot ensure our cell "batteries" are fully charged using drugs. Drugs will never keep the cellular "lights" on. *Drug management without comprehensive nutritional support is a disaster.*

Blood biomarkers won't be measurable in the early part of this acute phase but will gradually increase and become obvious in the chronic phase. With technological advances, we may be able to pick up extremely early signals of cells undergoing bioenergetic stress. As an individual, you have the power to avoid the vast majority of these inputs (insults), driving cell energy decline, which increases entropy. You can put a halt and reverse the ***biological rot*** that has its beginnings in this acute (early) phase. Drugs never stop this rot but only fumble to control the complications of this rot. Women planning pregnancy and our children must be protected from these early insults with long-term effects.

2. ***The chronic (long-term) phase*.** The acute phase becomes a chronic phase as chaos decay (increasing entropy) dominates cells. The crossover from acute to chronic can arguably be seen as a point when measurable effects can be detected, whether in the blood or blood flow dynamics or tissue and vascular damage. Multiple animal model studies have shown that epigenetic programming can "***potently impact***" metabolic dysfunction later in life ***without*** further insults (stressors) (Sales, Ferguson-Smith et al. 2017).

   The acute to chronic phase may take decades, but we are seeing that this may take just a few years as we see obesity, fatty liver and Metabolic Syndrome (MetS), and Type-2 Diabetes Mellitus (T2DM) occur in children and rise at a rapid pace. In fact, diabetes will increase four times (4x) the current level in the next few decades with a rapid rise in children 4 – 5 years old (Xue, Gao et al. 2016). It is epigenetics, not genetics, driving this risk. It is from all the cellular insults to mother and baby in the womb and after birth. Epigenetic programming wreaks havoc with energy pathways and can severely handicap mitochondrial ATP production. This mitochondrial handicap is discussed in the dedicated cell starvation chapter. Such epigenetic mitochondrial handicaps at the population level are poorly researched, but considering the vast extent of metabolic risk, it probably affects 100s of millions of people. These individuals are far more susceptible to the acute insults we will discuss, and they are prone to early acquired chronic metabolic diseases.

   It is so deplorable that the vast majority of these risks can be prevented. Epigenetic transmission of metabolic risk is poised to explode dramatically worldwide as gestational (pregnancy) diabetes rises to unmanageable levels out of sheer neglect. Countless millions shift from the acute to chronic phase every year, filling that metaphorical "prediabetes" balloon I will discuss in the next chapter.

In this chronic phase, we will see an increase in blood biomarkers such as glucose, LDL, VLDL, triglycerides, and others, and we will see an increase in inflammatory markers. Structural damage in cells, tissues, vascular systems and organs will become more and more obvious as the biological rot caused by metabolic biomarkers and inflammation takes its toll. It is in this phase that we will also be able to measure microcirculation network damage, which is our ultimate driver of biological rot and the silent assassin of multiple organ systems simultaneously. We need technological advances to test these small vessels in the very early chronic phase. I discuss some of these emerging technologies later. Most people in their 30s, 40s, 50s and beyond will have well-established chronic metabolic disease and biological rot, which has not been addressed—total neglect.

Our after-eating (postprandial) staple food insults become even more damaging in this chronic phase, and these ignored after-eating impacts will ensure we continue to see disastrous prevalence rates of chronic metabolic disease skyrocket out of control. As an individual, you have great power to self-control these after-eating insults to your biological system.

Instead of supporting cells with the nutrient resources they need to address diminishing cellular energy reserves, we use drugs with zero nutritional value to target the overt signals of cells in bioenergetic and structural distress. When this rising structural damage reaches a point of very high entropy (high chaos, decay and degeneration) in our biological systems, we will have overt organ failure manifesting as the many chronic diseases and complications that our healthcare infrastructure struggles to control. Organ failure is the very late stage of this chronic phase. The seeds are set to magnify and accelerate in this phase for mental health disorders, Alzheimer's, neurodegeneration, heart and vascular decline, and multiple organs failing simultaneously.

Our metabolically induced "biological rot" that is never addressed

I will talk about our ever-increasing biological damage from cells to blood vessels to ultimate organ failure as "***biological rot***". This description is hard-hitting because it needs to be. Tens of millions every year and hundreds of millions every decade die because of this biological damage that ultimately takes their lives. Using polite terms to discuss a truly ugly process that has destroyed 100s of millions of lives over recent decades is a travesty that will never get across the seriousness of this problem. *It would be best if you imagined this biological rot as an accelerating process throughout your lifetime.*

The result of our acute and then chronic phases of the "mother" of chronic metabolic diseases is our increasing entropy in biological tissues. This biological damage or rot is the total of all the metabolic dysfunction effects plus after-eating impacts that cause the slow and unrelenting deterioration of cells, tissues, vascular networks and organ systems. Biological damage or rot is driven by:

1. All the changes that are associated with insulin resistance, metabolic dysfunction, bioenergetic decline, and increasing entropy.
2. Every meal and every snack causing after-eating (postprandial) blood changes, leading to food-induced incremental and cumulative biological damage (rot) over time, which magnifies and accelerates the effects of point (1) above. Points (1) and (2) are deadly buddies in this game.

No disease or tissue is unaffected by these processes in points (1) and (2), whether from a true dominant genetic disease to asthma or musculoskeletal risk and chronic lung or skin problems. All diseases, bar none, are affected by points (1) and (2) above. Ongoing biological rot is why losing weight makes no difference to heart and vascular disease outcomes (Powell-Wiley, Poirier et al. 2021).

The after-eating impacts magnify the many metabolic changes created by the insulin resistance-metabolic dysfunction process, from biomarkers to oxidative stress and inflammation. We have downplayed and essentially totally disregarded these after-eating impacts to protect the staple food economy. We will look at how our focus on so-called "healthy" staple foods has had a huge impact on driving biological decay. A drug-centric model never addresses this food input in driving biological damage, and hence, we ignore a major reason why ongoing biological damage is never controlled, halted or reversed until death stops this process. It is no mystery at all that we progress to more and more complicated disease presentations. It is blatantly obvious why biological rot runs rampant because we never focus on points (1) and (2) above.

In this chapter, we discuss the tight link between energy and entropy. Ultimately, it is vascular damage, and specifically microvascular (small vessel) damage, that produces all the undoing we see in chronic diseases. Most people will never have heard of the damaging effects of food after eating (postprandial effects), and doctors downplay or are most likely unaware of this highly significant after-eating problem as a major driver of biological damage and ongoing chronic metabolic processes. The many parts of this after-eating damage are shown in Appendix-18, adding to this slow, incremental and cumulative damage meal by meal, snack by snack. How is it that we have ignored food-induced damage to our biological tissues multiple times a day and throughout our lifetimes?

No drug stops this biological rot, and dietary advice only makes this biological rot worse. Damaging dietary advice must change!

No organ fails all on its own: Misery loves company

So, live a long, healthy life, die fast and
leave a good-looking corpse.

The quip above is a neat thought, but in this day and age, we will all live a short life, riddled with multiple diseases, ageing fast, and, as mentioned, looking like plump and shrivelled prunes and hunched due to bony and muscle weakness. Who then will have any chance of leaving a good-looking corpse?

Multiorgan failure is what ultimately takes us all out, as there is no such thing as ***one*** pure chronic illness that sees just ***one*** organ fail, leaving the others untouched. 100% of our older population have multiple organ diseases before death, and ¾'s (75%) of those with diabetes have multiple diseases (Khunti, Chudasama et al. 2023).

I have to say it is truly comical that statistics are based on in-your-face disease characteristics or biomarker cut-offs. If we used ultra-early markers of metabolic disease in people, then we would see absolutes like 100% to indicate universal disease – the ***Metabolic Singularity*** discussed soon.

88% of the US population are metabolically unwell. Does this sound like we are getting closer to universality? More on this later.

Multimorbidity: Our clue to the single-thread continuum

According to the Australian Institute of Health and Welfare (AIHW) 2024 report on causes of death, this report commented on the problem of multimorbidity, where we will have more than one disease occurring simultaneously in our lifetime:

> *"The report shows that 4 in 5 deaths involved more than one cause, and almost one-quarter of deaths had 5 or more causes recorded." (AIHW 2024)*

Multiple diseases that occur at the same time are termed ***multimorbidity***. These diseases, as an added insult, often occur prematurely in our lifetimes. Once these diseases kick in, often in the most productive and enjoyable time of your life, then life changes forever. ***Multimorbidity is a huge clue that we have one process that links all our organs.*** We will look at how later. Your life may end suddenly and prematurely with a catastrophic heart attack or stroke. Cardiovascular disease is the number one killer in the world, making up a whopping 32% of ***ALL*** global deaths and where 85% of these deaths worldwide were due to heart attacks and strokes (WHO 2021). Our blood vessels are the victims of this metabolic process (our "mother") and the ongoing and untouched biological rot that occurs very early on in our lifetime.

Despite having the means to prevent or delay these illnesses until a ripe old age, we often fail to act. Beyond the metabolic diseases mentioned above and on the back cover, cancer is something we all fear happening in our lifetime and yet a vast majority can be prevented. In fact, over a third ($1/3^{rd}$) of cancer cases can be prevented by changing one's diet alone (Anand, Kunnumakara et al. 2008).

Cancer rates are booming in younger and younger populations under the age of 50, and, in fact, rates are 2 to 3 times that of the older age groups. According to a paper published in the British Medical Journal, up to 80% of cancers in the breast, bowel and prostate can be prevented (Cummings and Bingham 1998). Bowel cancer in those under 50 years of age is increasing at an alarming rate. So, where is all of this coming from? Weird cosmic rays from Mars? How absurd!

Cell energy decline and poor nutrient availability can impair DNA repair, increasing the risk of cancer. We neglect epigenetic programming that occurs in the womb, driving widespread metabolic disease and cancer as well. So, this growing burden of many diseases in younger groups has come from the epigenetic programming by previous generations and the failure to deal with this, all for the sake of drug sales and food economics.

We think mental health disorders just happen out of thin air and that, somehow, everyday factors don't count. We ignore the fact that metabolic disease is tightly associated with all mental health diseases, but we are at last waking up to the bioenergetic declines in brain cells causing mental health problems (Palmer 2022).

After all, where are mental health diseases coming from? It is our brain's right that we need to focus on. Do we have brains somehow immune to all the dietary, bioenergetic, environmental, and epigenetic impacts? I will explain brain energy in more technical detail later. It is worth reading again and again, if necessary, to get your head around this as your chances of getting through life without a mental health issue are becoming slim indeed.

Parents need to understand that the choices they make for their children will determine the health of that child in the long term, including their mental health. From dietary choices to toxic exposures, it all matters in that child's life. It is amazing how an ancient Ayurvedic proverb can sum up a 21st-century crisis of chronic metabolic diseases that we are all facing now. We have a misguided and highly dangerous fantasy that views drugs as the only answer to complex (wicked) diseases and wicked outcomes:

> ***When diet is wrong, medicine is of no use.***
> ***When diet is correct, medicine is of no need.***

Massive molecular shifts occur in our 40s and 60s. Stanford medical research

This 2024 study at Stanford is vitally important as it shows that ageing is not a gradual and linear process. The surprising finding was that dramatic molecular changes occurred in ***bursts*** in our mid-40s and then 60s. From the 60s on, carbohydrate metabolism takes on a special significance (Shen, Wang et al. 2024).

This finding means we must manage high blood glucose spikes from carb-rich foods. Why? Our metabolism changes and diminishes, so we don't burn as much glucose. Our livers can produce more glucose for various reasons, and our highly active skeletal muscle would normally "chew up" this glucose, but as we all know, lean muscle mass diminishes as we age (sarcopenia), so less glucose is being used up for muscle energy. So, keeping all this in mind with regard to decreased glucose utilisation, consuming foods that spike glucose levels after eating is not a clever thing to do, especially when insulin resistance increases as we age.

As the title suggests, in this Stanford University research, we have major genetic and molecular shifts making after-eating glucose impacts dangerous, thus increasing biological rot as we age. High glucose levels, even after eating, are a huge vascular risk for everyone. We discuss this soon. Good dietary advice should never be a sales pitch for staple foods that don't take hormonal, age and molecular shifts into account.

A massive amount of research has shown an undeniable link between high glucose levels and cardiovascular risk in ageing. It has been demonstrated that glucose is associated with accelerated ageing in several animal models (Lee, Son et al. 2017). Keep this in mind as you approach your 60s or are in your 60s and beyond.

If you are approaching your 40s, then it is a shock to learn that the prevalence of cardiovascular disease (heart attacks, strokes, vascular disease) is around 40% from 40 – 59. It is 75% between 60 – 79 and a whopping 86% from age 80 years (Yazdanyar and Newman 2009). Does this reek of a continuum of biological rot and risk?

Glucose is the primary fuel of our cells and is avidly used by our brain cells. It can be denied entry into cells due to insulin resistance, creating cell energy distress and bioenergetic decline. Glucose is but one part of this equation, but a major one at that. As an individual, you can make a huge difference in terms of acquiring a chronic disease just by focusing on the dietary factors that elevate blood glucose levels and avoiding them.

So, what is our major source of glucose? Grains are at the top of the list of foods that will significantly increase glucose levels after eating, but many processed and ultra-processed foods have high grain-based components and high sugar levels, which are 50% glucose and 50% fructose. Both these sugars (simple carbs) have specific risks, which I will discuss, that accelerate biological rot.

A recent Yale University finding shed light on the glucose to fructose shunt in our brains, with each high-carb meal threatening brain cell energy levels and increasing dementia risk. High grain-based, carb-rich foods chip away at our delicate glycocalyx, which is the inner lining of blood vessels with every meal and snack, setting the scene for our biggest killer on the planet – cardiovascular disease. I will also show how high-carb intakes can increase your risk for diabetes. This high carb intake–diabetes-triggering connection is well established.

The take-home message is that high-carb intakes need to be managed throughout our lives, including from childhood. We have all been conned by vested agricultural and food interests since the Green and Farming Revolutions of the 1960s and 70s, which produced a massive glut of cheap grains as a commodity that was twisted into horror foods. The name of the game from the 1960s on was to sell grains and the food derived from them at all costs, even if that involved producing the greatest medical disaster of all time, which we now have to deal with – our pandemic of chronic metabolic diseases.

Has dietary advice made even a slight dent in this pandemic? Dietary mismanagement has seen these diseases explode globally.

Cereal Grains: Humanity's Double-Edged Sword

Let's now expand on the inadequacies and adverse impacts of grains and grain-based foods. The foods we consume are packed with cereal grain foods made up from grain-based flour, and as Professor Loren Cordain states in his excellent review of grains, we have become so dependent on grains as a food source that humans have become "canaries". Just think of grain-based flour in the many things we eat, from bread, buns, cakes, fried foods, pizza bases etc.

The title of Prof Cordain's brilliant article, as shown in the heading above, warns of the potential harm of a grain-based diet and our dependence on grains in the food chain (Cordain 1999). This amazing paper outlines the inadequacies of grains as an antidote to the gaslighting by nutrition experts who argue about the necessity of grains to feed us and the world population. Grains do have nutrients and food energy but also anti-nutrients that decrease nutrient availability for absorption. Grains are also carb-rich, with the potential to spike blood glucose levels in the after-eating period.

Imagine your day starting with a huge hit of a grain-based breakfast poured out of a colourful box, those pancakes dripping with maple syrup, toast with jam, and pastries or during the day consuming rice or pasta dishes or bread, baguettes or that oat and mixed grain "energy" bar and on it goes where we peck at grains throughout the day like a canary would do.

But in doing this, what are the consequences of consuming such a high intake of grain-based food sources that are so deficient in many nutrients, let alone the glucose-spiking starch (carbs) in these grain-based foods? Each glucose surge in our blood chips away at the critical glycocalyx of blood vessel linings - our death by a thousand food cuts. In fact, there are tens of thousands of food cuts over a lifetime. Grains are low in the critical nutrients needed for cell energy (ATP) production, such as magnesium, iron, zinc, Vitamin-B12, Vitamin-D and Vitamin-A, and grains are not a great source of calcium. The bioavailability of Vitamin-B6 and the loss of other B-group vitamins in the processing and cooking of grains are major problems for the energy-producing enzymes in our cells and mitochondria (Cordain 1999).

A lack of Vitamin-B6 and Vitamin-B12 can result in high homocysteine levels, a very underappreciated risk for vascular disease and blood clotting. Countries like India, which are dependent on rice and legumes such as chickpeas and lentils as a food source, commonly suffer from B12 deficiencies. Nutrition experts gaslight the B-group vitamins in grains, but in reality, after milling, processing and cooking, the availability of B-group vitamins can be stripped away. These B-group vitamins, as you will see in the cell starvation chapter, are absolutely critical to energy (ATP) production, which would come crashing down if we lacked these vital B-group vitamins in the amounts needed for health.

Most of these nutrients are lacking in grains and are essential for energy production in cells, so is it any wonder that as "canaries" continually "pecking" at high-grain diets, we have a pandemic of people feeling tired all the time? The dietary causes are blatantly obvious, but we must support the grain economy at all costs, right?

It may be true that grains feed the world, but it is no excuse to put individuals in harm's way by pretending that grains and other starchy glucose-raising foods are harmless. So, we produce masses of grains as food energy for impoverished populations, keeping their bellies full, but all the while pretending that such foods cause no harm to all of us metabolically long-term, all because there is a financial reward for farmers and grain export dollars.

Grain-based diets in low-income countries are associated with high rates of blindness due to Vitamin-A deficiency or osteoporosis due to calcium deficiency, and iron deficiency is staggeringly rife around the world, affecting 1 in 3 people. If our diets are so incredibly high with grain-based products and we give no thought at all about nutrient adequacy, then is it any wonder that grain-based diets help drive our chronic metabolic disease pandemic?

It is unbelievable that one of the most critical vitamins for our mucosal lining of lungs, sinuses, eyes, ears, bowel, urethra, vagina, and the genitourinary tract is Vitamin-A. It is stated that "***no micronutrient deficiency is more synergistic with infection than that of vitamin A***" (Semba 1997). In fact, it is also stated that "***Vitamin A deficiency is a nutritionally-acquired immunodeficiency disorder***" (Semba 1997).

So, why is it then that Vitamin-A deficiency is never thought about when children or adults present to a doctor with one infection after another in these anatomical locations? Do doctors or nutrition gurus **even** think about this connection between Vitamin-A-poor cereals and recurrent infections? Children can present with dreadful recurrent middle ear infections that can damage their hearing, not to mention some deadly complications, and yet we don't discuss Vitamin-A through Cod Liver Oil molecularly distilled to remove harmful contaminants like mercury. Cod liver oil can provide both preformed Vitamin-A and Omega-3s, which are also sadly lacking in diets. Is this too much to ask? We would rather bombard a child with antibiotic after antibiotic and destroy their gut microbiomes rather than even think of a nutrient intervention.

The same happens with regard to recurrent urinary tract infections (UTIs) or lung and sinus infections. We would rather destroy our microbiomes with countless antibiotic courses than consider a nutrient intervention, which seems beneath drug intervention despite the crushing evidence as to the importance of that nutrient. This mockery of food and nutrient approaches to management has elevated drug-based approaches, but to what effect? Drugs have done nothing to halt or reverse chronic disease prevalence, which is poised now to overcome us.

This book looks at health at the level of an individual who is not caught up in politics or agricultural imperatives but is concerned about their health and the health of those they love around them. Why should individuals sacrifice themselves for these big-picture economic imperatives when they can tweak their own food inputs to dodge a chronic health bullet?

No cereal contains Vitamin A, and no cereal apart from yellow maize contains beta carotene, the precursor for Vitamin-A, and grains contain no Vitamin-C or Vitamin-B12 (Cordain 1999). The bioavailability of many minerals in grains, including calcium and iron, is low, impacting cell energy and immunity.

Suppose food surveys and the type and amount of food consumed determine nutrient adequacy. In that case, the results will be way off all because it is not nutrient content but the anti-nutrients or nutrient bioavailability that counts. There is, thus, a disconnect between indirect ways of determining nutrient adequacy in populations, often painting a rosy picture that is not deserved.

Iron is critical for cell energy production as a component of heme in the Electron Transport Chain (ETC) of mitochondria, and iron is a cofactor in many energy-producing enzymes. All these deficiencies in pregnancy are a disaster for mum and baby, and yet cereals will make up a large part of the diet of pregnant women and then the child after birth. Once born, a baby is presented with one cereal mash or gruel after another, producing one glucose spike after another after eating. Each spike of glucose or other after-eating biomarker is a dagger that adds to biological rot over our lifetimes.

However, in wealthy countries, grain-based foods make up a large part of food energy intake and are packed into processed and ultra-processed foods, which are a huge part of food intake in wealthy and developing populations. Developing countries have massive intakes of carb-rich food from legumes, rice and other grains, as well as highly processed sugary foods and drinks. Is it any wonder that developing countries are seeing colossal prevalence rates of "diabetes", strokes and other chronic diseases? Iron deficiency is rife in wealthy countries as well, so why would it be a surprise when wealthy countries have as many "canaries" pecking on grain-based foods as developing ones?

We have carb-rich, energy-rich grains that are relatively nutrient-poor, spiking up blood glucose levels after eating, and as you will see, a high carb intake has many negatives, including high blood triglyceride (fat) surges after eating carbs as well, along with creating a high Insulin/IgF-1 spike. Let's not forget the ability of high carbs and corresponding high glucose spikes to modify blood fats like LDL in this postprandial state, increasing vascular risk.

The high carb hits, I will note, damage the delicate glycocalyx lining our blood vessels with every high glucose spike. We then have high blood glucose spikes after consuming high carb loads from grain-based products, leading to a 30% shunt of blood glucose to fructose in the brain, where fructose can rapidly deplete our brain cells of ATP energy. We have often wondered why people feel so flat and sleepy after a high-carb meal and need a siesta. We now know that the brain's energy dimmer switch is turned down by high blood glucose levels being shunted to fructose in our brains, turning the "lights" out in many brain cells or where they are suffering a marked energy reduction after glucose spiking in the blood. No wonder people have brain fog and need to nap after a high-carb-loaded meal.

I will categorically state that there is NO such thing as healthy food. ***ALL food has the potential to harm us in the after-eating period.*** There is no such thing as an essential carb, as glucose can be created in many ways in our bodies, so we don't require carbs to produce glucose. Carbs as well are just one source of food energy.

I do not shy away from supplements as to think highly damaged cells, tissues and organ systems from decades of dietary and other neglects can ever be reversed without supplement support is downright naïve and foolish in the extreme. Drugs are not nutrients, so how can they help cells create ATP or repair damage? Yet drugs are all we offer cells damaged over decades that need nutrient resources to repair damage and survive. Cells cannot use alien pharmaceutical compounds devoid of nutrient value to repair any cell component or build organelles like mitochondria or enzyme systems. Cells cannot survive on drug support only!

Postprandial impacts on our vulnerable GLYCOCALYX damaging vascular systems

Ancient warfare would have armies surrounding a city and cutting off supplies to its inhabitants, who would get weak and die before any battle ensued. In a biological sense, our organs are the "cities", and the "inhabitants" are the cells that make up the organs. Our damaged microvascular networks are the "armies" that cut off energy, nutrients, cell building blocks (amino acids, fatty acids) and oxygen supplies, and when this happens, it is the end for these organs; as the "individuals", our cells in that "city" have all these critical components for cell energy (ATP) production and cell repair blocked off. However, cellular waste builds up as these microcirculation networks also remove cellular waste. So, our organs (our "cities") and the inhabitants (our cells) are immersed in a cesspool of waste. So, what chance do these organs have? Our microcirculation networks become the organ "assassins", and every time we have a high-carb meal, causing glucose levels in the blood to surge, we chip away at a critical barrier that prevents arteries from becoming damaged – our glycocalyx.

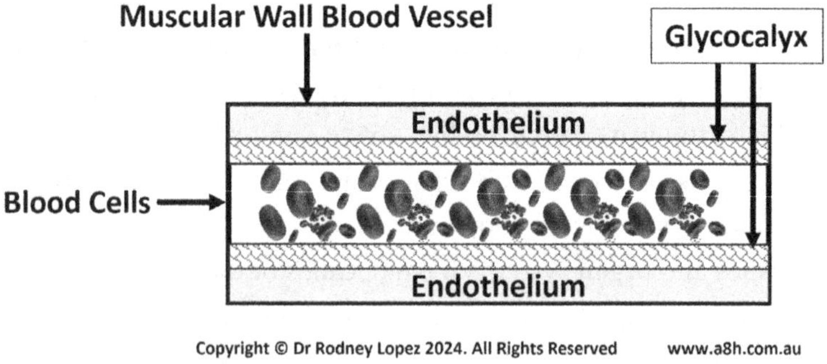

The glycocalyx can be seen as a "cloak" or barrier that helps keep risks in blood away from the lining of our blood vessels – our delicate endothelium. If the glycocalyx is damaged, the endothelium cells become vulnerable to glucose toxicity, inflammation, modified LDL, and other factors floating in our bloodstream that will set the stage for vascular disease, which is the biggest killer on the planet.

The best way to protect your glycocalyx and endothelium is to pay strict attention to the composition of the food you eat to prevent surges in glucose or triglycerides and inflammation that occurs as a result of transporting these digested components of food in the bloodstream. I discuss supplements such as Chondroitin Sulphate and Hyaluronic acid that can provide the elements needed to repair any damage to the glycocalyx.

It is a truly toxic "soup" in our bloodstream after we eat food. Digested food components such as glucose and triglycerides (fat) are carried to our cells and organs as fuel or building blocks for them. What is vital to remember is that changes after eating (the postprandial state) are considered a significant threat to the body, as stated in the quote below. In this quote, "***our organism***" means us as human beings. Each meal and each snack is indeed seen as a threat by our bodies, and each meal and snack adds to vascular, tissue and organ damage over our lifetime —exogenous means coming from outside the body, such as food or other environmental impacts.

> *"Indeed, it now appears that our organism perceives each meal as an exogenous 'threat' stressful enough to mobilize homeostatic mechanisms to adjust to the stress of the postprandial state." (Margioris 2009)*

The high glucose and blood triglyceride levels and subsequent high inflammatory state after eating changes the very nature of lipid fractions like LDL, changing them to oxidized LDL (oxLDL) or glycated LDL (gLDL), which are dangerous to the blood vessel lining (endothelium and glycocalyx). So, food composition matters greatly.

These highly destructive effects after eating have powerful, harmful impacts on our blood vessels, where the changes in our bloodstream after a meal can linger for 6 hours or more (Ceriello 2003). In fact, the changes in our blood after eating may never come back to normal if someone is insulin-resistant. We must remember that insulin resistance is a deadly and highly ubiquitous problem that is a global issue getting worse and worse in prevalence as the decades pass by. Why hasn't dietary advice been adapted?

High blood glucose levels after eating a high-carb load are like a "***mini diabetic episode***". High blood glucose (hyperglycaemia) in diabetes or hyperglycaemia after eating can thin the glycocalyx "***profoundly***", with fragments of the glucose-damaged glycocalyx floating around in the bloodstream once glucose levels rise, even after a single meal. So just think of this: each meal has the potential to profoundly damage your blood vessel lining and increase your risk for heart and vascular disease, which is the biggest killer on the planet. As stated in a scientific paper:

> *Glycocalyx volumes were profoundly decreased during hyperglycemia. (Nieuwdorp, van Haeften et al. 2006)*

The oxidized LDL and glycated LDL also produced in the after-eating period take advantage of this damaged glycocalyx to begin the plaque-forming process. A blockage to an artery doesn't happen overnight but incredibly slowly over years or decades of food neglect, with every meal and snack building on the damage caused by all the meals and snacks before it – hit after food hit.

The glycocalyx of the endothelium is highly vulnerable to increased glucose levels after eating meal-by-meal and snack-by-snack. People think the skin is the largest organ in the body, but it is the endothelium that takes the prize, far surpassing the size of the skin (Aranda, Morazan et al. 2023). The vast majority of the endothelium resides in the microcirculation networks. More on the staggering size of the endothelium will be discussed in the dedicated section on our critical organ microcirculation networks.

What is also well known is that ***N-acetyl cysteine (NAC)***, a safe, inexpensive form of L-cysteine, has been used for decades in emergency departments in medicine to manage paracetamol poisoning. Cysteine is a natural and vital amino acid that can boost glutathione levels. Glutathione is an abundant and important antioxidant in the body. This amazing supplement can protect against food-induced high blood glucose damage to the glycocalyx. NAC given at the same time as the high glucose levels not only abolished the thinning of the glycocalyx but actually decreased the damage and shedding of glycocalyx components into the bloodstream due to glucose damage. (Nieuwdorp, van Haeften et al. 2006). Glycocalyx components themselves can increase vascular damage (Villalba, Baby et al. 2021).

Carbs, dairy, and fat in animal flesh can all increase blood triglycerides greatly. Triglycerides can cause a "***soaring***" inflammatory response when high after eating (Margioris 2009). This food-induced inflammation takes advantage of glucose-derived damage to the glycocalyx. It is also important to understand that one of the most powerful causes of high blood triglyceride levels is a high carb load. So much for foods and carbs not causing any harm. So much for an "optimal diet" riddled with staple foods.

What lay nutritionists and trained dietitians always seem to forget is the strikingly high prevalence of insulin resistance and metabolic dysfunction in populations who cannot utilize and tolerate high blood glucose levels. Glucose is highly toxic to someone with insulin resistance. The wrong food advice will seal the fate of these individuals, and this is reprehensible.

Food (all food) is far from benign, and to think if you add "whole foods" to your diet, you will dodge this bullet is pure fantasy. It is these very "whole food" staples that cause fundamental harmful effects after eating. It is a very simplistic notion, then, that without looking at the after-eating impacts of poor food composition, you will avoid a chronic metabolic disease sooner or later. If you have a chronic illness, then these after-eating effects will hasten your fate.

A healthcare crisis of monumental proportions is only on the horizon. Are "healthy" foods that healthy?

Our medical, dietetic and public health professionals shake their heads in disbelief as to why we are losing this metabolic disease war. After all, we have a bagful of drugs to fight metabolic disease, and we follow trusted dietary advice to eat "healthy foods" as guided by the dietetic industry and endorsed by government bodies. So why are things going pear-shaped with metabolic diseases heading skyward? Typically, "healthy" foods comprise volumes of staple foods.

So, if these staples that we have all embraced from childhood and come to love and drool over using master chef recipes are so healthy, why are we not seeing these diseases come crashing down to very low levels if they are so great for our health? Something is very rotten with our core assumptions about staple food inputs.

It is interesting, then, that "diabetes" was almost unheard of before 1960, making up a fraction of 1% of all medical presentations (Heidemann and Scheidt-Nave 2017). However, from 1960 on, it exploded in prevalence on this planet, and as someone working in general practice, this problem of "diabetes" has a frightening prevalence. This take-off point can be seen in the CDC graph in Appendix-30.

The long-term impacts of "diabetes" are overlooked as the sheer numbers involved overcome those in medical practice, making them numb to these deadly health outcomes. You can't blame doctors as their Pharma buddies have come up with nothing that can cure this problem, and the nutrition industry, which is caught up as salespeople for Neolithic staple foods, is just fuelling these numbers. Why haven't we moved far beyond the foods of primitive man in the 21st-century? However, watch this space as, over the next decade and beyond, what we consider as staples will undergo dramatic changes, and I discuss some of these later.

If we think we are doing all the right things but seeing disease rates backfire on us, don't you think we are missing something blatantly obvious in all of this? We have assumed drugs will save us, and we have assumed that staple foods have no impact on disease prevalence. We have been totally wrong in both **of these** assumptions.

Powerful primal urges drive food consumption. We either dramatically change behaviour around food consumption, or we better well change the very nature of the food being consumed. If we don't, then all we can do is wait for the monumental healthcare crash headed our way that will take a toll on 100s of millions of people.

What's the difference between "bad foods" and "good foods"? Absolutely nothing. Let me explain

This book is all about challenging norms, especially in the face of monumental failure in chronic disease management, which will affect everyone sooner or later. If we do not challenge our perceptions of food as the principal driver of chronic disease, then we are all doomed to suffer the same fate as previous generations. Do nothing, and history repeats itself.

Suppose you asked the man on the street about food and how it relates to health outcomes. In that case, they would, in all probability, indicate that there are "bad foods" and "good foods", and the only way to stay healthy is to avoid those "bad foods" and all will be fine. Everyone will tell you that these "bad foods" will lead to a heart attack, stroke or other terrible health **complications**. Yet, a hot topic battle is raging on between experts who say "bad foods" like processed and ultra-processed foods (UPFs) seem to be just as bad as unprocessed whole foods in terms of health.

We are so confused about the negatives of unprocessed (whole foods) versus ultra-processed foods (UPFs). As stated in the July 2024 New Scientist magazine – "***The trouble is that simply opting for foods with fewer and less processed ingredients doesn't guarantee a healthier diet"*** (Wade 2024)

It is important to note that many research papers are not in favour of UPFs, showing higher risks of cardiovascular and metabolic diseases and high mortality rates. It is interesting, then, that a British Medical Journal (BMJ) article in 2024 stated the following about ultra-processed food (UPF) consumption and its consequences:

> *Higher ultra-processed food intake was associated with slightly increased all-cause mortality. (Fang, Rossato et al. 2024)*

In reading this from a highly reputable medical journal, I thought you have to be kidding that there is only a "*slightly increased*" all-cause mortality, i.e. death from any cause from consuming a diet riddled with ultra-processed foods. You would have thought the comments would have been "dreadful risk findings", "warning, warning, highly significant UPF risk", or "catastrophic findings" with high UPF consumption. But no, just "*slightly increased*" mortality.

How can this be? The fact that outcomes are not that different from ***ultra-processed*** versus ***unprocessed*** (whole) foods must mean that whole food staples are just as bad in damaging health. Just imagine nutrition experts going red in the face when reading this. This reaction may be that they have been brainwashed from their university days, or more sinister, that they are the warriors for the agricultural and food manufacturing industries. Yet, like it or lump it, we can't throw away decades of research on food-induced biological damage meal after meal, snack after snack, whole food or not.

However, to put this argument into context, many findings have found significant adverse effects of UPFs on health outcomes. Yet some researchers continue to argue that there are "good UPFs" and "bad UPFs," and this creates even more confusion among populations that are already highly confused about dietary matters. ***My argument is that both types of food, processed or unprocessed, have the potential for great harm if that food does not meet the requirements for nutrient density fibre diversity, has a high level of bad fats (Omega-6s, trans fats), high food energy, glucose spiking potential and where that food can have significant and damaging after-eating (postprandial) impacts.***

For example, you can crush wholegrains into a wheat biscuit, and this is an undeniable act of minimal food processing, but some would argue that this kind of processed food is fine. But for me, this is not fine as this is a carb-rich, nutrient-poor meal that will have a high impact on blood glucose levels in the after-eating (postprandial) period. Are dry wheat biscuits ever eaten as such? No, it will be consumed with insulin-demanding dairy (the GI-Insulin Disocciation we will discuss later) or added sugar or honey where the fructose content of these sweeteners can rapidly deplete cells of energy and let's not forget that orange juice or other fructose-rich fruit juice consumed with those wheat biscuits will add to the energy depleting fructose effects of this meal on top of the carb-induced glucose and triglyceride (fat) surge that will occur in the after-eating (postprandial) phase—so much for whole foods being benign.

Also, where are the vast number of nutrients, omega-3s, phytochemicals and diversity of food fibre in a crushed wholegrain biscuit made up of grains that are notorious for nutrient deficiencies? To take a crushed grain biscuit out of context of how these wholegrain biscuits will be eaten is laughable, and yet this is the argument being put forward about UPFs. I will expand on what I mentioned above, so don't worry if you are unfamiliar with these food effects just yet, as all will be revealed in the coming chapters. I discuss ***Toxic Breakfasts*** under the ***Fiendish Fructose*** chapter.

But what if the "good foods" were almost as bad as the "bad foods?" If this were the case, then you wouldn't expect to see a big difference in negative medical outcomes if UPFs were compared to "healthy" staple foods that are just as damaging. Both kinds of foods will be associated with negative medical outcomes due to inherent deficiencies or harmful after-eating (postprandial) effects.

It all sounds like food-related heresy, you must be thinking. It seems unbelievable and far-fetched that many of these foods used over millions of years and since the Neolithic Revolution could be harmful in any way. It all sounds like a step way too far to suggest that "good foods" or "healthy foods" can actually cause harm. I did mention that I would challenge you. Keep reading, and all will unfold. You will be very surprised to find in the BIG-10 Womb-to-Tomb list at the end of the next chapter how our cherished staple foods can be so damaging to our bodies with every meal.

Yet what I must point out is that food harm caused by "healthy foods", our staples, has been known for decades through intensive research on their undeniable negative after-eating (postprandial) impacts by dedicated researchers who have devoted their professional lives to unwrapping how food damages us in the after-eating phase. If everyone is following the "good food" advice and consuming staple foods they are told to for health, and yet population disease continues to skyrocket globally, then something is very wrong with this dietary message.

There is research galore indicating that ***excluding*** dairy, eggs, animal flesh, and fish has been associated with a significant reduction in many of the chronic diseases confronting us (Thompson, Tresserra-Rimbau et al. 2023). A non-processed plant-based diet that excludes many staples and grains is the way forward. Other considerations regarding dietary management must be discussed. We simply cannot ignore food-based biological damage anymore.

Research on the biological damage caused by all food may be indisputable, but it is also an inconvenient truth as it threatens our mega industries and food corporations, from the agricultural complex to food boards and food and beverage corporations and governments as well, because governments have their greedy little fingers in all these pies and pretend they are angels and are beyond this disease crisis. Absolute hypocritical political shame, but what's new in this 'Game of Thrones'?

It is redundant to argue about processed, ultra-processed, and unprocessed whole foods if we ignore how these foods impact us on a meal-by-meal basis. Food impacts and food composition matter greatly. What is necessary for this argument is that we need to take into consideration the after-eating (postprandial) effects of food or the inadequacy of nutrients and fibre within that food and, importantly, the energy impacts of any food being consumed as excess food energy can surprisingly shut off cell energy production (nutri-stress). Do people consume far more food and food energy in any given meal and do this multiple times a day? You bet!

Energy cannot be produced in cells if the food consumed is micronutrient deficient, as are most processed and ultra-processed foods, but unfortunately, the same applies to staple foods like grains or legumes packed with starch (carbs) and where these staples are not only deficient in many critical nutrients but are also full of anti-nutrients that block nutrients from being absorbed. Thus, micronutrient-deficient foods will not have the necessary co-factors (minerals) or co-enzymes (vitamins) for the enzymes needed to produce ATP energy. Other factors to consider in foods are preservatives, emulsifiers, artificial sweeteners or sugar and fructose loading. Fructose, as you will learn, is a " ***Weapon of mass destruction***" and a major "***energy bandit***" for cells. If we ignore these critical factors regarding food, then what's the use of superficially assessing one food versus the other unless we see all food in a far larger sense? Yet this is exactly what researchers or lay "talking heads" do in discussions on nutrition.

Arguments that pit 'bad' against 'healthy' options put populations at risk, leaving them blissfully ignorant of the dangers. In effect, the research is merely comparing apples with apples. I want to show you in detail how food harms us in many ways, irrespective of whether they are seen as "good" or "bad". This distinction is truly embarrassing, and any research is superficial unless it views food from a vastly different perspective, i.e. that all food has the potential to cause harm. It is food composition and adequacy that counts.

Marion Nestle, Paulette Goddard Professor of Food Studies and Public Health emerita at New York University, like me, has been a staunch critic of nutritional reductionism. She stated that we need to view nutrients in the context of food and food in the context of diet, lifestyle and culture. ***To this end, I can add that we need to see food as a destructive input depending on the composition of a meal.***

Meal composition is pivotal to producing good health

We desperately need to shift our thoughts from individual foods to ***meal composition***. Truly understanding the impacts of that particular meal on our bodies is the only way forward if we are to defeat these chronic metabolic diseases. Even our most revered diets, such as the Mediterranean, MIND, or DASH diets, are packed with staple foods because researchers know the storm that will follow if they dare to suggest that people should avoid staple foods. These legendary diets can be made so much better by avoiding the staple food propaganda embedded in them.

Our food inputs make up the greatest threat to all of us in terms of health outcomes. When the proof is laid bare in this book, it will dawn on you as it has for me that food composition and impacts that we have ignored have been the ***missing link*** to explain this unimaginable healthcare disaster threatening all of us and putting our nations on the edge of a steep and dangerous precipice.

That food is helping drive this metabolic disease nightmare for all of us seems like a paradox. However, it is only a paradox because we don't understand the dangers of food, and we also have many corporations and interests pulling the wool over our eyes. Compelling evidence should make it absolutely clear that poor food inputs of any kind are the powerful driving force behind our miserable failure to halt these diseases.

Unfortunately, food, as the fall guy, rubs many corporations the wrong way. You are made to believe you will die if you don't consume staple foods, but as you will see in the final chapter, this thinking is far from the case. In fact, you are getting sick and will die through the consumption of the very staple foods being hyped as our saviour and yet driving the metabolic dysfunction continuum in so many ways to unimaginable heights.

Our current medical (or dietetic) models are not fit for the 21st-century era

Medicine has waged a war against metabolic diseases and metabolic markers with drugs suited to another era and an outdated mindset. 21st-century diseases "laugh" at these drug-centric attempts. I have already noted how dietetics is adding fuel to this fire.

It has taken 100s of millions of lives lost to strip away this façade, and yet we have seen the writing on the wall for a very long time but ignored the warning signs of impending doom to satisfy the needs of many vested interests. The arrogance of the use of drugs as our only tool in this fight against metabolic diseases that have totally disregarded critical dietary inputs is a less than useless strategy, as witnessed by relentless, ever-increasing metabolic disease prevalence globally in over 60 years. No fantasy drug will save us. It is pointless fighting a pharmaceutical war ***individual by individual*** while we leave populations totally vulnerable and where we are reaching the ***Metabolic Singularity*** of universal disease. Believe me, we are not far off Aldous Huxley's prescient quip used at the beginning of this introductory chapter.

Drugs will be vigorously defended to the hilt by medical gurus. They will discuss how Drug-X is so much better than Drug-Y in this or that medical situation used at the level of an individual regarding the management of aspects of chronic disease such as high blood pressure or high glucose or lipid levels. But what we must consider in all of this gaslighting is the following:

The comparison of drug versus drug "benefits" is an unbelievably redundant argument if ALL drugs have failed to cure ANY of these chronic diseases in existence in over six (6) decades.

So, overall, if one pointless drug is better than another ineffectual drug that fails long-term to cure anything, then what is the use of presenting that drug research other than to con people?

Drugs, however, keep pouring out as novel tools, each as ineffective as the other as the drug war on metabolic disease was lost a very long time ago. Preventing an immediate medical risk short term by a drug approach is a bandaid approach for preventable diseases caused by absolute neglect in the first place.

Regulatory bodies fuel drug centricity by declaring doctors must achieve a certain number of points over a triennium (over three years) as Continuing Professional Development (CPD). Yet independent, unbiased avenues to get these points are few and far between. CPD intentions have backfired and failed. Pharma are masters at delivering CPD points for doctors painlessly. And so we have a group of doctors as nerds absorbing everything medical gurus say to them. Pharma trains gurus in "speaker programs" to be influencers in meetings, conferences, and webinars. And so drug-centric management continues, and we throw doctors to the wolves.

Dietitian CPD is no different, as dietitians are also thrown under the bus. Dietitians get their knowledge through agriculture and food corporations or gurus dictating the "huge benefits" of this or that staple food, blowing out of all proportion any positives seen in research on dairy, eggs, animal flesh, carbohydrates, fats, legumes, and cereals foods when any staple food thrown at individuals with underlying horrific food inputs to start with would obviously show some benefit. Thus, anything with even marginal nutrient benefits will show positive outcomes in sick populations with awful food inputs. Nutrients matter. Food components matter, and after-eating food impacts matter, not individual staple food types.

The monumental clash of two synergistic metabolic effects damaging all of us

(1) *The insulin resistance-metabolic dysfunction (IR-MD) continuum*

(2) *The after-eating (postprandial) effects of food*

Points (1) and (2) above are synergistic. These are the titans of metabolic dysfunction, as discussed previously, that are propelling chronic metabolic diseases to dizzying heights. Point (2) tremendously magnifies the metabolic disease processes produced by cells suffering insulin resistance and metabolic dysfunction. These after-eating impacts add salt to the wound. The majority of staple foods consumed greatly piggyback on and magnify what happens in the IR-MD continuum of biological change and damage towards organ failure. Point (2) becomes vitally important, considering the Stanford University findings on metabolic shifts in our 40s and 60s discussed previously.

The Stanford Univerity findings make point (2) above a crucial factor at all ages but particularly so from your 60s on when our carbohydrate metabolism changes, and this now puts these individuals at great risk by consuming a high-carb glucose-spiking diet supported by the dietetic industry as a "healthy" thing to do irrespective of age, insulin resistance or metabolic disease.

In the graphic below, the insulin resistance continuum (IR Continuum) is created in the acute (early) phase by multiple cell shocks discussed throughout this book. As cellular energy levels drop, insulin resistance kicks in, and we then see progressive metabolic dysfunction as cells become damaged. We can test all the adaptations and metabolic biomarkers, such as high blood pressure or an increase in glucose, etc. All these factors are enough to damage our delicate vascular networks, particularly our smallest blood vessels, which make up our critical microcirculation networks.

However, to make matters many times worse, there are endless hits, one after the other, multiple times a day, throughout our lifetimes. These after-eating hits (Postprandial Impacts in the graphic) add to this barrage of insults, worsening biomarker changes with every meal and hence increasing damage potential to our blood vessels. For those with well-established insulin resistance or diabetes, to not consider such after-eating damage by food is unbelievable negligence. To push damaging staple foods just to sell agricultural products and not warn these at-risk individuals is unforgivable.

Microcirculation damage is armageddon for our organ systems. It is the ultimate cause of the biological rot, and for this reason, I will discuss our microcirculation networks in far more detail in the "prediabetes" chapter. Notice the arrow in the graphic leading from the microcirculation to the larger blood vessels. Later, we will discuss how large vessel disease actually originates from small blood vessel damage.

Allostatic load is the total of all the harmful factors to our cells. Food is a major player in driving chronic metabolic disease prevalence, but it doesn't act all on its own. It has many harmful "buddies" in the 21st century that can hammer and impair cells simultaneously. Metabolic marker changes such as blood glucose or triglycerides (blood fat) are both increased by the underlying insulin resistance-metabolic dysfunction continuum, and these very same biomarkers are also magnified in the after-eating period, with both inflicting a great deal of damage to our blood vessel linings – the endothelium/glycocalyx.

That food has dramatically changed from our primitive hunter-gatherer beginnings millions of years ago is blatantly obvious. Major changes in farming and food production occurred during the Neolithic Revolution (Agricultural Revolution) around 12,000 years

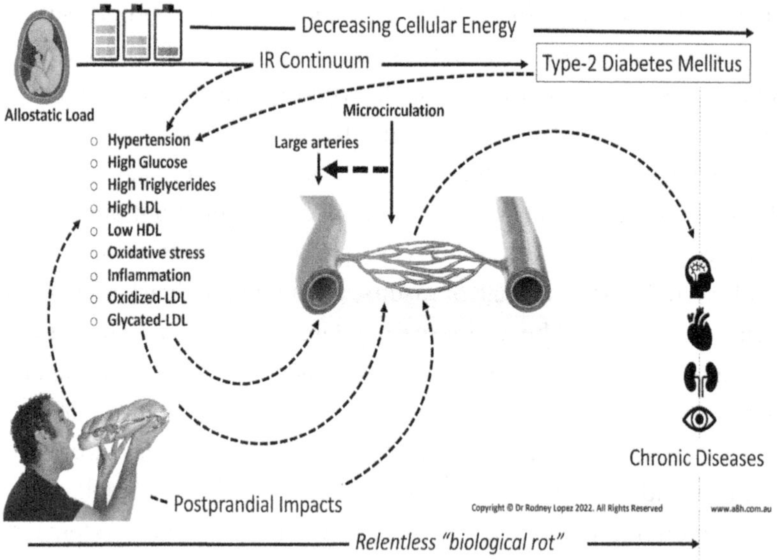

ago when grains, plants, and animals were domesticated. and this revolution changed farming and food practices ever since. The Green and Farming Revolutions of the 1960s and 1970s can be seen as the Neolithic Revolution on steroids.

The revolutions of the '60s and '70s produced a glut of cheap grains, which was hijacked by greedy corporations whose only concern was making money by converting this cheap grain commodity into "value-added" Frankenstein foods that started our descent into a chronic metabolic disease nightmare from the 1960s on. Let's hope that our 4th Agricultural Revolution, which AI and big data will drive, will create food that is fit for health and not disease. I hope our bumbling politicians recognise that it is pointless creating food that harms all of us and then scramble to prevent healthcare systems from crashing and burning due to the disease burden caused by pathetic food inputs.

What causes point (1) above, i.e. insulin resistance and metabolic dysfunction, is something that is argued until "experts" are blue in the face, and yet they seem blind to all the harmful acute impacts I outline in this book that hammer our cellular energy-producing enzymes in pathways prior to our mitochondria or slam our multienzyme complexes in the mitochondrial Electron Transport Chain (ETC). Energy is King, and if energy declines, then the kingdom within cells comes to a crashing halt as chaos takes over.

We have a powerful link in the ***energy-entropy loop*** that I will expand upon soon. As energy declines, cell decay increases, and we have growing entropy if cellular energy is not restored.

Historically, the nutrition industry has seen food as energy (food calories) and nutrient resources only, thus ignoring the very fact that food has profound ***metabolic, physiological, neurogenic, vascular, blood pressure inducing, blood clotting creating, hormonal effects, glycating properties, LDL-modifying, oxidative stress producing and inflammatory generating impacts*** after eating (the postprandial state) as shown in Appendix-18. We ignore this after-eating (postprandial) period to our peril.

Stop-gap measures such as managing high blood pressure and lowering blood glucose do nothing about the relentless biological rot that continues untouched. How does adding a stent prevent the vulnerable arterial lining above or below the stent from being damaged by ongoing biological rot and blocking off blood supply? We concentrate on biomarker wars and treating high blood pressure, etc., but forget that biological damage (rot) will continue without a focus on providing nutritional resources for cells to create energy to reverse entropy (decay). Will treating biomarkers or high blood pressure or lipids put an end to the ongoing biological insults from after-eating and other impacts?

The Two Golden Rules About Food Intake

There are ***two golden rules*** with regard to meal composition. Meal composition is the only game in town, and if we want to stay healthy, our meals need to address the following to minimise biological damage:

1. ***After eating (Postprandial), Damage*** is caused by the wrong type or combination of food being consumed—the composition of every meal and snack counts. The biological damage after eating is summarized in Appendix-18. Every meal and snack can chip away at our blood vessel linings and damage the vulnerable glycocalyx discussed previously, and all surges in blood glucose can damage our brains through the glucose-to-fructose shunt that occurs after eating. All will be revealed as we progress in this book. I will discuss how the insulin resistance and metabolic dysfunction process synergise with the impacts of food after eating.

2. ***Nutrient Density Including Fibre Diversity:*** Do we ever consider the nutrient adequacy of any meal or snack? Taste usually takes priority. We really need to be mindful of the nutrient density of all food about to be consumed. Staple foods can be deficient in many critical nutrients for cell energy production and health. The question about any food input is whether I can meet all my nutrient resource needs for vitamins, minerals or trace elements needed for health and the production of energy (ATP) from those food sources. Does it have the thousands of plant phytochemicals or

antioxidants needed to protect cells, tissues and organs from oxidative stress and inflammation? What is the Omega-6 to Omega-3 ratio of that food? Does that food have enough provitamin-A carotenoids to protect the mucosal surfaces in our gut, lungs, sinuses, renal tract, ears, eyes, etc.? What about the diversity of food fibre needed by our gut microbiome as a food source? Do we even think about our gut microbiome in food planning and composition?

That up to 90% of daily energy input in many societies and groups of people can be from energy-rich, nutrient-poor, ultra-processed foods is shocking (Gibney 2019).

The two points above are critical if your quest is to keep away from deadly chronic diseases. Most dietitians would fail dismally to achieve the balance of these two points even with all their knowledge, so why do we expect lay people to pull off nutrient adequacy without detailed knowledge about food composition?

We are crushing the health of future generations

We must wake up to the problem of epigenetic programming in pregnancy and stop this metabolic epigenetic issue occurring in the womb that insults the health of generations to come. As you will see, one mother affected by gestational diabetes will affect four generations – herself and three future generations (the child, grandchildren, and great-grandchildren) all condemned to a life of metabolic disease. How nice of us to destroy future lives and generate exponential metabolic disease growth through avoidable effects in the womb. The mother's life may be cut short by cardiovascular disease as a result. Shame on us!

> *"The medical profession and its leadership did not recognise or respond appropriately to the rising prevalence of chronic disease. As a consequence, a health care crisis emerged, with inadequate access to care and quality of care together with excessive costs."* *(Holman 2020)*

We discussed the alarming increase in cancer in younger individuals under the age of 50. As mentioned above, this rate is 2 – 3 times that of the older group in a population, and so we have an "unknown factor" driving this rise in cancer in young individuals. There are obvious reasons for such a generational shift in cancer rate as a 30-year global trend described as a "***Dramatic rise in people under the age of 50***". As stated in ***The Harvard Gazette***:

> *"We found that this risk is increasing with each generation." (Harvard-Gazette 2022)*

So, is this dramatic rise in cancer that hard to understand? We have the following factors occurring that will ensure this "dramatic rise" in cancer will snowball and that we pretty well screw up the health risks of future generations:

1. Risk is transferred to three (3) generations ahead through epigenetic programming by a mum affected by metabolic disease that will handicap mitochondria and energy production.
2. Decreased cellular energy is a product of epigenetic mitochondrial handicapping, and on top of this, all the other factors ("energy bandits") I mention in this book rob cells of energy. Not having enough energy to go around in cells means less energy is **available** to reverse damaged DNA (increased DNA entropy), which can lead to cancer—more on entropy below. Micronutrient deficiencies add to this DNA damage and cancer risk (Ames 2001).
3. Ongoing microcirculation damage in metabolic dysfunction as a part of the biological rot will further decrease fuel supplies and cell-building materials, accompanied by reduced oxygen delivery needed for ATP production. Micronutrients delivered to cells will decrease due to ongoing decay in blood supply.

Why don't we see the obvious cause of generational cancer driven by blatantly obvious metabolically-based reasons with all the points above conspiring to this intergenerational cancer risk?

Our mini-diabetic episodes after eating can modify proteins or lipoproteins

Every spike in glucose or triglycerides or the inflammatory surge after eating has the potential to change proteins or lipid fractions, damaging them or making them more pathogenic (more destructive, more damaging). Not only is glucose elevated by a high carb load, but also triglycerides (fat), small dense LDL (sdLDL) and glycated LDL (gLDL) that can damage blood vessel networks with each meal, in particular our vulnerable microvascular networks, which are the silent "organ assassins" and you will learn why throughout this book.

Insulin resistance (IR) followed by metabolic dysfunction is primed in the womb, and babies can be born obese and with insulin resistance. As you will see, it is very easy to trigger IR through food impacts and other factors that hinder cell energy production, leading to metabolic dysfunction (cells and organs behaving badly). There is an almighty clash between these two titan pathological processes numbered above every day and multiple times in a day in 100s of millions of people, driving all the greatly damaging after-eating processes outlined in Appendix-18.

There is a way out, though, but it needs deep structural change. As an individual, you can undertake rapid change to make a personal difference. Please read this book with an open mind and question everything I say. I do, however, back up what I say using references you can check. The only hope for individuals now who have the power to change their lives is through the right information, not to buy into deception, and to move forward with meaningful knowledge.

An "Optimal" Diet?: There is no such beast

Ask any expert what an optimal diet consists of, and you will soon find a mess of ideas, but most will be riddled with staples that we have consumed since the Neolithic or Agricultural Revolution around 10,000 - 12,000 years ago. These staple foods, as I have discussed, are grown now for yield and not nutrient density on topsoils, eroding at an alarming rate (Koch, McBratney et al. 2013).

Staple foods are deficient in many ways, and these deficiencies are magnified in many ways. I will now expand upon a quote earlier. Professor Loren Cordain highlights our narrow food choices:

> *"Most of the 195,000 species of flowering plants produce edible parts which could be utilized by man; however, less than 0.1% or fewer than 300 species are used for food. Approximately 17 plant species provide 90% of mankind's food supply, of which cereal grains supply far and away the greatest percentage." (Cordain 1999)*

We produce food for food's sake and not because it promotes health. Over 3 billion people on this planet suffer from debilitating and life-threatening nutrient deficiencies, with iron, zinc and Vitamin-A deficiency accounting for 2/3s of childhood deaths.

> *"Inadequate consumption of even one of these nutrients will result in adverse metabolic disturbances leading to sickness, poor health, impaired development in children, and large economic costs to society." (Welch and Graham 2004)*

Being born in a Western country is no shield to a micronutrient deficiency. In fact, we are riddled with micronutrient deficiencies. These nutrient deficiencies are simply gaslighted as we don't want to alarm people, which may affect staple food sales – gasp! Our health is impacted by nutrient inadequacy long before we can even measure it. Experts are calling for transgenic approaches to modify the nutrient content of staple foods. We have depended upon these staples, and yet they cause so much harm. Bring on the staple food revolution, which is not too far away. ***We MUST change the very nature of staple foods.***

Our staple food con game: *All* foods can cause harm

Each staple food, whether cereals (wheat, oats, rice, rye, millet), vegetable oils, dairy, eggs, animal flesh, sugar or starchy foods like legumes or potatoes, fructose all have specific impacts (metabolic fingerprints) on our bodies and waistlines that I will discuss in the ***BIG-10 Womb-to-Tomb*** list at the end of the next chapter. Just sugar itself, made up of 50% fructose, can rapidly deplete your cells of ATP (cell energy). Remember, no cell energy means no power to build or repair things in cells and no power to reverse entropy.

Please make no mistake: these effects are NOT just caused by staple foods being mangled into processed and ultra-processed foods. ALL foods, processed or not, cause these after-eating impacts! No food is benign or perfect. Staple foods are not benign in the least. All food has the potential to harm.

Our accepting mindset of embracing staple foods as harmless has to shift now. We are driving horrendous diseases with this thinking.

We must keep in mind the number of times we consume food in a day, a week, a month and the rest of our lives. Eating the wrong foods at the wrong time of day can heighten damaging food effects just by the impact of circadian rhythms.

A dietary strategy that does not address insulin resistance is less than hopeless

The level of insulin resistance in populations is striking. We have discussed that around 88% of Americans may have insulin resistance, along with 50% of those in India, China and Mexico and around 33% of those in Europe and Canada (Bikman 2020). These statistics, as impressive as they are, do not reflect the huge prevalence approaching universality worldwide.

To ignore this massive insulin resistance prevalence globally when dietary advice is handed out is, in my mind, totally out of whack with the current reality. The wrong advice in this massive group with insulin resistance shapes their medical destiny. This risk is pretty well in most of us now or will be. I will discuss how we approach the universality of insulin resistance as we age.

Critically, a diet with any meaning needs to bypass the fact that glucose is not getting into cells due to insulin resistance. Thus, we need to ensure that an alternative fuel in the form of ketones will give struggling and damaged cells a fighting chance. If any diet doesn't overcome the dominant and rapidly increasing problem of insulin resistance (IR) that is engulfing humanity, then any dietary approach will fail without a doubt.

It has been gross negligence that we have not recognised that our cells are starving of energy because our primary fuel (glucose), so vital to cells, is being denied entry all because the "boss" of glucose entry into cells (insulin) is not behaving as it should. If glucose as the primary fuel is being denied, then don't you think the bright thing to do is side-step this glucose cell entry problem and use another fuel that virtually all cells with mitochondria (the vast majority including our heart and brain cells) can burn to create ATP?

Cellular energy and structural decline and rising metabolic biomarkers

> *"There is abundant evidence that insufficient energy, or energy failure, contributes to the pathophysiology of many inherited and degenerative diseases, cancer, and ageing." (Mendelsohn, Bennett et al. 2018)*

We have an incredibly weird notion that blood biomarkers, such as glucose, triglycerides, LDL, etc., somehow occur for no rhyme or reason. Blood biomarkers are not a gift from the gods for Pharma to declare war on. This viewpoint is astonishingly naïve and overly simplistic. Nothing happens in the human body that has not been honed through evolutionary history, and you can bet your bottom

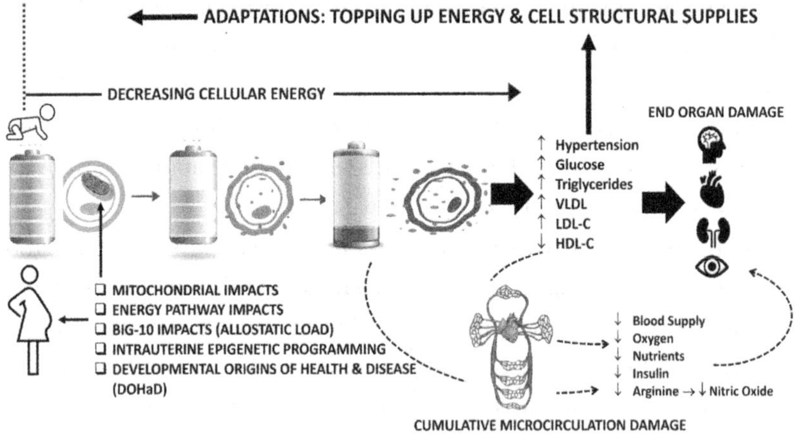

dollar that it will have something to do with survival. These biomarkers, like glucose, LDL, etc., also do not exist just for Pharma to create a drug so that a doctor can end a 6-minute consultation with a script of one drug or the other to attack these biomarkers.

So, glucose, lipids, and hypertension can all be seen as survival mechanisms that try to provide direct fuel resources (energy) or structural support resources for repair. You will learn that hypertension, as I see it, occurs to ensure blood gets through our increasingly choked microcirculation network. To think that high blood pressure is "essential", i.e., it just happens, is truly naïve as hypertension in most cases now is driven by worsening microvascular disease. More on hypertension later. These evolutionary adaptations to cells undergoing energy and structural decline are Janus-faced (two-faced) and will ultimately damage us – i.e., lead to biological rot. This damage or rot eventually happens as we negligently ignore those early biomarker flickers and fail to extinguish them by nutritional means. More on metabolic biomarkers in the chapter "***That's no way to treat a metabolic marker.***"

We have been blind to this process and totally ignorant of these biomarkers as adaptations and friends in the early stages of cellular distress. Thank goodness for the brilliant mind of Professor Beatrice Golomb, who saw through this metabolic mess to provide clarity on a process and see all of this through the lens of the cell starvation model and see all of this as an adaptive process (Golomb 2011).

> ***"The concept of intracellular starvation compliments these mechanisms by providing valuable insights into the pathophysiology of seemingly unrelated processes and offers hope that research addressing the phenomenon of insulin resistance will yield new therapeutic modalities to prevent or treat type II diabetes, hypertension, atherosclerosis and coronary artery disease."*** *(Fournier 1998)*

Energy: The fundamental currency of the universe and biological systems

It should be self-evident that energy propels everything in the universe, at the unimaginably vast cosmic scale, to the intricately complex world operating within our cells at the micro, nano, biochemical, molecular, and ***quantum biology*** scales.

We have a mind-numbingly complex biological universe within our cells that ***HAS*** to behave according to the laws of physics and thermodynamics that govern the whole cosmos. Energy is fundamental to how the cosmos or biological systems work, so why, then, have we neglected the one critical factor that cannot be ignored – ***ENERGY?***

> *"Mitochondrial dysfunction, as well as disruptions of cellular bioenergetics, have been shown to be ubiquitous in some of the most prevalent diseases in our society, such as type 2 diabetes, cardiovascular disease, metabolic syndrome, cancer, and Alzheimer's disease." (San-Millán 2023)*

If cellular energy drops, then it will affect the building of signalling molecules, receptors and other organelles in cells, as these components cannot be created without energy expenditure. Energy decline will thus affect insulin signalling. Even our ATP energy-producing powerhouses in cells, which amount to trillions of mitochondria in the body, can't be built if cellular energy is low, let alone being able to create the vast number of energy-producing enzymes in the Glycolytic and Krebs Cycles and all the trillions of enzyme complexes along the inner membranes of our mitochondria. If signalling molecules are affected, it means that insulin signalling will be affected, as mentioned above, and if this happens, we will then have insulin resistance, which in turn limits fuel (glucose) entry into cells, thus worsening ATP (energy) production many times more. Cell energy decline sets off a domino effect that spirals out of control. Ironically, we have cell starvation in the midst of plenty of fuel (glucose) outside of our cells that simply cannot get into cells.

It is shameful that "experts" are blind to what is incredibly obvious. Insulin resistance, as we will discuss in far more depth, has a monumental effect on cell energy production and cell structural decay. Insulin inaction (insulin resistance) blocks not only fuel (glucose) from entering cells but also blocks cellular building supplies (amino acids, fatty acids) from getting into cells—more on this in the dedicated cell starvation chapter.

These universal laws of physics are not up for negotiation as they are what they are and have to be obeyed irrespective of commercial interests that make money out of disease prevalence and management that side-steps what must be done in metabolic diseases, and that is to ensure our trillions of cells are well supplied with ***ALL*** the necessary nutrients to create ATP.

The amount of ATP energy needed every day is phenomenal. An average person needs around 40 kg of ATP each day to stay functional. Yes, you read that correctly – a whopping 40 kilograms. I will expand on this later. Without a constant supply of energy, our cells will crumble.

Keeping our "***cellular batteries***" fully charged needs to be our absolute focus. Our cellular "lights" need to be kept on 24/7 to prevent entropy (cell structural, biochemical, signalling, molecular chaos, decay, deterioration) from overwhelming our cells, thus leading to organ failure.

Entropy: Fundamental, inevitable, relentless cellular disorder, chaos, decay, degeneration. Chaos loves company

> "***A living cell requires energy not only for all its functions but also for the maintenance of its structure***" *Albert Szent-Gyorgyi.*

Energy and entropy are tightly linked. Energy is vital to keeping order in cells and preserving cell structure. Without enough cellular power, as night follows day, our biological systems will start to crumble, and the ***biological rot*** begins. Stopping this biological rot is not hard. All we need to do is ensure that our cells have all the nutritional resources they need to power up, keep the cell batteries fully charged, and enable the cellular "lights" to stay on 24/7.

Our medical and dietetic models have never considered the need for cells to maintain balance through energy resources. It has always been about drugs that only deal with the aftermath of cells in distress and biomarker signals and biomarker wars. As far as current dietary advice is concerned, our cells have no hope, as the concern here is the sale of staple food with no regard for the many food impacts we will discuss that completely undermine the needs of cells that are always involved in a life and death struggle against multiple factors that threaten cell energy production that allows entropy to flourish.

The ***Second Law of Thermodynamics*** predicts that our cellular and biological course will always move towards disorder, chaos, decay, and deterioration, and all these terms can be applied to entropy, which is the degree of disorder in systems, including our cells and entire biological systems. Our cells undergo a tight regulation of order within them. Without enough energy in cells, they will spiral into decay, where damage will accumulate (our relentless biological rot) unless energy systems are restored. It is entropy, after all, that drives biological rot throughout our bodies, and thus, without a focus on cellular energy and the provision of all the nutritional resources needed by cells, there is no hope of holding back entropy. Medical arrogance about supplements is outdated.

Drugs don't hold back entropy; they are designed to hold back an immediate threat, such as a heart attack or stroke. So drugs are concerned with immediate threats but have failed to halt the ultimate danger, which is ongoing entropy leading to organ failure. This multi-organ failure happens despite ANY drug treatment, as the fundamentals of energy and entropy are never addressed. This Second Law of Thermodynamics can't be ignored, but what have the medical and dietetic professions done? They have completely disregarded the laws of physics and the cosmos.

Our human cells are remarkably organised and normally have low entropy. But to maintain a highly ordered state with low entropy, our cells need to invest vast amounts of energy to maintain order. Hence, there is a need to produce around 40 kilograms of ATP in an average human, as I have mentioned above (Acuña-Castroviejo, Martín et al. 2001). I think you will agree that this is a colossal amount of ATP needed daily for all our cellular, biochemical, molecular and housekeeping functions.

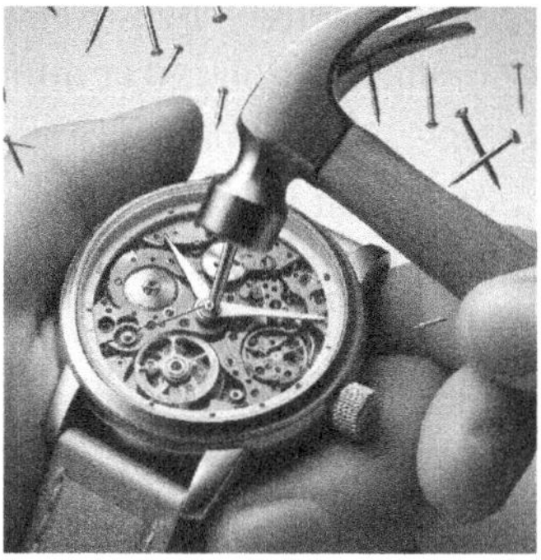

In comparison to the finely sharpened and immense cellular complexity created by billions of years of evolution, drugs are crude instruments and are like using a hammer and nail to fix a precision Swiss watch. It is no wonder then that we have so many devastating drug-induced side effects as there are no laser precision biochemical or molecular hits a drug can execute, and thus, drugs can create a lot of collateral damage – our ultra-common, often devastating and sometimes deadly Adverse Drug Reactions (ADRs).

We may need drugs in various circumstances, but this should never be a ***set-and-forget*** knee-jerk reaction. We should ***never use a drug totally isolated from dietary and nutrient support for metabolic diseases*** or, indeed, any other disease.

Trying to stop or contain entropy is like trying to capture Niagara Falls in a teacup. If it wasn't for entropy, though, life as we know it wouldn't even exist. However, it is uncontrolled entropy with no brakes to slow the process that will determine organ failure. Our brakes for the biological rot in action in chronic metabolic diseases is nutrient support for biochemical energy production. As I have pointed out, it is the biological rot that continues despite drug use that is hijacking and destroying our healthcare systems through the burden of chronic metabolic diseases. Drugs are a tool that can be used to prevent an impending medical disaster only. By not supporting cellular energy production to reverse entropy, drugs are next to useless in halting this monumental disaster that keeps skyrocketing despite the many drugs used in managing chronic metabolic diseases.

Chronic metabolic disease is the result of an insulin resistance, metabolic dysfunction continuum that stirs up a high entropy state in its wake, where this entropy gathers momentum to eventually result in organs that fail due to the high cellular entropy level. What's the use of putting a label on an organ failing as a "disease"? We must now see all of these diseases emanating from one metabolic process producing bioenergetic and structural decline – increasing entropy!

One main branch, multiple side branches, and various medical "faces": Insulin resistance, a major "energy bandit", and a Metabolic Storm

Insulin resistance and metabolic dysfunction are bi-directional problems reinforcing each other and driving the smaller branch adaptations. Insulin resistance is humanity's nemesis.

> *"Insulin resistance has been called a "metabolic storm" in the body, where normal function breaks down." (Cucuzzella and Teicholz 2022)*

When the hormone insulin doesn't work, the body pours out more insulin to try and overcome what it sees as a hormonal obstruction that needs a "surge of troops" (more insulin) to overcome. This extra or high insulin level in the body is termed ***hyperinsulinaemia***:

> *"Hyperinsulinemia, directly and indirectly, contributes to a vast array of metabolic diseases, including all inflammatory conditions, all vascular diseases, gestational and type 2 diabetes, non-alcoholic fatty liver disease, obesity and certain cancers and dementias." (Crofts, Zinn et al. 2015)*

The main branch of insulin resistance and metabolic dysfunction becomes our singular thread or the main continuum that binds all the branches you see in the graphic, then leads to all our chronic metabolic diseases through our damaged microcirculation networks –

our silent "organ assassins." Once our small vessels are affected, then this has an even bigger impact on cells already struggling with insulin resistance (IR). On the one hand, we have insulin resistance, which is robbing cells of energy and structural (building) supplies. On the other hand, we have a diminishing blood supply created by ever-increasing damage to our small blood vessels over time (our microcirculation networks), leading to blood supply blockade of cells, tissues and organs, robbing cells even further of fuel, oxygen, nutrients and building supplies—a huge double-whammy.

As you can see, overfat, overweight, and obese are mere branches stemming from this main insulin resistance and metabolic dysfunction continuum triggered by the acute impacts mentioned above in the womb and from childhood. Our cells are starving and giving off famine signals. Obesity, in this regard, should be regarded as simply an appropriate adaptation to starvation pressures in this circumstance to store energy as fat as a survival mechanism.

Because insulin resistance and microcirculation blockade are doing essentially the same thing, i.e., robbing cells of fuel, nutrients, and building supplies, they are both tightly linked with powerful bi-directional effects, with each worsening the impact of the other. Our metabolic disease drugs have zero nutrient value. Thus, drugs can't be burnt off to produce energy (ATP), drugs can't be used to build cell membranes or cell organelles like mitochondria, and yet we use them

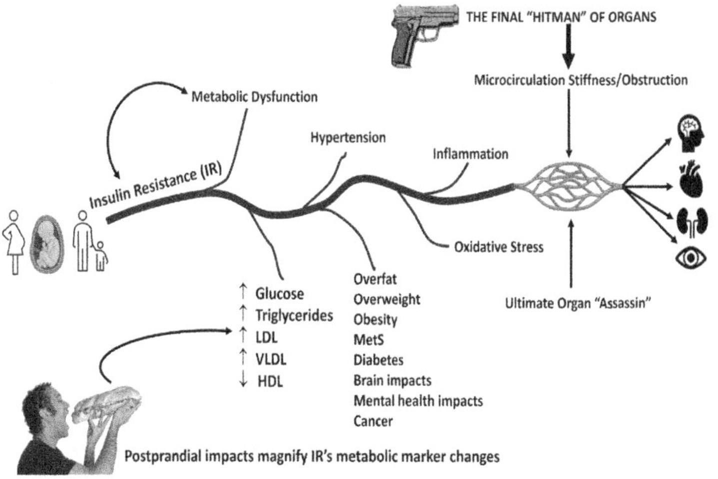

as the only therapy, ignoring critical nutritional resources needed to generate the power they need to fight entropy by building or repairing damaged cellular components. All these anabolic (building) processes require vast amounts of energy, and this is not arguable. Drugs ***without*** nutrient resources are a bankrupt concept that should be thrown into the trashcan of medical history.

All roads lead to microvascular damage over decades of cellular insults, as I point out in the graphic. Please keep this branching image in mind as you read through this book. We forget that from prepregnancy through pregnancy and childhood, our medical destiny is set by the many factors that rob cells of energy and cause damage to our cells. It all starts in your mother's womb and childhood and manifests later in life. All of the harmful impacts of the 21st-century are lifelong and not just when we get older. They don't just happen, and these impacts are slow yet relentless in every human being unless we are fully aware of the factors at play.

Dualism: The disastrous gift to medicine from philosophy and religion over centuries

Our understanding of medicine has evolved over centuries, and this journey has been fraught with numerous obstacles. Philosophers, scientists, and early medical practitioners often had to exercise caution in their pursuits, as they risked persecution or even death, particularly from religious authorities.

René Descartes (1596-1650) was a highly influential French scientist, mathematician, and philosopher best known for his phrase '***Cogito ergo sum***' ('I think therefore I am'). He was a seminal figure in philosophy and regarded as the father of ***Cartesian Dualism***, which led to the idea of duality (mind-body dualism) that shaped medicine and psychiatry at the time and is still shaping how we think today in medical matters.

This mind-body dualism is where we have a separation of the body and mind (brain) known as the ***Cartesian Divide***. So why, then, did philosophy and religion want to divide the body and mind? Well, here is where the religious influence of the time comes in. How can a pure soul and spirit that was thought to reside in our brains ever be associated with the vile, ignoble functions of our bodies? And herein lies the problem. This dualist approach separating the pure and divine brain from the body led to the church taking over care of mental health disorders while medicine and science took over diseases of the body.

This separation of body from mind and the religious influence in mental health disorders is the reason why psychiatry has been held back so much from the rest of medicine for so long. When clinical problems are guided by religious doctrine rather than scientific rigour, it inhibits progress as belief systems dominate thinking. It is why psychiatry has been seen as the lesser cousin of other medical disciplines. But did the rest of medicine truly progress? The idea of dualism or separation, which we can view in a larger sense as "divide-and-conquer" or compartmentalisation of diseases, puts each disease or mental health disorder in a specific box, keeping the spirit of duality or fragmentation alive in the modern era of medical science. This divide-and-conquer thinking has been a disaster for acquired chronic metabolic diseases, now exploding in populations worldwide.

Echoes of duality persist in how we think about metabolic disease. Can we truly separate the heart from the liver or the gut from our brains, and can any one of the estimated 37.2 trillion cells in our body ever operate as a solitary cell that functions in isolation from the trillions of other cells? We have a similar number of gut microbiome cells. Are these gut cells not connected to the cells and organs of our body? We know how ridiculous this even sounds, but it is amazing how such rigid thinking has dominated medical thought and influenced medical management.

It is only recently that we have recognised how our gut microbiomes influence all our organs and immune cells and profoundly affect our brains through the gut-brain axis. Hotly investigated is the link between our gut microbiome and neurodegenerative diseases like Parkinson's disease.

An amazing book by Professor Ed Bullmore, who was the Don of Psychiatry at Cambridge University until 2021, discusses the futility of duality and is an overview of how inflammation can profoundly affect brain function, symptoms and signs. The book is called ***The Inflamed Mind*** and is well worth a read (Bullmore 2018). Ironically, it is psychiatry held back for so long by religious thinking that now seems to be leading the way to a better understanding of the universality of metabolic disease and the critical nature of bioenergetic decline that is leaving other medical disciplines behind in the dust. Psychiatry, ironically, now leads the way.

Enter Harvard's Professor of Psychiatry, Christopher Palmer, who has written a book called ***Brain Energy (Palmer 2022).*** This book is a huge step in the right direction and shows you a revolutionary new way of thinking about mental health problems that should not be put in their respective boxes but seen as a bioenergetic decline in brain cells. The decline in energy affects all our body cells and our brain cells. No surprise here. Medical research gurus have been "screaming" out on the issue of cellular bioenergetic decline long before Professor Christopher Palmer, but their revolutionary thoughts were ignored as the agenda in medical care has always been to support Pharma with a drug-centric approach. Self-interest and vested interests stifle real medical care. No surprise here, either. What good is getting cells to a normal state by boosting cell energy levels? Who makes money out of that?

We have a huge overlap with all our metabolic disorders of the body, affecting the brain. What this all means from a mental health perspective is that there is no such thing as depression, schizophrenia, anxiety, delirium, ADHD, or manic depression. All of these are simply different manifestations tied together by that one abnormal metabolic thread, a process that I will reveal to you caused by bioenergetic decline triggered by and driven by all our cell "***energy bandits***" from the womb to the tomb.

Our cell energy crisis sends signals to the body that demands a response. The cells are saying *Save Our Souls* with crisis SOS signalling

Low cellular energy is an existential threat to our cells. Low cellular ATP levels are not tolerated, and thus, the body will be called upon to respond to this enormous survival threat. This call to action occurs through cell starvation signals that will amplify and demand a response from the body. The response will obviously be to supply resources of energy (glucose, lipids, amino acids, ketone bodies), and thus, these energy resources and lipoprotein (lipid) carriers will rise in the bloodstream, which we can measure.

Insulin resistance restricts critical supplies from entering cells, thus starving cells of fuel and anabolic (building) supplies. The Save Our Souls (SOS) signalling in the graphic is essentially famine signalling. I will discuss some of these signalling molecules later. From an evolutionary perspective, humans are used to famine throughout their evolutionary timespan. So it is no mystery that over millions of years, we have developed a starvation signalling system and an adaptation response to supply cells with the nutrient resources needed to re-establish energy stores along with cellular building blocks required for cellular repair and the creation of cellular components.

If you look closely at all the metabolic biomarkers, you will see that they are either energy (fuel), nutrient or structural resources. All these biomarkers will change in a highly predictable way.

Biomarkers as "frenemies" can cause biological damage if left uncontrolled. They can be seen as friends on one hand and enemies on the other. It is because we ignored the very early rise of these biomarkers and did not apply the right non-drug approaches using nutrient support that we allow these biomarkers to "bite" us. They become our enemies out of sheer neglect.

This cellular signalling is vital to human survival. The body's response is appropriate, and that is to provide nutritional resources in their various forms to struggling cells, from glucose or lipids (our measurable biomarkers) as energy supplies as well as cholesterol and phospholipids and amino acids for structural repair and reversal of cellular disorder (entropy). Thus, these blood biomarkers are not just convenient targets for medicine and Pharma as this is simplistic thinking in the extreme. Ignoring the other friendly side of biomarkers becomes a gold mine for Pharma, who produce drugs to fight the "enemy", and drugs provide a quick-fix solution for time-strapped medical practitioners who are baffled about the intricacies of nutritional management of abnormal biological processes. It is intervention madness and not prevention that guides doctors.

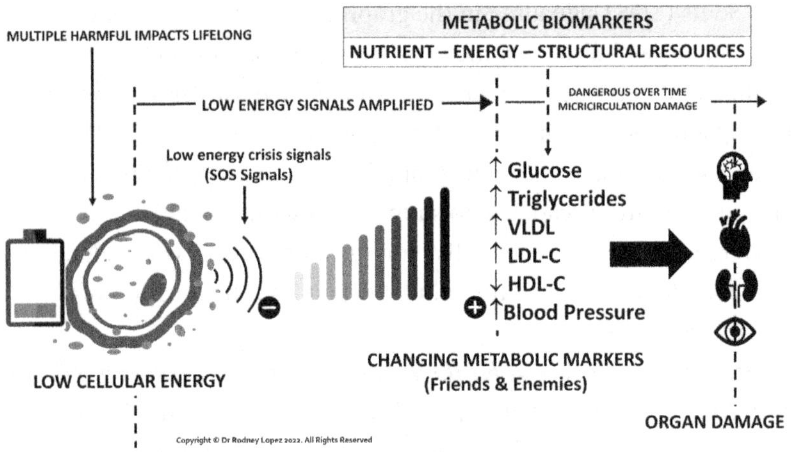

Drugs can work counter to what the body is trying to achieve, at least in the early stages of metabolic dysfunction. After eating effects that distort and magnify these metabolic markers can simply make matters worse by driving most of these biomarkers higher and higher with each meal than is safe for our biological systems.

Fix the cell, fix the problem.

The Gordian Knot does NOT need to be unravelled one microstrand at a time

It is said that using a complicated scientific reductionist approach is like trying to appreciate an intricate orchestral symphony by listening to each musical instrument on its own. The symphony as a whole needs to be heard in all its glory. The same is true for metabolic disease. We must view the big picture and not fragments.

Why do we bother with reductionism if the causes and fixes are blatantly obvious? Do we really need to understand the exact mechanism? We need a heuristic approach that incorporates observable, pragmatic, empirical, intuitive, a priori methods, and common-sense management of metabolic diseases. We use drugs in practice, and more often than not, we don't even know how drugs work in-depth. Does this stop the medical profession or Pharma from creating or using these drugs? Such a double standard is extreme. What seems fine regarding incomplete knowledge about drug action becomes damaging if we use food or nutrients in the same way. Yet, even a monster drug group like the statins used for lipid lowering have their mechanism of action still hotly debated since lovastatin was released in 1987. Did this lack of knowledge stop the sales pitch for statins? Typical arrogance and conceit for the sake of money-making drug sales while 100s of millions will die through the contemptuous promotion of drugs for chronic metabolic diseases that have never responded to drugs at all in over 60 years! Holding back a catastrophic medical event is not brilliance in terms of drug action, as the disastrous medical event being held back in the short term is only delayed in the life of an individual.

We can liken chronic metabolic diseases to the Gordian Knot. The Gordian Knot is legendary and a metaphor for highly complex problems where a knot of rope is so intertwined that it becomes nearly impossible to untangle. It existed in an ancient town square in Asia Minor during Alexander the Great's military campaign to conquer Egypt. If only medicine were as smart as Alexander, who tackled this knot with great simplicity. When he came across it in the town of Gordium, he just wielded his sword to slice through it. He thus solved this complex problem using one thrust of his sword.

Taking apart this knot one micro-strand at a time is known as ***scientific reductionism***. To me, this is not only foolish but downright deadly.

All our metabolic diseases and mental health disorders need to be thrown into one box

What medicine has always struggled with is finding a common thread that binds all of these diseases together. We must now take these seemingly different diseases with all those fake disease labels out of their specific boxes and put them all together collectively in one box labelled "*Acquired Chronic Metabolic Diseases*". Into this one box, we need to throw in all our mental health disorders as well and perhaps add another label to it - "*Courtesy of cellular bioenergetic and structural decline*".

We will look at all these cellular impacts that drive bioenergetic decline, metabolic disease and ageing.

The *Metabolic Singularity*: Are we there yet?

> *"...the rapidly increasing prevalence of metabolic disease is now viewed as a global health emergency." (Lee, Park et al. 2022)*

I have coined the term ***Metabolic Singularity*** to get across the fact that we are fast approaching a point where 100% of the population globally will suffer from insulin resistance and metabolic dysfunction. Why I am saying this will become entirely apparent when I discuss the prevalence statistics.

As mentioned, 88% of Americans (almost 9 in 10 people) are not metabolically healthy (Araújo, Cai et al. 2019). Such a prevalence figure of abnormal metabolic health should send a shiver up the spine of those involved in public health initiatives.

This fact of universal disease may seem so unbelievable, but it is a reality fast approaching humanity, making Aldous Huxley's prophetic quip - ***"Medical science has made such tremendous progress that there is hardly a healthy human left"*** - an almost fulfilled prophecy.

You can build a powerful case for saying that the ***Metabolic Singularity*** is a stone's throw away and is inevitable soon.

If we look at the statistics in the British Medical Journal that 96% of the world's population is sick, then the metabolic singularity is already here! That only 4% of the world's population is possibly healthy is startling (Vos, Barber et al. 2015). In my mind, if we look hard enough at this 4% of seemingly normal people, we will find a metabolic dysfunction signature for very early disease in all of them.

The main culprits for such extensive world population ill health include chronic disease and multimorbidity (many chronic diseases occurring simultaneously). The authors of the British Medical Journal (BMJ) paper went on to say:

> *"If true, health is not the norm, but an anomalous state and only a tiny fraction of the world's population could meet the WHO's exacting standard." (McGrail, Lavergne et al. 2016)*

It is an undeniable fact that metabolic dysfunction can lead to multimorbidity. One process with many disease labels or "faces".

> *"Multimorbidity, recently described as the "most common chronic condition," affects at least half of the population over age 65." (McGrail, Lavergne et al. 2016)*

So, multiple diseases will occur in our lifetime, all at the same time, unless we get this right. If we accept the following Australian study as exposing the extent of insulin resistance in the population depending on the definition used, it showed that a massive 56.1% to 91.1% already have insulin resistance based on the ATP III or the European (EGIR) definitions, respectively:

> *"Insulin resistance was detected in 56.1, 69.7, 50.9, and 91.1% of those meeting the ATP III, WHO, IDF, and EGIR definitions, respectively." (Cameron, Magliano et al. 2007).*

Even if we took the lower figure of 56.1%, can this be dismissed as insignificant when over half (1 in 2) of the population have insulin resistance? How incredibly disappointing that medical and dietetic care is oblivious to the vast numbers of individuals in populations whose cells are energy deprived all because glucose is denied entry to those cells by insulin resistance.

Yet dietetics and dietitians, as the great staple food salesforce that they are, push high starch grains and other carbs when most people can't clear glucose in the blood due to insulin resistance.

A United Nations (UN) global health report published on 19th May 2023 stated that:

> *"...by around 2050, chronic diseases such as cardiovascular diseases, cancer, diabetes and respiratory illnesses – will account for 86 per cent of the 90 million deaths each year: a staggering 90 per cent increase in absolute numbers, since 2019." (UN 2023)*

Chronic bi-directional inflammation processes drive chronic metabolic and respiratory diseases.

Our pointless focus on Type-2 Diabetes Mellitus as an endpoint

Medical gurus unwisely state with great authority that these metabolic markers may not reach the state of Type-2 Diabetes Mellitus (T2DM). This focus on T2DM, or just "diabetes", is the biggest blunder of all. This focus on "diabetes" as an endpoint is irresponsible and dangerous, as it should never be our focus.

It is NOT "diabetes" we need to worry about, but the incremental damage to cells, tissues, organs and vascular systems – our "mother" driving ***biological rot*** that we need to target as early as possible. Our focus on T2DM, a late point on the insulin resistance continuum, has destroyed lives all because biological damage (rot) has begun to accumulate long before these very high blood glucose signals for prediabetes, Metabolic Syndrome (MetS) or Type-2 Diabetes Mellitus (T2DM) that tells us we have arrived at these fake metabolic states. 100s of millions of lives will be saved by moving on from this highly flawed medical construct of biomarker cut-off points.

Metformin given to many with insulin resistance is a pathetic and token gesture when outcomes are never ultimately changed.

MetS, our fake disease "exploding" worldwide

"Metabolic syndrome (MetS) has been termed the "epidemic of the XXI century". Its prevalence is exploding, not just in overfed developed nations but worldwide." (Golomb 2011)

MetS and Type-2 Diabetes Mellitus (T2DM) are the two most common metabolic problems worldwide. However, these labels and the others we use are not quite what they seem to be. Such labels are, in fact, imposters used to try and make sense of a complex problem. ***Occam's Razor,*** a philosophical principle, states the simplest solution to a complex problem is usually the correct one. We are, in fact, being held back by these fake labels and complexity, which makes no sense. If this fragmentation of a continuum using cut-off points actually worked, we would not be seeing an unimaginable explosion of chronic metabolic disease worldwide.

> *"Complexity is your enemy. Any fool can make something complicated. It is hard to keep things simple".* Richard Branson

Let's consider the staggering prevalence of insulin resistance (IR) globally, ranging from 15.5% to 46.5% (Fahed, Abou Jaoudeh et al. 2020). This IR prevalence means that in a world of around 8 billion people as of 2024, around 1.24 billion to over 3.72 billion people are affected by insulin resistance, making up almost half of the world's population. The Australian Institute of Health and Welfare (AIHW) has declared chronic disease the greatest health challenge, accounting for 90% of all deaths in 2011 (Health and Welfare 2014).

We need to see MetS and diabetes merely as stepping stones towards chronic diseases. As you will learn, MetS is a mash-up of various medical problems we put under this one designation. All of these MetS components, such as high glucose, high blood pressure, increased waist circumference, etc., are simply metabolic problems (adaptations or branches) generated by one metabolic dysfunction continuum – our "mother".

Thus, MetS is definitely not a distinct medical entity but a fake mash-up of adaptations and biomarkers, although a high cardiovascular risk for those with this problem, bogus as it is.

If you search for a list of complications of MetS, one of them will be "diabetes" or Type-2 Diabetes Mellitus (T2DM). How can this make sense at all when these labels are only stops (glucose cut-off points) along the same journey towards chronic metabolic diseases? It is a continuum of change and risk, plain and simple. Thus, "diabetes" is not the be-all and end-all of this journey. Even a flicker of metabolic dysfunction should be regarded as a dangerous signal, as even this flicker sets us on the journey towards chronic diseases.

A metabolic continuum is something we can halt and reverse but not divide and conquer. Our motto should now be "unite & conquer"

"It is now time to focus on obesity and the metabolic syndrome, which require more a public health than a pharmacologic approach." (Cheung 2010)

> *"...the physiological continuum of risk can indicate the need for resolution rather than waiting until diagnostic measurements go beyond a cutoff point or are outside a normal range." (Preuss 2018)*

Suppose we take blood glucose levels as an example. If we do another blood glucose test close to the first one, say in a week or a month, you won't see much of a difference. However, if you choose two points farther apart in time, doing a blood glucose level, say in a year or two years after the initial test, you would then likely see a significant difference in glucose levels, and this applies to other biomarkers in an insulin-resistant state getting worse.

The Cambridge Dictionary defines a continuum as:

> *"...something that changes in character gradually or in very slight stages without any clear dividing points."*

The moral of this story is that a continuum is a super-slow process with a painfully gradual change that will not be noticed until a significant amount of time passes by. What we must realise now is that in the early stages of a continuum of risk, our biomarker test results may be entirely normal, at least according to our current definitions and our current technological limitations to find extremely early metabolic dysfunction. The current testing is crude and cannot detect the very early signals of cellular distress – our very early flickers of biomarker signals.

Each and every point on this metabolic continuum has significant risk, not just the cut-offs we choose to add fake significance to.

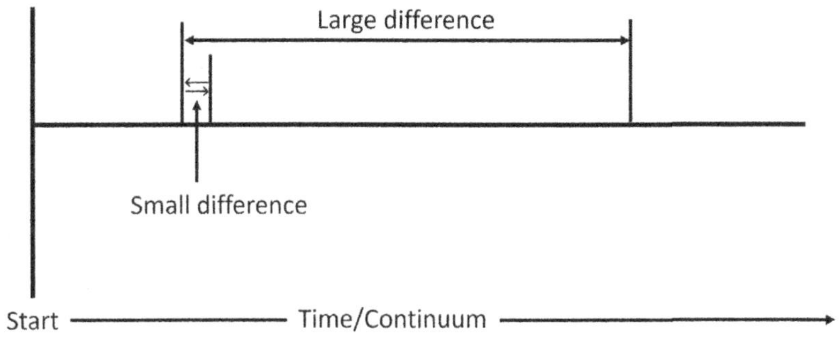

Multiple continuums from one underlying "mother" of a metabolic dysfunction continuum

Clinical trial data, landmark clinical trials and evidence of new pathophysiological mechanisms have validated that coronary artery disease (CAD) is a continuum (Dzau, Antman et al. 2006). Furthermore, not only is CAD a continuum, but peripheral vascular disease (PVD), cerebrovascular disease, and renal disease are also continuums (Dzau, Antman et al. 2006).

All these continuums start in the womb and after birth; hence, the baby in the graphic below indicates that harmful factors in childhood trigger these continuums over our lifetimes.

Fatty liver can now be added to the list of continuums. Not surprisingly, all these continuums can be traced back to the primary insulin resistance continuum (IRC) and metabolic dysfunction

(MetD), which leads to ongoing damage where IRC/MetD are, in fact, the "mother" of all the other metabolic continuums that branch out of this central metabolic process. Fix this main continuum (main branch), and we will put an end to these other branching continuums and end this mess of chronic metabolic diseases.

Dzau et al. rightly state that basic scientific analysis has "*rendered obsolete*" the thinking that some specific or single impact is the cause of cardiovascular disease (CVD). We have "*common and overlapping mechanisms*" involved across the cardiovascular disease spectrum.

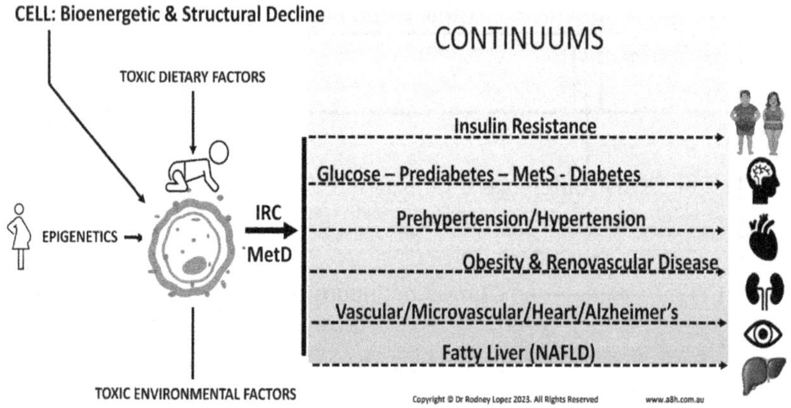

Remember, our continuums in microvascular beds leading to Alzheimer's Disease, heart failure, kidney failure, blindness, and many other diseases affected by vascular disease can all be halted and reversed with early action on the underlying IRC/MetD process. Concerning the CVD continuum, the authors state:

> "*...intervention at any point along this chain can modify CVD progression" (Dzau, Antman et al. 2006)*

Insulin resistance is now well and truly viewed as a continuum, i.e. a ***S***low, ***I***ncremental and ***C***umulative (***SIC***) continuous progression (a continuum of change) with a beginning and an end (Levy-Marchal, Arslanian et al. 2010) (Bagchi and Sreejayan 2018). Dropping a tag or "GPS marker" on the glucose continuum is absolutely meaningless when ***any point*** on that glucose continuum is a progressive and cumulative risk for cardiovascular disease and many other diseases.

Metabolomics, mitochondrial transplants

The research race is ongoing in Metabolomics to find chemical (biomarker) fingerprints of disease, and we are now talking about mitochondria transplants to drive cellular energy (Hill, Shiva et al. 2019). This research is all about moving towards precision medicine, but it will take decades to become a reality. All the while, you will put yourself at risk, and you will see family members and friends suffer and die needlessly from preventable diseases, waiting for a sexy scientific solution that will, without a doubt, make a few mega pharmaceutical companies unbelievably richer while nations crumble under the costs of magical interventions that deliver no solution.

Ultimately, these approaches will all fail if fundamental principles with regard to inputs and nutritional resources are not met. After all, what is the use of revving up the engine with fuel becoming increasingly choked off and engine parts crumbling?

What about those poor souls in developing countries where metabolic diseases are exploding? How will they afford these sexy medical "solutions"? Why do we think about mitochondria transplants rather than using nutrient-based approaches, including NAD^+ boosters, to maximise mitochondrial function and mitochondria numbers (mitochondrial biogenesis) along with a wealth of critical nutrients to keep our energy-producing pathways "well-oiled"? Mitochondria are our cellular "engines" that can't create energy as ATP without supportive nutrient supplies, and where after-eating impacts, epigenetic handicaps or environmental toxicities impair them. Why are we looking at complicated solutions and not readily available nutrient interventions as our answer? What's the use of injecting mitochondria into cells and yet ignoring the fact that they won't work at all without nutrient resources?

San-Millán, the author of the paper quoted under the energy section above, is far more astute than others I have read. Most place great emphasis on mitochondria as if they work in a vacuum to the other cell processes that come before the mitochondrial stage. As he stated, "*Mitochondrial dysfunction, as well as disruptions of cellular bioenergetics...*" can severely impact ATP production.

Mitochondria do not work independently of the multiple biochemical steps that go before the mitochondria to produce ATP. You can see this in action in Appendix-29, and you don't have to understand this in-depth, but this one graphic shows we have a Glycolytic Pathway, Krebs Cycle and then the Electron Transport Chain (ETC) in mitochondria working in concert to produce copious amounts of energy in the form of ATP. All these stages need copious amounts of micronutrients to work. Multiple steps before the ETC in mitochondria can't be ignored when we are talking about bioenergetic decline.

I challenge all medical and dietetic gurus to answer the following questions

Both the medical and dietetic models are bankrupt. Society should demand answers to the hard questions below that need to be asked of any medical or dietetic guru wanting to deny this unfolding tragedy of chronic diseases. These hard questions are:

1. Why are metabolic disease rates skyrocketing out of control? If your models were that brilliant, shouldn't disease rates be plummeting?
2. Why are younger and younger individuals getting chronic diseases such as MetS, diabetes, obesity, kidney disease or fatty liver, where many young people may need liver transplantation?
3. Why are we seeing an explosion of ***preventable*** cancers in those under 50 years of age?
4. Why is it that after 60 years of a metabolic disease pandemic, we don't have a cure for any of these chronic diseases, only "patch-up" jobs at the level of an individual in medical trouble?
5. Why is it we target individuals where we only buy them a little more time before a medical complication strikes

them and ends their lives? Why are we not focusing our attention on population health instead?

6. Why is it that massive sums of money are spent on healthcare, yet healthcare systems are crashing and burning?
7. Why are we expecting an "explosion" or "tsunami" of chronic diseases, including cancer, in the coming decades if drug management or dietary advice actually works?
8. Why are we targeting the expressions of cells in distress, i.e., biomarkers and blood pressure and not targeting the factors that drive cell distress and biomarker abnormalities in the first place?
9. Why does it seem that drug research is more valid than nutritional research, especially when drugs have been a dismal failure in halting this pandemic and where nutritional research has been so amazingly positive?
10. Why haven't you bothered to look for and deal with very early signs of metabolic disease, and why do you cling to outdated glucose cut-off points, leaving people condemned to increasing biological damage and disease?
11. Why are you not screaming for a change in medicine and dietetics to adopt nutritional modifications in the face of soaring insulin resistance and metabolic dysfunction?
12. Why are you not accepting you have failed and continuing with a lie?

Finding early risk. Early, early early detection is vital. Technological advances, AI and the discovery of microvascular disease

The authors of a study that used multiple early markers for paediatric MetS, which, as we have discussed, is an advanced insulin resistance state, found metabolic dysfunction marker signatures in children as young as five (5) years old (Azab, de Souza et al. 2021).

Finding early metabolic signatures and early microvascular disease that rob cells of all the things they need to survive will be a game changer. We are now moving into a technologically advanced world of non-invasive tests where AI will have a big role to play. These tests: "*...provide data on a variety of biomarkers, which include height, weight, body mass index, systolic and diastolic pressure, oxygen saturation, body temperature, heart rate, insulin sensitivity, immune response, recovery capacity, fat mass control, mental stress, artery condition, lipid control and an overall wellness score" (Rao 2019).*

Forward-looking infrared (FLIR), along with non-invasive flow velocity measuring devices, will enable us to get an insight into early vascular disease and endothelial (lining of blood vessels) dysfunction. These technologies will move us truly forward in recognizing early metabolic and vascular disease so that food-based, nutrient-based approaches can be implemented. A drug to end chronic metabolic diseases seems like a pipedream. However, a ***pharmaconutrient*** such as a long-acting L-arginine or, better still, L-citrulline or a transcutaneous delivery system that can boost Nitric Oxide (NO) may be of tremendous benefit to those with more advanced microvascular disease.

Many compounds can help the vital Glycocalyx, a carbohydrate-rich gel layer on the endothelial surface facing the interior of a blood vessel. Research has shown we can repair this essential part of blood vessels with supportive nutrients. Nitric Oxide (NO) is a vasodilator (opens up blood vessels, allowing more blood through), and we see diminished NO in early vascular disease, worsening microcirculation delivery of blood, fuel, oxygen and micronutrient supplies.

There is a tremendous amount of nutritional support we can provide cells and vascular networks that we ignore in favour of already failed drug-centric approaches.

The train and railway track analogy of chronic metabolic diseases

We need to be mindful that we have one thread or process represented by a railway track from the womb to the tomb that winds its way through all the fake metabolic labels to end up as an organ failing, which we then label as this or that chronic disease or a mental health problem.

> *"...the physiological continuum of risk can indicate the need for resolution rather than waiting until diagnostic measurements go beyond a cutoff point or are outside a normal range."* (Preuss 2018)

We can consider this insulin resistance – metabolic dysfunction ("mother") towards chronic illness as a railway track.

ANY point on this railway track, from womb to tomb, will have a lower medical risk below it and a higher medical risk above it.

All points on this railway track would have some level of biological damage (biological rot) at that particular point if we had the tools to see extremely early damage. All our blood biomarkers will increase along this railway track from glucose, triglycerides, etc., where after-eating effects magnify these biomarkers many times a day. No point on this track should be emphasised in comparison to any other as the terminus of this railway journey from that metabolic flicker on will be our chronic metabolic diseases, and the whole railway track can be viewed as progressive ***biological rot*** to multiple organs failing simultaneously.

By dividing this railway track into stops (railway stations) using fake constructs like glucose cut-off points, this thinking ignores all the damage that occurs between the railway stations (cut-offs).

The brakes on this train, however, are failing, and populations hurtle towards the ***Metabolic Singularity*** all because we do nothing to stop the factors that propel this runaway freight train on its tracks. It is thus no wonder that metabolic disease continues to skyrocket with no end in sight.

Our railway journey leads to the terminus: Microcirculation damage, our final stop and the silent microvascular assassin of organ systems

Years and often decades of biological damage happen **in between** the glucose cut-offs, i.e. between those railway stops we call "prediabetes", "MetS", and "diabetes".

The journal Cardiovascular Research states that:

> *"Coronary microvascular disease may be part of a systemic continuum of microvascular disease, with multiple affected organ beds." (Berry and Duncker 2020)*

What is also unequivocal is that we can protect our microcirculation networks through better glucose control.

> *"As noted, in contrast to macrovascular disease, the impact of better glycemic control on microvascular disease is unequivocal." (Orasanu and Plutzky 2009)*

Macrovascular is a term used for our large blood vessels. It is well established that microvascular disease leads to large vessel disease and cardiovascular risk (Stokes and Granger 2005).

> *"Moreover, epidemiological evidence shows that the relationship between plasma glucose concentration and CVD extends well below the glucose level defined for diabetes and even impaired glucose tolerance." (Gerstein 1997)*

Our microcirculation networks, with their vast endothelial surface area, are highly vulnerable to glycocalyx damage from high glucose spikes after eating.

We can view this metabolic process as essentially three (3) vital components that form a continuum of risk and biological damage:

$$\textbf{IRC} \rightleftarrows \textbf{MetDc} \rightleftarrows \textbf{MVDc}$$

This "equation" of sorts is easy enough to understand where the Insulin Resistance Continuum (IRC) can lead to a Metabolic Dysfunction Continuum (MetDc), and these processes will snowball throughout our lifetimes, damaging our small blood vessels to cause the Microvascular Disease Continuum (MVDc).

Once these components have been set into place, they are all bidirectional and self-perpetuating.

Type-2 Diabetes Mellitus (T2DM) is described as the "mother" of chronic metabolic diseases. Yet it is the insulin resistance continuum that is the "mother" of T2DM

A paper was published in the World Journal of Diabetes in 2015 titled: "***Diabetes Mellitus: The Epidemic of the Century***" (Kharroubi and Darwish 2015).

> ***"Diabetes mellitus, long considered a disease of minor significance to world health, is now taking its place as one of the main threats to human health in the 21st century. The past two decades have seen an explosive increase in the number of people diagnosed with diabetes worldwide."***
> *(Zimmet, Alberti et al. 2001)*

The focus, as I have mentioned, needs to be on the metabolic continuum that leads to diabetes if we are to tackle the ever-increasing and relentless march of chronic diseases. Our focus on "diabetes" is now completely redundant and highly embarrassing, considering the wealth of knowledge refuting this construct.

> *"While only a few things can be predicted with certainty, one thing that seems certain is that the future of health care will be dominated by the challenge of complex chronic disorders."*
> *(Nolte, Knai et al. 2008)*

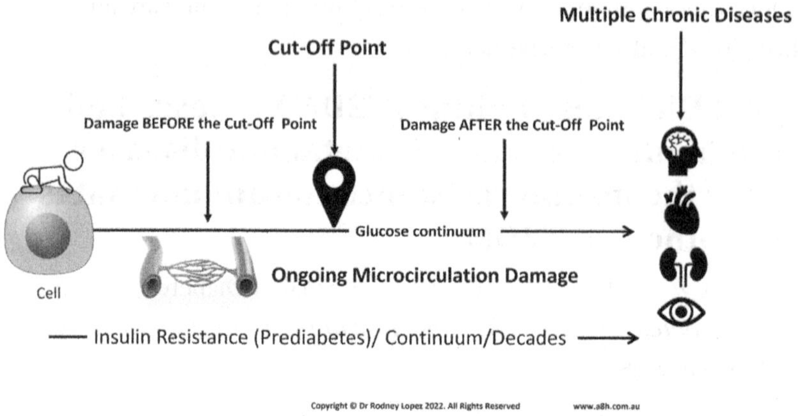

The death toll of chronic diseases is far greater than ALL wars and ALL pandemics in history combined.

The death toll as a result of chronic diseases in 2019 was 42 million (AIHW 2021). So, one would think that in a decade, this death toll will be 420 million. However, this will not be the case as this number will be far greater as disease levels increase exponentially due to the ticking time bomb of pregnancy-induced epigenetic programming affecting future generations.

The estimated human cost of all pandemics in history is approximately 1 billion if we include the potential loss of lives due to COVID-19 (Dasgupta and Crunkhorn 2020). So, just think that in one decade, we lose almost half of all lives lost in the entire history of pandemics on this planet.

The lives lost in all wars in history have been estimated to be somewhere between 150 million to 1 billion (Hedges 2003) (Hedges 2007). Suppose we use that figure of 42 million deaths in only ONE year and take it back six decades when this metabolic disaster started to explode. In that case, you will be able to calculate that 2.0 billion to 2.5 billion deaths will have already occurred due to chronic disease. But we need to remember there was a gradual loss of life from the starting point around 60 years ago, which accelerated at a tremendous pace since 1960 and is set to soar even more rapidly in the coming decades– see Appendix-30.

However, we are moving into a super-accelerated pace of metabolic diseases doubling or tripling over recent decades. We need to imagine the death toll of the next few decades but consider that these diseases are now exploding in numbers, and you will see that the human cost of chronic diseases makes the loss of life from all pandemics and all wars in history pale in comparison.

The Obesity Continuum (OC): Are anti-obesity medications (AOMs) a blessing or a medical disaster unfolding? Two studies sound loud alarm signals

Obesity is not a standalone problem, and we only treat it as such. Fatness is tightly tied to all our metabolic diseases, so why do we target the accumulation of body fat and not its causes? As I have discussed, we have multiple "energy bandits" robbing cells of energy, and thus, we must see increasing body fat as a response to the energy crisis that the body perceives as a survival threat –cell starvation (famine) signalling. Fat has far more energy calories than glucose or protein, and so it is the ideal storage vehicle for energy in the body.

If we now add fructose from glucose and fructose-rich foods on top of the other "energy bandits" like fructose from sugary foods, fruit juices, honey, agave, etc., we will add to this fatness problem as fructose is a fat-generating "machine". This fat-making "machine" that is fructose will be further discussed in the ***Fiendish Fructose*** chapter.

On top of the "energy bandits" and the inevitable regular daily hits by fructose, if we consume foods that push blood glucose and insulin/IgF-1 through the roof in the blood (think carbs, dairy, protein and even fat), we now choke off fat-burning as there is no way fat will be burnt off as energy when we have plenty of fuel in the form of glucose for cellular energy and where we boost the most powerful anabolic hormones in the body (Insulin-IgF-1) by these same foods whose sole job is to support the building of things in the body from proteins, glycogen to fat. If insulin levels are high, then the door for fat burning as an energy source will be slammed shut. So, it is no wonder that our staples prevent us from decreasing body fat as all our staples will either spike blood glucose or trigger insulin release. Dairy is notorious for spiking insulin levels.

One thing for sure is that overfat, overweight and obesity are not the cause of diabetes or metabolic diseases. It is the other way around. It is metabolic dysfunction that leads to fat gain through distorted famine signalling created by all our cellular "energy bandits", and fructose hits that make it appear that our cells are starving. It is paradoxical starvation in the presence of food plenty, but food plenty doesn't mean food adequacy by any means.

We can greatly dampen down insulin responses created by food inputs, decrease fructose impacts, improve cellular energy levels through ketones and nutrient resources, and feed our gut microbiome the dietary fibre foods they must have, and then body fat levels will decrease naturally. Weight loss should occur as a byproduct of taking care of cellular energy and nutritional needs.

Our new anti-obesity drugs work due to the fact that we are starved by reducing our appetite. The weight loss due to these drug measures that ignore nutrient-dense dietary inputs will come from fat loss, muscle loss and loss of organ size. So, we lose lean body mass, which is never a great thing in the long term. By ignoring detailed dietary inputs, we are just creating ***medical malnutrition***. Imagine the long-term harm of medically induced malnutrition. Pure drug-induced weight loss is dangerous when dietary inputs and the fundamental needs of cells are totally ignored.

We absolutely underestimate the number of individuals that are "***overfat***" in the absence of being overweight or obese. Overfat is the common chubbiness we see in vast numbers of children and adults over time and is a problem that is considerably underestimated (Maffetone and Laursen 2020). The magnitude of this issue of being overfat vs overweight or obese becomes apparent when we see that the estimated prevalence of being overfat is as high as 76% worldwide (Maffetone and Laursen 2020). Our nutrient-deficient staples, fructose hits, and all the robbers of cellular energy will promote overfat, overweight and obese individuals who then struggle to lose this body fat.

Overfat is defined as a high body fat level that can impair our health. Just think how overfat changes even your appearance as your face fills out as you age. Overfat is a problem rising in parallel with our insulin resistance-metabolic dysfunction continuum, our "mother" of chronic illness. But a glance at people walking on the street, in shopping centres, food malls, etc., will show the staggering number of people who are overfat, overweight or obese. With up to 40% of these overfat individuals regarded as normal weight, what are we going to do? Do we start treating normal-weight yet overfat individuals with anti-obesity medications?

The extent of this obesity problem is simply staggering. It is expected that if trends continue (as they have for decades), by 2035, 51% or 4 billion people, equating to 1 in 2 individuals on Earth, will be overweight or obese (WOF 2023). Far more will be overfat. The World Obesity Federation (WOF) also stated that the economic impact of obesity by 2035 will reach 4.32 trillion USD. Ouch! What a sickening loss of money going down the drain. In a mere 15 years, from 2020 – 2035, there will be a 100% increase in childhood obesity (WOF 2023). Strikingly, 80%-90% of those with Type-2 Diabetes mellitus are obese (Nianogo and Arah 2022).

"Obesity is not a disease which you either do or do not have: rather, it is a continuum" (Bray, Kim et al. 2017)

That fat stores are fiercely defended in the body is not in doubt. This fat defence mechanism is understandable as energy stores are a precious commodity in the human body. Energy is critical for the survival of an organism. A 2023 paper published in JAMA Network Open stated the following:

"The principal finding of this study was that a weight loss of more than 10% was associated with higher all-cause mortality (including increased mortality from cancer, CVD, and noncancer non-CVD) among both men and women." (Hussain, Newman et al. 2023)

Two past studies have warned us of the risk caused by our obsessive focus on weight loss. The ***CHARM*** study looked at those with heart failure and found a stunning four-fold (4x) increased risk of dying short-term with a loss of 10% weight or more (Pocock, McMurray et al. 2008). Likewise, the ***TOPCAT*** study of individuals with heart failure showed that an even smaller 5% weight loss or more was linked with not only cardiovascular mortality but all-cause mortality (Vazir, Claggett et al. 2017). Now imagine a world inundated with cardiovascular risk due to insulin resistance, metabolic dysfunction, and a developing pandemic of heart failure!

Interestingly, a scientific statement by the American Heart Association stated that no reduction in cardiovascular disease (CVD) was seen with weight loss (Powell-Wiley, Poirier et al. 2021). How does weight loss stop the damaging after-eating effects if this input is not tightly controlled? How does the weight loss due to drug-induced malnutrition help cells already struggling malnourished cells to create energy, which was the underlying factor for fat gain in the first place?

We want quick fixes at any cost. How does injecting a fat-loss medication or taking a pill for it change all the inputs required to prevent biological rot and vascular damage if food composition is never addressed? So, it is no wonder that weight loss will still see ongoing cardiovascular and chronic metabolic disease risk.

So imagine that weight loss doesn't prevent CVD or may increase our risk for disease and death. Talk about a chaotic biological system. Weight loss without the necessary nutrient resources in place is a pointless exercise that makes Pharma a lot of money. Medical or dietetic gurus seem silent on these findings, wanting you to keep believing in the tooth fairy.

OBESITY

⇅

IRC ⇄ MetDc ⇄ MVDc

⇅

CHRONIC DISEASE

Essentially, we have the Insulin Resistance Continuum (IRC), Metabolic Dysfunction Continuum (MetDc) and the Microvascular

Disease Continuum (MVDc) as the central "engine" of metabolic diseases. Obesity is not separate from the IRC continuum.

Obesity should never be classified as a disease, although Pharma would love this idea. It is an adaptation to 21st-century inputs that threaten all our cells. Finally, please remember that it is calories-in not calories-out that matters and that ***you can't outrun a bad diet.*** In other words, diet and not exercise is the answer to losing fat. Don't think exercising strenuously without a supportive diet and nutrient plan will shed any fat. This thinking has been well and truly debunked by Professor Herman Pontzer (Pontzer, Durazo-Arvizu et al. 2016).

We are at a medical crossroads: A mea culpa moment for the medical and dietetic professions

We are now at a crossroads in medicine and dietetics. This chasm we are seeing in healthcare had to open up sooner or later, and we are seeing the effects of gross mismanagement now.

As Dr. Mark Hyman, an American champion of food and nutrient-based approaches to disease management and prevention, stated in a communique dated the 3rd of August 2023 and titled "***How Censorship, Corruption, And Greed Are Keeping Us Sick And Divided.***"

> *"We live in a country that claims to be based on science, goodwill, and policies intended to help people. But in reality, these things are often heavily influenced and manipulated by industry, particularly Big Food, Big Pharma, and Big Ag, which have corrupted many institutions, politicians, professional associations, and research entities. And it has, unfortunately, led to mass confusion and illness in the public."*

Dr. Mark Hyman's statement is absolutely true, but what he states is not the complete story, as you will see when you read the chapter ***Revolution Time.*** Corruption is not my focus in this book, but we must see corruption as a powerful driver keeping all of us sick or well on our way to chronic ill health. That a small group of individuals and corporations can hoard wealth while the vast numbers in the world suffer from their actions is beyond sickening. Self-interest, vested interests and corruption keep disease at groundbreaking levels, and unless we make a stand, this health disaster will continue to soar in populations. We get sicker, weaker and poorer while corporations keeping us sick get richer and richer.

Governments enable this disaster due to huge conflicts of interest due to the taxes they earn from the agricultural and food economies. When do they wake up to the role they are playing in this never-ending story of metabolic diseases? Seeing farmers in their moth-eaten hats on TV or in documentaries talking about their livelihoods and family traditions does not cut it. Why are their lives and family traditions more important than everyone else's? Why should we suffer and die for their livelihoods? Should populations keep on getting sicker and sicker so that these affable farmers can continue doing what they do? We don't want to take away their livelihoods, but we want to change what they do as farmers to create food that promotes health and stop farming practices that are destroying lives.

Complex chronic metabolic diseases (wicked diseases) are not genetic

Stanford Medicine states up to 90% of chronic diseases are not caused by a dominant genetic variant (Stanford-Medicine 2010). It is our diet, epigenetic programming, mitochondrial handicaps, harmful environmental exposures, exercise habits or other detrimental habits like smoking or alcohol, along with adverse medication effects that drive or worsen the chronic disease pandemic. Yes, many medications pull the rug from under cell energy production, making matters many times worse.

However, as pointed out in the Lancet, diet has the greatest impact globally on the prevalence of chronic diseases (Afshin, Sur et al. 2019). Dietary inputs are well in your grasp to do something about and easy to control as an individual. If dietary exposures are this impactful on chronic diseases, why do we tolerate the medical profession being so ignorant of nutritional concepts, and why do we accept dietitians being so clueless about the medical impacts of their dietary advice?

Minor genes are in play, but we don't have a powerful sledgehammer gene for any particular chronic disease. Genome-wide association studies (GWAS) since 2002 have been looking for those "killer genes" for chronic diseases but have not found any (Rappaport 2016). We have minor genes that have some impact but are not the answer to our pandemic of chronic metabolic diseases.

The Holy Grail has been trying to find a particular "killer gene" for any of the deadly chronic diseases, which means we have a blockbuster drug target, and once we do, think of all that money Pharma could make. Is the medical field truly considering this unrealistic approach? Is the dietetic profession equally misguided? There is no altruism here, only the thought of making money. ***As they say, our genes load the gun, but the environment pulls the trigger***, which is true.

So, suppose environmental factors like diet, epigenetics or toxic exposures are to blame, then why are we not tackling these highly modifiable global exposures meaningfully to change our food and other inputs? Why are we not changing the very nature of foods?

Cardiovascular disease (CVD) is a monumental global killer that is increasing in prevalence. The WHO states many "***die too young***". Food can strongly impact CVD. Child and adolescent obesity has unbelievably increased by 10-fold (Rao 2019).

Toxic wounds

We are, at last, waking up to the toxic soup we live in. This toxicity is hidden but deadly. The documentary ***Revealed: How to Poison a Planet*** is an eye-opener about the huge problem of forever PFAS chemicals. To think all these untested chemicals are not having an impact on cellular pathways, including our energy-producing pathways, is to be truly gullible indeed. Who in their right mind would permit a chemical producer to create something and then release it into the world without testing it for safety? Yet this is exactly what has been done around the globe without our knowledge or permission. Who do we hold responsible? Who do we lynch legally, strip them of their assets and throw them in a dark, gloomy cell for all the misery and death caused?

Our cells are constantly being assaulted daily by many of the 350,000 environmental chemicals out there. This gigantic number of chemical compounds released to the environment is derived from the 2020 chemical inventory (Pelley 2020). The vast number of these environmental chemicals have not been tested at all, but some bureaucrats out there have glanced over a document presented to them by the industry, superficially read it and stamped that document "Approved for release". How much money was exchanged for this approval? Were these officials so dumb that they accepted the false argument that states: "*How can an incredibly small amount of chemical exposure do any harm?*"

So, is it any wonder that we have a cellular bioenergetic and metabolic disease crisis, decreasing sperm counts ("spermageddon"), reduced fertility rates, autoimmune diseases rising, a cancer explosion, neurodegeneration such Alzheimer's or Parkinson's increasing where Parkinson's has doubled in just over two decades. What about the emerging cancer epidemic in younger and younger people? Toxic chemicals are a part of this chronic disease and cancer nightmare that cannot be denied or ignored anymore. They cannot be overlooked in this story. Why should we have to prove they are dangerous when the industry itself needs to prove they are safe and then bear a massive fine if what they say is not true?

Being surrounded by toxic chemicals is taken for granted. Do we ever consider all the poisonous compounds we inhale every second or those in our food and water? Some of us even run alongside roadsides packed with cars spewing out toxic fumes or even run through a haze of smoke when we have terrible bushfires, thus inhaling trillions of PM2.5 micron particles that then embed themselves in lung tissue for perhaps decades and maybe forever. Do these individuals even think about inhaling more and more toxic particles by their exertion and deep breaths? These small PM 2.5 particles become trapped in our lungs and elicit an inflammatory response that will then pour out inflammatory cytokines, eventually triggering a heart attack, stroke, dementia or cancer down the line.

This inflammatory response is no different from a foreign body response like a splinter in our finger where the immune system attacks these foreign lung particles unsuccessfully, leading to chronic inflammation and thus adding to the inflammation from chronic metabolic disease, visceral fat, damaged vascular endothelium, etc. This lung-derived inflammation is strongly linked to dementia.

Another hidden threat to our health has emerged in microplastics and the endocrine-disrupting chemicals in them. A published paper stated that there could be 11.6 billion microplastics and 3.1 billion nanoplastics in just one teabag (Hernandez, Xu et al. 2019). Yikes! All of these threats work their toxic "magic" over our lives.

Cell shock indeed! Many of these chemicals not only have powerful hormone-disrupting characteristics, but they are also carcinogenic. Imagine this combination of chemical activities in hormone-sensitive organs such as breasts or prostates at high risk. Imagine the devastation of hormone disrupters in the brains of a developing foetus. How many behavioural problems can you think of that can be caused by the chaos of hormones being disrupted in cells of the body and brain, especially during foetal development? What impact are these vast numbers of chemicals having on mental health prevalence on top of all the metabolic dysfunction issues I have discussed?

A breakthrough occurred in Minnesota, USA, all due to the courage of a young woman called Amara Strande, who suffered an extremely rare malignancy, ultimately paying the price of losing her life at such a young age of 20 years. As Amara stated, she lived in the "3M plume", as did many classmates also affected by cancer. This 3M factory in Minnesota produced many PFAS chemicals known as "forever chemicals". It is said that 9000 to 16,000 of these PFAS chemicals are floating around in our environment and affect all of us as they linger in this planet's air, food, water and soils. This unbelievably brave young woman selflessly went to the State Capitol to fight for legislation against dangerous chemicals. Ultimately,

Amara's Law was passed, limiting unnecessary use of PFAS in Minnesota. This law is a start, but there is a long way to go with regard to ridding us all of environmental toxicities. Where is the medical profession in this fight?

Amara's family fights on. Finally, we need to ban these chemicals and force companies to test them irrespective of the cost. It is their greedy mess that they should clean up. No new chemicals should ever be released without extensive testing and approval by an independent, untainted oversight board. It is not up to us to prove they are dangerous. It is up to the industry to establish that any chemical to be released into the environment is safe by stringently assessing safety through long-term testing. Why do we accept being slowly poisoned in our lifetimes?

The 3M company reached a USD$10.3 billion (AUD$16 billion) settlement in April 2024 to address contaminated water. Yet this sum is pathetic when we consider the enormous scope of this problem. In 2019, the movie *Dark Waters* was released, and it starred Mark Ruffalo. This movie was based on a true-life story about legal action against DuPont, a giant manufacturer of industrial and agricultural chemicals. Despite the fact that Mark Ruffalo starred in this movie, it was ignored by the Oscars and Golden Globes. How many quaint and forgettable documentaries are given an award, and yet, those who hand out the awards or are in the movie industry will all feel the brunt of these chemicals in the form of progressive damage to their cells, leading to early ageing or a multitude of autoimmune diseases, chronic illnesses and cancers?

We have been gullible to have been persuaded by companies that profit from these chemicals that they are safe. The hormones in our bodies work at infinitesimally small doses and yet produce the most powerful of biological effects in cells and tissues. So, small doses mean nothing as an argument against adverse effects. We also forget the huge potential for synergistic effects of these chemical compounds, and we forget they can ***bioaccumulate*** in our fat and tissues and embed themselves in these tissues forever. Think cancers, leukaemias, and autoimmune diseases emerging in time.

The extremely few environmental chemicals tested have shown toxicity to our energy-producing powerhouses – the mitochondria. However, other chemical toxicities, including common medications, can also affect the mitochondria and energy-producing biochemical pathways, thus causing an additive effect with toxic environmental compounds. Which medical practitioner ever thinks of their drugs acting in concert with poisonous chemicals to rob cells of energy, thus triggering insulin resistance and chronic diseases? This damage to cellular bioenergetic pathways and mitochondria is well documented.

It is easy enough to see how a gradual loss of cellular energy occurs throughout our lifetime through toxic exposures that can affect us in the womb. That these chemicals can pass from mother to child in the womb is not contested.

A multitude of chemicals act simultaneously, causing cell energy starvation, thus boosting the insulin resistance disaster we are seeing worldwide. Inflammation is due to an activated immune system, and we will look at these super systems in the cell starvation chapter that are "***energy and nutrient hogs***". An activated immune system will then compete for energy and nutrient resources, drawing these away from already struggling cells undergoing energy starvation pressures.

It is well documented that medications are a part of this toxic soup we have to contend with. Medications used for mental health problems can have powerful disruptive effects on cell ATP (energy) production. Thus, it is no wonder that drugs used for Schizophrenia or other mental health problems can trigger weight gain and the emergence of frank diabetes in these unfortunate individuals. We add to their misery by using toxic medications that undermine cell energy production and hence trigger cell metabolic dysfunction, diabetes and chronic diseases.

The PFAS forever chemicals mentioned have been targeted recently in the USA to remove a handful of these chemicals from water supplies. However, only six (6) have been chosen to be removed from a PFAS family of at least 9000 chemicals (NIH 2023). However, there may be up to 16,000 PFAS chemicals out there.

Tokenism right? According to the NIHs National Institute of Environmental Health Sciences (NIEHS), PFAS chemicals can bioaccumulate, i.e. stay in our bodies and increase in concentration in tissues like fat and organs the more we are exposed to them. Once in these tissues and organs, we will have a disruption of metabolism, adding to our overfat, obesity, diabetes, hormone disruption effects, infertility and the cancer pandemic. Is this even arguable? Just look at the horrific story of AETT in Appendix-32 and be prepared to be shocked at the negligence shown with just one fragrance chemical.

So, six PFAS chemicals will be targeted, meaning we only need to worry about the other 349,994 chemicals surrounding us in our air, food and water. How do you target any chemical already released into the wild that can linger on for centuries? PFAS compounds are called "forever chemicals" for a good reason, as they hang around like a bad smell. According to an article on the University of NSW's (UNSW) website in Australia, these chemicals may hang around for 1000 years before decomposing (Duong 2023). Lucky us! These chemicals are an intergenerational problem, and we have allowed this to happen.

One of the greatest dangers to everyone, particularly children, is using fragrances in everyday cosmetics, lotions, cleaners, shampoos, conditioners, perfumes, deodorants, reed diffusers and many other fragrance products that fill the air in the house, office or car. We have 24/7 fragrance dispensers in homes, offices, and vehicles. There is a wonderful book titled ***The Case Against Fragrance*** that is an eye-opener on the dangers of chemicals that smell nice (Grenville 2018).

Any baby or child in that home or car will then inhale these hormone-disrupting fragrances. Let's not forget the signature fragrances on the mother and father, who are also reeking of these fragrant chemicals. We expose babies and children to thousands of chemical scents in their lives as if they mean nothing, and we never think those exposures can lead to long-term harm. What are we doing for the future health of a child by using toxic scents personally and choosing scented products that contaminate their environment and even penetrate their skin? Always choose fragrance-free products. These non-scented products exist for a good reason.

Think of a child undergoing rapid cell multiplication during growth spurts after birth and their immune systems undergoing crucial developmental changes. Imagine a newborn being exposed to 1000s of fragrances (chemicals) around them, let alone the 350,000 other environmental and industrial substances they encounter in daily life. How does hormone disruption by fragrances, microplastics embedded with hormone-disrupting chemicals in their water and food, along with other ecological toxicities, affect endocrine (hormone-producing) organs?

These fragrance impacts have not been studied in depth. They smell nice, but does this imply they are safe? Incredibly naïve. The AETT story in Appendix-32 will show you how destructive a fragrance can be to biological tissues. This horrendous story about one chemical can be found in the Kate Grenville book above. For any doubters about the potential danger of any scent, this AETT story will put a shiver up your spine. How many millions of lives were destroyed by this one fragrance?

There are 4,000 chemicals used to create fragrances, and each fragrance may have 50-300 distinct chemicals (Guardian 2019). Many "hormone disrupters" can interfere with estrogen or testosterone action on cell receptors. Women can be heavy users, and in "super-users", common synthetic musk chemicals used in fragrances were found at concentrations 10,000 times greater than those who use scents far less (Roosens, Covaci et al. 2007). Yet regulators will reassure us that this is just fine! Why, then, are we seeing an avalanche of hormone-sensitive breast cancers and a tsunami of prostate cancer (Medscape 2024)? Add these toxic exposures to all the other "energy bandits" that cause chronic metabolic disease, and we have a recipe for a colossal healthcare disaster.

"***The exploding worldwide cancer burden***" was the paper's title on this concerning problem (Wilson, Tobin et al. 2004). Early onset cancer in those under 50 is another emerging pandemic (Ugai, Sasamoto et al. 2022). Is this really a surprise to anyone? But think about the burden of breast cancer, endometriosis, lower sperm counts, prostate cancer, and infertility, which are all hormonally sensitive problems.

That these chemicals can affect mitochondrial function is beyond doubt (Reddam, McLarnan et al. 2022). Energy is king in cells, as I have mentioned, and we seem determined to sabotage cellular energy through our diets, the irresponsible use of fragrances and the neglect shown in saturating our environment with toxic compounds that can significantly impact cell energy systems.

A snapshot of vital statistics & Important points

- A paper published in ***Circulation,*** an Americal Heart Association (AHA) journal, titled ***Avoiding the Coming Tsunami of Common, Chronic Disease*** stated:

"...we will face an enormous wave of death and disability as a result of common chronic diseases (CCDs), with cardiometabolic diseases at the crest." (Califf 2021)

- According to the Australian Institute of Health and Welfare (AIHW), in a 2024 report online, the top diseases causing death include – Coronary Heart Disease (heart attacks), leading to at least 1 in 5 deaths, Diabetes, Dementia, Hypertension and Cerebrovascular Disease (damaged blood vessels of the brain) (AIHW 2024). All these diseases will have microcirculation damage at their core, and the incidence reported is often pathetically inaccurate as we only now have non-invasive ways of detecting microvascular flow problems.

- An Australian Bureau of Statistics (ABS) report released on the 15th of December 2022 stated, "*...almost all (99.2%) people aged 65 years and over had at least one long-term condition.*" Long-term medical conditions are called chronic diseases. Long-term or chronic diseases don't just start at a particular age. They take decades to manifest. Yet another statistic backs up the concept of universality or ***Metabolic Singularity.***

- We think we can throw money at this healthcare mess, and miraculously, we will fix this metabolic disease nightmare. Of around 4.1 trillion dollars spent annually on health care in the USA, 90% of this expenditure is for chronic illness (CDC 2022). If you think this is an obscene sum of money and it is staggering, then between 2016 and 2030, it is estimated to balloon to 42 trillion dollars in a short interval of 14 years (Boyle 2023). So 4.1 trillion dollars to 42 trillion dollars in only 14 years is buying us what?

  > *"The U.S. spends more on health care as a share of the economy — nearly twice as much as the average OECD country — yet has the lowest life expectancy and highest suicide rates among the 11 nations" (Commonwealth Fund 2020)*

  It is no wonder that the life expectancy of Americans has diminished since the 1950s and is lagging behind many other countries (Woolf 2023).

- *"Thomas Kuhn, in his book The Structure of Scientific Revolutions (Kuhn 1996), argued that when a scientific endeavor invests increasing effort in a problem with diminishing returns, the difficulty may lie with the core assumptions (paradigms) on which the work was based." (Wallace 2011)*

  With undeniable failure slapping us in the face as metabolic diseases continue to skyrocket and where drugs and dietetics have done nothing to stop this tide of disease and death, shouldn't we be challenging our "***core assumptions***" and stop the medical and dietetic business-as-usual strategy even though they are failed professions in this war on metabolic disease?

- *"The present trend is not sustainable unless a magic cure is found (unlikely) or concerted global/governmental/societal efforts are made to change the lifestyle that is promoting it." (Saklayen 2018)*

We face a bleak healthcare future unless we dare to make monumental changes. This problem demands major changes in dietary intake and major investments in prepregnancy and pregnancy health. We must minimise the ongoing impacts of environmental harm on cells and understand that all this happens from birth.

- *"Astoundingly, it has been estimated that about one-third of medical care is of no value, while another 10 per cent is actually harmful." (Buchbinder and Harris 2021)*

  This quote comes from a recent book called Hippocrasy, written by two Australians: Prof Ian Harris, an Orthopaedic Professor and Epidemiologist at the University of New South Wales (UNSW), and Prof Rachelle Buchbinder, a Rheumatologist and Epidemiologist from Monash University. Imagine that 1 in 3 medical encounters is of no value, and in total, 4 in 10 are of no value or actually harmful. But these figures are too kind. Even going back almost two decades, the statistics were grim with regard to chronic diseases with the following stats then:

"They account for 81% of hospital admissions; 91% of all prescriptions filled; and 76% of all physician visits." (disease 2000)

As chronic disease always skyrockets, it would be safe to say that around 90% of GP and Specialist visits are of no value. Chronic disease dominates medical consultations. So, what is any consultation worth if we are witnessing chronic disease armageddon threatening healthcare systems? Biological rot continues despite drugs that attack glucose, LDL, etc. If no cure is being offered, then what is the use of these scripts if all we are seeing is explosive increases in chronic metabolic disease?

90% of all deaths in Australia are due to chronic disease (Health and Welfare 2014). We must address and fix these highly avoidable diseases flooding healthcare systems;

otherwise, where is the value of any medical and dietetic care? Do you want to be another statistic in this foolish game?

CHAPTER 1

A medical war we have already lost

"Every time you eat or drink, you are either feeding disease or fighting it." Heather Morgan

The "Tap" and "Sponge" analogy. Our metabolic dysfunction "balloon" of skyrocketing chronic metabolic disease prevalence

We will explore the many "***energy bandits***" wanting to slowly "dim the lights" in our cells over our lifetime in the coming chapters. However, in this chapter, I would like to highlight the many factors that condemn you and humanity to an ever-increasing prevalence of chronic metabolic diseases. Understanding the early telltale signs of metabolic disease is vital, and these metabolic marker flickers are abundant if we only open our eyes to them.

It is no mystery at all as to why chronic metabolic disease prevalence is skyrocketing and will continue to rise exponentially in the two decades to come. If we don't stop the very early signs of metabolic disease and biological rot, then we have a snowball's chance in hell of avoiding chronic illness.

A vast majority of adults will have had blood tests done for the metabolic markers medicine focuses on to determine metabolic dysfunction. Each laboratory test will have a specific "normal range" from a lower limit to an upper limit. A doctor may have told you that a particular biomarker result of yours is "in range" or "out of range". But reading these results is not so straightforward as what happens within that space we regard as "in range" is a treasure trove of information that, if you know what to look out for, can reveal highly significant metabolic risk well within the lower and upper limit of that range. Changes that occur within this "in range" space will determine your health destiny. Knowing what to look for can help you dodge a metabolic disease bullet. ***We must view a "normal range" as an early warning system for chronic metabolic disease.***

Identifying early disease is the Holy Grail for preventing chronic metabolic diseases. It is your right and in your interest to ask for a copy of your blood test results or request the ones I mention in this chapter and Appendix-31. I will describe what to look out for in a "normal range", and if you think you are seeing abnormal metabolic signals, then request further testing such as a ***Glucose Tolerance Test (GTT) + Insulin Levels*** or the ***Insulin Response Test***.

Doctors will almost invariably test glucose only in a GTT, but this focus on glucose is oblivious to the fact that it is elevated insulin levels (hyperinsulinaemia), which is the absolute hallmark of early diabetes. Glucose levels are, in fact, a late-stage marker of this insulin resistance process. It can take a very long time for glucose to become elevated, so testing glucose only and not insulin is essentially redundant in the early phase of insulin resistance.

So, a doctor who orders a GTT but forgets about the insulin levels will say your glucose is "in range" when, in fact, your insulin levels could be sky high. The doctor essentially has totally missed the diagnosis of insulin resistance by ordering the wrong test. Any test, however, will need corroborating evidence, and such evidence is easy enough to see perhaps in you, such as a big waist, being overfat, overweight or obese. If you have hypertension, raised uric acid, raised glucose, or raised lipids such as cholesterol, triglycerides, LDL, or lower HDL, then these additional markers of metabolic disease will all substantiate your insulin response test to support or disprove the lab findings and if you are in trouble metabolically.

As I have alluded to, we, in general, do not look for early markers of metabolic disease in medicine. The reason is political, as there is a cost to looking for early metabolic disease. The other issue is if we find any abnormality, then what do we do? Drugs have been hopeless in stopping and reversing metabolic disease, so why bother looking for telltale signs of metabolic disease when we are powerless to do anything? We wait for biomarker signals to slap medical practitioners in the face to wake us up that something is wrong metabolically. If you know what to look for, you can see alarm bells sounding in a "normal range" for glucose, triglycerides, LDL and other markers, let alone waiting for in-your-face biomarker signals. Waiting for a high-level glucose cut-off point to diagnose "prediabetes", "MetS", or "diabetes" is a disgrace because, as you will see in the coming chapters, we allow a tremendous amount of biological damage (biological rot) to occur to our bodies by waiting and waiting for this loud glucose or other biomarker signal to manifest. It is not acceptable in the least to wait for a glaring biomarker signal to warn us something is wrong because if we can see early signs of metabolic dysfunction, we can act urgently to prevent a chronic disease disaster through nutritional interventions.

We only have to look at the USA, where I mentioned 88% of its population is already metabolically unwell (Araújo, Cai et al. 2019). The rest of the world is not far behind. All of these individuals with abnormal metabolic biomarkers are primed for biological damage where the biological rot will eventually lead to a fatal heart attack, stroke, or slow death from dementia or the triggering of a mental health disorder or two. You don't die because you have reached a particular glucose cut-off point and a diagnosis of Type-2 Diabetes Mellitus. You, in fact, die from all the cumulative biological damage that occurs long before that diagnostic glucose cut-off and then long after that glucose cut-off point. The diagnosis of "prediabetes", "diabetes", or "MetS" is an unnecessary, useless, and outdated concept. It is a scar on medical thinking that puts all of us at risk.

The "tap" and "sponge" analogy

It is assured that no one will escape chronic metabolic diseases using the current medical and dietetic models. To understand what is happening visually, I will use the analogy of a ***tap*** that represents the flow of metabolically diseased individuals towards a healthcare system, represented symbolically as a ***sponge***. This flow of chronically diseased individuals from our "tap" towards healthcare systems, our sponge, started in the 1960s with the Green and Farming Revolutions. As I have mentioned previously, diabetes as a disease was unheard of before 1960, making up "***considerably lower***" than 1% of all medical presentations (Heidemann and Scheidt-Nave 2017). I need to state this fact time and again as some gurus seem clueless to this historical fact of "diabetes" rarity before 1960 historically and think all of this began in their lifetimes. Not knowing history means that the "guru" is not only ignorant but dangerous and deadly.

Type-2 Diabetes Mellitus baffled doctors at that time. The Green and Farming Revolutions of the 1960s and 70s triggered this deadly metabolic problem as a result of cheap grains flooding the market. Once we have a cheap commodity, all we need then is a rampant, greedy capitalist and marketing system, and voila, we have monster foods that "speak" to our primal brains, making us want more and more of these monstrous foods that make all of us incredibly sick. Let's not forget "energy" snacks created from cheap carbs with big profit margins in colourful wrappings that are found conveniently in every petrol station and every corner store.

The CDC graph (Appendix-30) on diabetes trends should make it absolutely clear how this dietary change caused diabetes rates to soar. Are there gurus out there pretending to be confused about how this pandemic of diabetes and chronic diseases started? Why are they confused? Our genes didn't change suddenly, did they? It would take over 1 million years for genetic change to "hit and stick" (OSU 2022). What changed dramatically is our carb load and food energy intake, and by this, I mean starchy carbs that produce horrendous postprandial (after-eating) spikes in glucose that can be likened to ***mini-diabetic episodes,*** as we discussed in the introductory chapter.

Let's not forget that the concept of adequate micronutrients and fibre simply went out the door. Ugly greed and capitalism took over.

You can view the USDA food pyramid created in the 90s in Appendix-38. At a glance, you will see how grain-based foods packed the base of this pyramid, advising people to consume large amounts of carb-rich foods. It is common knowledge that food industries that are either supported or highly subsidised, like grain, meat livestock, and dairy, become powerful lobbyists. Their agitation shaped what was included in this pyramid out of self-interest and not science or the health of populations, thus condemning all of us to a pandemic of chronic diseases. This twisted carb-packed pyramid still shapes the recommendations of dietitians. It suits governments that make monumental sums of money from the sales of grains and other staple foods. We have allowed food lobby groups to act as the foxes that guard the henhouse, and thus, we have enabled these food groups to damage all our lives for decades (Schaffer 2002).

It was cowardice from the medical and dietetic professions not to dig their heels in with regard to blatantly distorted food pyramids and dietary recommendations for populations. These professions will face the music in the coming decades as healthcare systems crash and burn and then justify why they allowed this killing machine of chronic diseases to flourish. You will need to understand how your thoughts on food consumption have been based on flawed food pyramids and food recommendations built on the vested interests of agricultural and food economic imperatives. Your health was never a consideration. Only self-interest and greed were.

So, from the 1960s on, the number of people with diabetes exploded, and initially, this flow was a trickle from our "tap". It does take a decade or so for high-carb intake madness from our food revolutions to manifest as diabetes. This surge in diabetes didn't start immediately. This lag time is shown beautifully in the CDC graph of diabetes prevalence, seen in Appendix-30.

Over time, this flow accelerated from a trickle (drips) from our disease "tap" to a downpour and then a torrent flooding our healthcare systems, which we are witnessing now. The mind boggles to think of the torrent becoming a ***tsunami*** of diseases in the next two decades, producing such volumes of diseased individuals that nations start to crumble. It is now sheer madness to argue against this association between dietary inputs and diseases that are crushing healthcare systems. We have been gaslighted enough and blind to dietary impacts for far too long, and this makes sense only to gurus and corporations with twisted agendas driven by vested interests.

The medical profession has long dismissed the profound positive impacts of nutrition with the right nutritional advice and belittled the use of nutrients as if to say these approaches are rubbish and that drugs are our only hope. It is easy enough to see why this propaganda against nutrition began. The medical profession is driven by pharmaceutical interventions, and medical professionals unquestioningly accept the dogma of its profession without challenge. So if food and nutrients are rubbish practices, it then leaves us to depend on drugs, drugs and more drugs and yet this rubbish drug-centric approach has categorically failed in over 60 years to protect us and has seen the emergence of a dreadful pandemic of metabolic disease of unprecedented historical proportions.

So, instead of abandoning drug-based approaches that have unequivocally failed, they want to persist with them as it suits the quick-fix agenda that ends consultations fast to move forward with a busy medical schedule to add more and more to the bottom line at the end of the day. But if we consider all those millions of consultations amounting to absolutely nothing over the decades where drugs have cured ***NOTHING***, then that money doctors have earned in their 6-minute consultations has simply gone down the drain. Money lost means other important agendas in society suffer.

My solution to solving this confusion is to have all these confused gurus locked in a clinic with no escape and to provide them with meal after meal of high-carb grains until they emerge out of their ears and then check their bloodwork and weight in 1 to 2 months. We should do the same for those gurus now trying to gaslight the "virtue" of ultra-processed foods by feeding them copious amounts of horrific ultra-processed foods. At the end of this exercise, these gurus would be overweight, look absolutely sick, feel as grimy as can be and full of abnormal metabolic markers, signalling they are extremely unhealthy and at risk for a catastrophic medical event. Which guru will ever take up this challenge?

In reality, this exercise was carried out in volunteers given ultra-processed foods in a controlled metabolic ward with a staggering increase in energy intake of 500 calories per day, and the individuals who were on the processed food diets "***gained commensurate amounts of weight*** (Nestle 2022). It's a pity these were research subjects and not gaslighting medical or dietetic gurus locked in that controlled metabolic ward that Professor Marion Nestle the Paulette Goddard, Professor of Nutrition, Food Studies, and Public Health Emerita at New York University stated was one of the most important nutritional studies she knows. Remember, it is not just ultra-processed foods that are a problem; it is all our staples considered "healthy" that adversely impact all of us with each meal. These "gurus" should be forced to prove to us that what they say has any meaning whatsoever by being locked in that metabolic ward so there is no cheating and show the world how ugly and disingenuous their rantings are by consuming vast amounts of processed or unprocessed staple foods as they expect everyone else to consume.

So, initially, our chronic disease burden was low, and our sponge (our healthcare systems) could absorb these diseased individuals because, in the early decades, it had plenty of capacity to absorb this flow as diseases were in the process of forming and slowly accelerating to become the disaster it now is. However, as the drips became a torrent, the health system sponge became saturated with diseased individuals. Once this torrent of diseases saturated the sponge's capacity, it naturally triggered an overflow where complicated disease problems constantly occupied hospital beds, preventing other severely ill patients from getting a bed in a hospital setting. Severely complicated patients are not easy to boot out of the hospital, and so there they linger in hospital beds, full of multiple organs failing and too complex and fragile to move out to make place for new patients reaching an advanced stage of disease where they too will present with their complex medical problem/s needing hospital admission for stabilization. Notice I mention "stabilize" as there is no cure. The biological rot continues no matter what medical practitioners do.

In fact, we really don't need to lock medical or dietary "gurus" in a metabolic ward. Look at these "gurus" or your doctors as they, too, believe in their propaganda, so just look at their waistlines, check their skin to see if it is healthy and match their known chronological age with what you see in front of you. Most of these "gurus" or doctors look downright sick, overweight and unhealthy.

These complex medical problems produced by the insulin resistance metabolic dysfunction continuum where "diabetes" is simply a fake point on this journey constantly fill the appointment books of doctors who can only offer already failed drugs to individuals who will ultimately develop a chronic disease or die of organs failing. Handing out drugs to individuals is incredibly deceptive, and this is done out of ignorance by doctors who are lemmings who never question their failure and never truly understand the metabolic dysfunction processes at all. In fact, after reading this book, you will have far more knowledge than the majority of doctors out there. I, too, was once a medical lemming.

When beds are full of very damaged people with complicated (wicked) metabolic outcomes, we can then expect to have ambulance "ramping". Ramping is where ambulances wait in a parking queue outside an Accident and Emergency Department, waiting for a bed to become available through the discharge of a patient. So, we have individuals in need of urgent "patch-up" jobs to stabilize them who simply wait in those ambulances in a parking line waiting for someone to get booted out of emergency or wards back to their homes so they can take their place.

Where, then, does this leave the huge numbers out there in suburbia that are also affected by this abnormal metabolic continuum, reaching a crisis point on their metabolic timeline, having a heart attack, stroke or collapsing on the street out there somewhere?

Where are the ambulances for these people? Oh, wait, the ambulances are ramped outside hospitals, acting like a substitute for a hospital bed.

What can we expect when we have done nothing to stop these chronic diseases from exploding on this planet? What have we done to prevent horrific foods from being produced that are soaked with sugar, salt, fructose, carbs, bad fats, low in good fats and nutrient-poor high-energy foods? Have we stopped foods being researched for "bliss points" that hook people into consuming these highly addictive foods? Such food alteration and manipulation is a modern curse. Have we done anything whatsoever to support our distressed cells or to restore their energy levels and restore balance? What do we do to reverse the entropy (decay, chaos, degeneration) in cells due to pathetic nutrient inputs?

So, what should we do? Turn off the tap by modifying food and other harmful inputs, or should we build a bigger and bigger sponge and then complain of staffing shortages or not enough hospitals as those bigger sponges become saturated as well with complicated metabolic diseases? It is stunningly ignorant, but mindless governments want to make bigger sponges by building more hospitals, churning out more nurses, and recruiting quasi-medical wannabe medical practitioners like pharmacists and even allied health practitioners without medical degrees to do what doctors should be doing, all in the name of attempting to absorb more and more diseased individuals. It is political cowardice that has created this crisis by not dealing with the inputs that cause disease in the first place. What could go wrong with wannabe doctors who maybe didn't get the marks to get into a medical school or haven't walked on fire like doctors have to do to get their experience? Experience doesn't come easy.

Shouldn't we be turning off this darn tap rather than building bigger and bigger sponges? We can turn off this tap easily if only politicians and professionals give up their self-interest and then cut the strings from vested interest puppeteers for the sake of population health and the health of future generations. Medicine and dietetics can be so much more if their focus is on health and not on their own and corporate bottom lines.

Health professionals need to take heed of this Latin phrase: ***Primum non-nocere*** – which means first, do no harm.

The metabolic dysfunction "balloon" about to explode

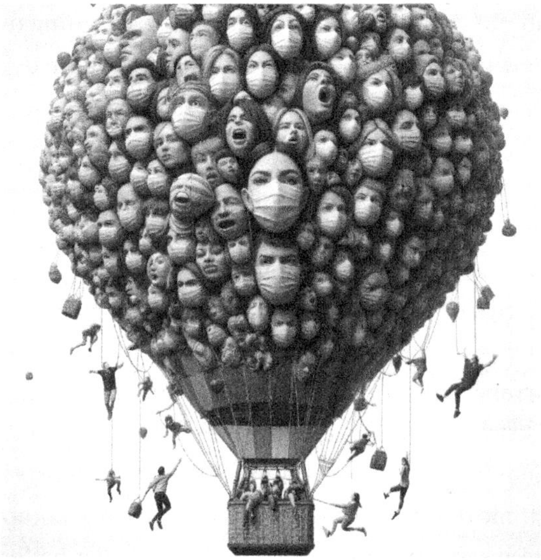

I will expand on this concept of a symbolic metabolic dysfunction balloon, expanded upon in the "prediabetes" chapter next. Like it or loathe it, we are all destined to be crammed in this balloon sooner or later unless there are drastic changes as outlined in this book.

This balloon represents the masses of people around the world with early, middle or late insulin resistance and metabolic dysfunction, where these numbers are increasing by the minute. They are all crammed into a metaphorical balloon that keeps on expanding, with more and more metabolically diseased individuals filling this balloon daily. They all have the ***biological rot*** I have discussed that is never fixed, and where this biological rot continues in the background of all of these crammed individuals within this metaphorical "prediabetes" balloon.

This balloon is set to burst in the not-too-distant future. It is a crushing number of people who get sicker and sicker decade after decade and then develop more and more complicated diseases as time goes by, as the metabolic dysfunction continuum and the ensuing biological rot is never interrupted by any drug at any time in its course and thus simmers in the background of the lives of those crammed in this ever-expanding balloon. No drug and no medical patch-up job at the individual level does anything to halt or reverse this continuum of rot, and thus, this balloon becomes incredibly stretched. Dietetics does all it can to fire up and accelerate this process with its outdated staple food dietetic advice for a monumental problem that seems to be going over their heads.

All we are focused on is to stop an acute event as much as we can, such as delaying a heart attack or a stroke. Our aim is never to fix the underlying metabolic problem from forever progressing until death. It is all about piecemeal approaches individual by individual that simply buy that individual a little more time on this planet.

This focus on drug interventionist approaches is our downfall and the reason why this balloon is expanding at a dangerous rate right now. As mentioned, the prevalence of diseases emerging is now a torrent and about to become a tsunami. Stabilization of chronic diseases is the name of the game, and then once stabilized, we throw them back into this crammed balloon, waiting for another inevitable but more severe life-threatening medical complication to occur in these same people that spilled out of that balloon into our healthcare system and then thrown right back in because this is no fix. The problem is that individuals by the millions are being added to this ever-expanding balloon yearly. Newly diagnosed insulin resistance (IR) sufferers are being squeezed into a tight space with old-timers with IR, all never cured and all waiting for increasing medical complications to manifest. GPs and hospitals are clueless about halting biological rot, so the balloon keeps on expanding.

Individuals are continuously falling off this balloon in increasing numbers all because a cure is not an option or not a focus. The individuals falling off that balloon are what I describe in my tap analogy, where medically damaged individuals continue to fall from that metaphorical balloon onto a "conveyor belt" headed for general practice or a hospital, thus stretching healthcare systems to their limits. All of this accelerated from the 1960s on as a legacy of the Green and Farming Revolutions that produced high-yield grain varieties that only needed the "magic touch" from corporations who didn't care less about health outcomes and only sales of their damaging food products, making those products more and more desirable but uglier and uglier in terms of health impacts. When does dietary management wake up to their disastrous food recommendations? By becoming proxy salespeople for grains, dietetics has fuelled this metabolic disease fire, which is now a raging inferno.

"Prediabetes", "MetS", and "Type-2 Diabetes Mellitus (T2DM)" are all fake labels. Have these false medical constructs stopped a deadly chronic disease pandemic?

It is no wonder we have lost this medical war against metabolic chronic diseases. My goal is to equip you with the comprehensive background knowledge needed to spark a profound realization that if you hand over your life to failed medical and dietetic models, then you don't stand a chance of dodging a chronic disease bullet. Additionally, I aim to delve into the intricate details explaining why our cells are driven towards a state of bioenergetic and structural decline. The trick is to avoid these cellular declines.

We point the finger at blood glucose as our nemesis, but then we seem to conveniently ignore the fact that glucose increases along a continuum of risk. As I have indicated, all points on this glucose continuum, from the earliest flicker to the Mt Everest of blood glucose levels we call "diabetes", will have a certain risk at those cut-offs. But the risk of something like glucose gets higher and higher the longer and higher glucose levels get. Each point anywhere along this continuum has a medical complication risk. The final result of the glucose and other metabolic continuums is all our horrific chronic illnesses given enough time. The extent of this risk is determined by:

1. Time along this continuum – how long has this biomarker been allowed to linger and cause biological damage (rot)?
2. The Level of the Biomarker – how high does this biomarker rise in the blood?

If we limit the time and level of biomarkers, we could make a huge difference in the extent of biological damage they cause. Yet this charade continues. We continue dishing out drugs, and Pharma continues to make billions out of a fake system of disease biomarker cut-off points. Has this system of cut-off points made any dent in the prevalence rates of metabolic diseases? The answer is a resounding ***NO*** over 60 years. When we reach a glucose cut-off point, it is not as if an amazing cure awaits any of us at that point. There is no cure at any point of this continuum towards chronic metabolic diseases! The biological rot gets worse and worse until death. No drug stops this rot, but we keep pretending we are doing something by ending a medical consultation with a script.

"Normal" Ranges: Not so normal after all

Most of us will have had blood tests done, and we may be told our results are either in or out of the "normal range". Falling in between the goalposts does not mean all is well. We can apply our railway continuum analogy between the normal range goalposts, i.e. the continuum of risk between the lower and upper limit. Thus, getting higher and higher in this continuum between lower and upper limits within a normal range indicates the risk is increasing (Preuss 2018).

Hopefully, you will have recent results to look at in light of the knowledge ahead. Risk can begin long before even the lower or upper limit of this range. So, normal ranges can give you a false sense of security, and these results need to be expertly assessed.

Glucose cut-off points are ineffective in identifying this increased risk within a normal range. Let's look at the risk for glucose levels between a so-called "normal" range of glucose provided by the WHO, with a level of 3.9 to 5.9 being regarded as normal.

If this WHO range is correct, and if we assume that we fall anywhere within this range, we will be fine, then this is a false sense of security. Why, then, does a high heart mortality risk start from 4.7 mmol/L, as shown below (Bjørnholt, Erikssen et al. 1999)? Breast cancer risk and spread increase from a glucose level of 4.8 mmol/L (Contiero, Berrino et al. 2013), and we have a high heart failure risk from a glucose level of 5.6 mmol/L (Wu, Liang et al. 2021). Go figure!

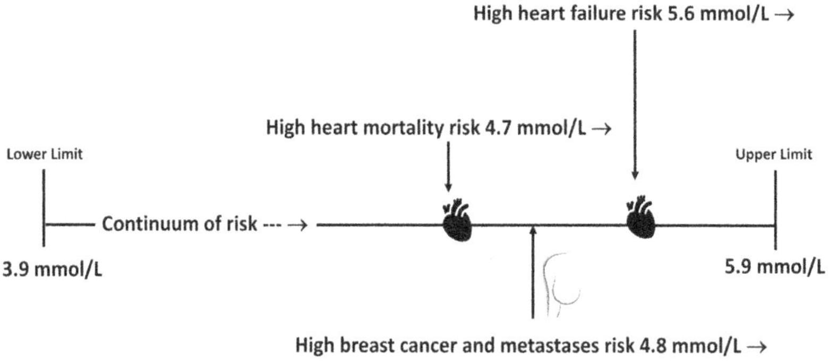

WHO Reference range for fasting blood glucose

From these incredible risks ***within*** the normal range of fasting glucose, you can see the dietetic madness to recommend high-carb intakes mindlessly, especially when insulin resistance is so prominent in populations, with the potential of high-carb intakes keeping blood glucose (and insulin) levels high throughout the day. We increase risk in individuals to protect agricultural economics.

Let's look at the WHO definition of classifying someone as having diabetes when they reach a fasting blood glucose level greater than or equal to 7.0 mmol/L. If medical risk starts far lower than this very high glucose cut-off level for diabetes, then our classification system is completely wrong. I use this diabetes-centric approach adopted by the medical profession to illustrate a point and show how flimsy and confusing this model is. Diabetes should never be our focus, as I have mentioned, and glucose cut-off points are totally outdated. Preventing diabetes from emerging in the first place should be our absolute focus, and we must take action from very early signs of metabolic disease.

So, we designate 7.0 mmol/L as a significant fasting glucose cut-off point to define a diabetic state. And yet, with a fasting blood glucose level of just 5.3 – 5.5 mmol/L, we have a 2.3 times (2.3x) increased risk of becoming "diabetic" than those with a fasting glucose of less than 4.8 mmol/L (Kiat 2020). Suppose there is a risk of transitioning to diabetes well within this normal range. In that case, we will also have an accompanying risk of biological damage (rot) occurring in this normal range continuum as well.

These high-risk levels of 5.3 – 5.5 mmol/L are way below the WHO diabetic cut-off of 7 mmol/L, as you can see. It is important to know that a fasting glucose level of 5.3 – 5.5 mmol/L is considered within the "normal" range of 3.9 mmol/L to 5.9 mmol/L. Thus, think of the huge damage done to people who had their results dismissed as normal when, in fact, they had a very high risk of developing heart failure and other chronic diseases over time.

The other fact to consider is that for every 0.1 mmol/L rise above a very "normal" glucose level of 4.8 mmol/L, there is a huge 12% increased risk of "diabetes" (Nichols, Hillier et al. 2008, Kiat 2020). This 0.1 mmol/L incremental and cumulative risk reinforces that we have a risk continuum and that "diabetes" risk begins way below the incredibly advanced glucose cut-off points used in medicine.

We are primed for insulin resistance in our lifetimes. Once again, I am not in favour of seeing "diabetes" as an end-point, only the biological damage or biological rot that occurs before and after this fake diabetes cut-off point, but historically, this is what medicine has done.

The Quintile-Climb: Danger increasing within a normal range divided into five parts

I have coined the term ***Quintile-Climb*** out of concern for poorly interpreted laboratory tests and the need for early signals of metabolic dysfunction. What follows is the concept of a ***Quintile Climb*** (***QC***) within a normal or reference range for a laboratory blood test. This ***QC*** does not apply to all tests, as a quintile climb may either be a positive or a negative thing. For example, with vitamins, we may want to see an increase from the lower to the upper end. However, such a rise in other blood biomarkers can indicate you are in deep trouble and headed towards metabolic dysfunction, which, if left alone, you will end up with a deadly chronic disease.

Quintile Climbs are nearly always ignored in medical care. For example, a quintile means one of 5 parts, and thus, a reference range can be divided into five equal parts termed quintiles, with each quintile being one-fifth ($1/5^{th}$) or 20% of that range. So, each quintile contains $1/5^{th}$ of the total population studied from the bottom to the top quintile. Risk exists along these quintiles from the bottom to the top quintile as a continuum.

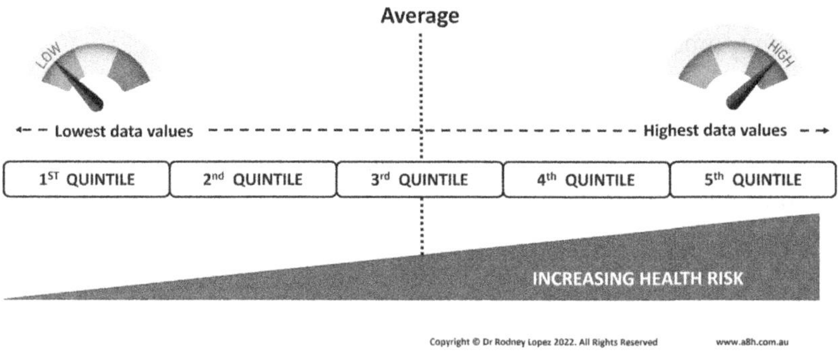

It is your right to ask for your laboratory results, which are often provided in chronological order along with the reference range for that biomarker. This way, you can "eyeball" these results to see if they are getting higher from the lower to the upper end. You can then single out the common metabolic biomarkers such as glucose, LDL, VLDL (if measured), HDL, Triglycerides, uric acid, and inflammatory markers like CRP or ESR. If you notice a Quintile Climb for these biomarkers is happening, then you will need to use other markers as confirmatory evidence. It is interesting that, with HDL, in metabolic dysfunction, lower levels of HDL are less of a risk than higher levels. Trying to raise HDL with drugs has been an absolute disaster. More on this later.

Consider any ***Quintile Climb*** of your biomarkers in light of perhaps high blood pressure diagnosed in you or if you are putting weight around your abdomen (visceral fat). Other clues that you are undergoing metabolic dysfunction include a strong family history of diabetes, a diagnosis of Metabolic Syndrome (MetS) in a family member or if close relatives have had premature heart attacks or strokes. You then have powerful supportive evidence of underlying metabolic dysfunction that is more likely than not to proceed to chronic metabolic disease. It's time to take action if you have multiple points of substantive additional evidence.

This need for early action is all about healthy outcomes. It will be risky to take a drug with a huge potential for an Adverse Drug Reaction (ADR). Drugs may be needed to stabilize metabolic dysfunction until nutritional action kicks in, but not with a view to keeping someone on this drug or drugs long term.

The view should always be to stabilize an individual with a drug or two and then move heaven and earth to provide meaningful nutrient support and then deprescribe.

It is never OK to dismiss a biomarker climbing up a reference range. We must avoid this simplistic interpretation of reference ranges concerning disease risk. Damage to biological systems will occur throughout the climb from the lower quintile to the upper quintile. Laboratories can easily determine this creep or ***Quintile Climb*** upwards as a red flag for doctors to draw attention to potential early warning signs for metabolic risk. However, this climb up the quintile ranks is often never highlighted by laboratories, thus ignoring an early red flag—a missed opportunity. Only advanced biomarker signals that go beyond the upper limit grab attention and are flagged by laboratories when results are truly "screaming" out that they are abnormal. Doctors only pay attention to advanced biomarker signals.

We need to look at the rate of increase within a reference range as we do with other biomarkers like Prostate Specific Antigen (PSA), which we call the "PSA Velocity", to warn us that rapid change is happening and that there is a prostate cancer risk. We should do the same for the rate of change in metabolic signals, perhaps as a "***Metabolic Dysfunction Velocity (MDV)***". Rapid changes can and do happen in many metabolic disease states. We must remember that rapid metabolic change will mean a rapid deterioration in blood biomarkers, causing accelerated biological damage and adverse medical outcomes.

This linear increase in risk along a range applies to LDL (the "bad" cholesterol), triglycerides (almost always raised in insulin-resistant states) and blood pressure (Shaye, Amir et al. 2012). All these markers are hallmarks of insulin-resistant diseases that will undergo ***Quintile-Climb*** that we can and should recognise to enable us to act early in the process. Acting late seals our fate.

This linear risk for an adverse outcome across a "normal" or reference range was derived from the CARMA study of 10,913 men and women designed to look for cardiometabolic risk in normal men and women. Not only was there a linear risk along the quintiles, as shown in the CARMA study, but there was also a significant independent risk of developing Type-2 Diabetes Mellitus (T2DM) in young adults well within the reference range within six years (Shaye, Amir et al. 2012).

> *"Similar to observations with other risk factors such as elevated blood pressure and cholesterol, CVD morbidity and mortality were suggested to progress as a continuum across blood glucose concentration, from levels well below the conventional cutoff values used for the diagnosis of DM." (Shaye, Amir et al. 2012)*
> *CVD = Cardiovascular Disease, DM = Diabetes Mellitus (T2DM)*

Cut-off points have failed all of us, but a Quintile climb is like an early alarm bell saying loudly - "wake up" - there is risk happening here, so pay close attention. Like all other test results, Quintile-Climb should always be seen in a clinical context, along with other disease markers, and not in isolation. We should never assume people don't want to be warned and that they will not take action. It is not a decision for a doctor, dietitian, specialist or government to make for an individual. It is unethical that they are not warned about the early signs of disease.

> *"Elevated CVD risk is strongly and independently associated with glucose levels within the normoglycemic range. Fasting plasma glucose may help in identifying apparently healthy persons with early metabolic abnormalities who are at increased risk for CVD before progression to prediabetes and overt diabetes mellitus." (Shaye, Amir et al. 2012) Normoglycemic range = normal glucose range, CVD = Cardiovascular disease*

Fasting insulin levels. A powerful predictor of future metabolic dysfunction

Beyond what has been mentioned above, a high quintile fasting insulin level powerfully predicts later metabolic dysfunction. Elevations in insulin levels can then become chronic and trigger self-perpetuating insulin resistance (Del Prato, Leonetti et al. 1994).

What we never take into consideration is the great demand for insulin from the beta cells of our pancreas, not only by high starchy carb intakes such as rice, potato, bread, pasta, etc. but also by high protein and fat intakes. What is also never on our radar in our rush to support the dairy industry is the huge insulin demand caused by the ***GI-Insulin Dissociation*** that is never on the radar of professionals trusted to care for our health. We will discuss this dissociation at the end of this chapter.

Why don't we mention this exaggerated insulin effect caused by dairy to our patients or clients? Because it will affect dairy sales? It seems we would rather preserve dairy sales and damage lives than stop an industry from producing a food source that is gaslighted as being "essential" to our health for various superficial reasons but then puts us at risk for insulin resistance. Flimsy rebuttals are seen, but there are no definites from gurus that state categorically that dairy will not cause insulin resistance and beta cell burnout. After all, we have 100s of millions consuming dairy on a daily basis, so why are populations going down the gurgler with metabolic diseases that increase decade after decade? Such gaslighting rubbish.

Only nutrients in foods are crucial, and you can always get these nutrients from other less damaging foods. It is disingenuous and dangerous to suggest that people will perish by not consuming a particular food such as dairy or carbs.

It is interesting that they point to benefits and yet ignore the risks. One paper stated:

> *"Conversely, milk intake might be associated with a higher risk of prostate cancer, Parkinson's disease, acne and Fe-deficiency anaemia in infancy." (Zhang, Chen et al. 2021)*

We can add Type-1 Diabetes Mellitus (T1DM) to that list above and many other problems like allergies, lactose intolerance, etc. It makes you wonder, in studies that have shown benefits on blood pressure or metabolic outcomes through dairy consumption, whether they excluded those with insulin resistance at higher risk of adverse outcomes, thus skewing the risk. Shonky research, indeed. Most of these studies are short-term, while long-term studies are costly and require dedicated researchers and funding. It is much easier to produce short-term industry-funded papers that can be used in propaganda to support an industry. Is any of this justified for a food like dairy that is not essential for any nutrient?

So, what we haven't recognised in the past is that consistently high insulin levels can lead to insulin resistance (Del Prato, Leonetti et al. 1994). This situation of persistently elevated blood glucose and insulin elevations after eating is easily caused by high carb and dairy intakes that will put us at risk for metabolic diseases.

What follows is research that shows why you do not ignore fasting insulin levels. There is no "touch of diabetes" or "mild" diabetes or "your levels are only just beyond the higher level". These are profoundly uninformed and dangerous statements made by professionals that seal the fate of millions of individuals. Millions have died miserable deaths as a result of this mythical and dangerous thinking of a "mild" metabolic dysfunction problem. The term "mild" has no meaning on a continuum of risk where mild progresses to severe along this continuum eventually. We seem clueless about a ***continuum of risk*** and a need for a ***continuum of care***.

Let's take a look at research on 515 men and women tested and found to have an insulin level in the upper part of the "**NORMAL**" reference range – i.e. in the upper quintile range - the upper 5th quintile. So, in grassroots medicine, doctors would have commonly ignored a fasting insulin level in the upper 5th quintile, and why? Because doctors are trained to see a figure that falls anywhere within this range as normal, so they ignore it if it does.

It is foolhardy to dismiss any early biomarker signal in an individual that has hypertension, a wide waist, a strong family history of early heart attacks, strokes or metabolic disease like diabetes. All these factors must be taken into account even with an early flicker of a biomarker signal, even if it is in the high quintile range. These individuals found to have high normal fasting insulin levels were then studied again, but impressively, the follow-up was 24 years later using another Glucose Tolerance Test (GTT) to check their metabolic status.

The follow-up study showed fasting insulin levels predicted "prediabetes" or "diabetes" **24 years after initial testing**. Thus, a high quintile insulin level is like a time machine that predicts an individual's future health. In addition, the results on follow-up for people with fasting insulin levels in the upper quintile were the following:

- **Half of the participants developed dysglycemia (abnormally high glucose levels)**
- **11.1% progressed to impaired fasting glucose (IFG),**
- **9.9% progressed to impaired glucose tolerance (IGT),**
- **4.5% progressed to both IFG and IGT and another 24.3% to type 2 diabetes.**

You can now see how we have mindlessly used IFG and IGT to label someone as having "prediabetes" when even a high quintile insulin level within the "normal" range can predict disease.

This quintile fact once again shows that fake glucose cut-off points are meaningless and dangerous. A high quintile fasting insulin level warns us of medical trouble ahead. It would be pointless to use drugs as they do nothing to halt and reverse this metabolic process. We falsely think those in the lowest part of a normal range have the same risk as those in the upper ranges of a reference range (Dankner, Chetrit et al. 2009). This thinking is false as risk increases through this range. Our risk of a complication climbs higher and higher as we progress along a continuum, and we allow this metabolic dysfunction continuum to run rampant and cause biological damage.

Using a drug of any kind in the early stages of metabolic dysfunction will provide a false sense of security because these drugs do not stop the multitude of factors that create a bioenergetic and structural decline in cells, allowing biological rot to simmer and increase in the background of anyone with a chronic metabolic disease. If we serially followed results over time, we would see a quintile climb as an early marker for all the diseases crushing healthcare systems.

We ignore early warning signals to our peril.

Endometriosis

Endometriosis, or "Endo", affects a staggering 10% of women globally. It can be severely debilitating for women who suffer from this gynaecological disease, where endometrial tissue (cells lining the inside surface of the uterus) can embed themselves outside the uterus and pelvis. Endometriosis is a complicated disease that has baffled the medical profession for decades, but the picture is becoming much clearer now. As this paper states: "***There is compelling evidence regarding the progress of endometriosis in the context of severe metabolic dysfunction.***" *(Lu, Ling et al. 2023)*

There are significant causal associations between Gestational Diabetes Mellitus (GFM) and Fasting Insulin (FI) with endometriosis that we cannot ignore (Xin, Li et al. 2024). High fat and high dairy intake can increase the risk of endometriosis (Lu, Ling et al. 2023). That fat and dairy are implicated is no surprise, as both can cause insulin to shoot through the roof, worsening metabolic dysfunction. Every woman with endometriosis needs their glucose and fasting insulin measured. The best way forward is to adopt a diet, as suggested in the final chapter.

We have been unbelievably foolish and irresponsible not to see insulin resistance and metabolic dysfunction driving such a wide range of diseases that we have not associated with metabolic dysfunction. After all, insulin resistance is an absolute curse for humanity, inflicting so much harm we are ignoring.

Our fairytale use of fake blood glucose cut-off points and fake labels: *Once upon a time*

Professor Edwin Gale, a UK specialist in diabetes, endocrinology, and metabolism, and many colleagues were bewildered about the path that medicine took regarding blood glucose levels. His paper "***The Myth of the Metabolic Syndrome***" began with a story tale opening: He stated:

> *"Once upon a time, no one knew what diabetes was... but a line had to be drawn between those who had diabetes and those who did not, and no one could agree where to draw it." (Gale 2005)*

The thought of continuums didn't exist in the early stages of trying to understand metabolic disease. Type-2 Diabetes Mellitus (T2DM) was almost non-existent, as I have pointed out, before the 1960s. Over my 40 years of practising medicine, it baffled me that we didn't see this connection between prediabetes, MetS and diabetes. It was like mass delusion being passed on to everyone in the medical profession.

How amazing is it that the diabetes prevalence rate was so rare before the 60s, and now almost everyone seems to have it? And so the false assumption arose that we needed to draw a line in the sand – our arbitrary glucose cut-off points that we artificially label as a "disease" entity. This line or cut-off has been a true medical disaster. It has gone unchallenged and is firmly entrenched in the minds of doctors. As you know, it is hard to shift an embedded idea from the minds of individuals, but this is unforgivable when it comes to the medical profession, as it becomes very dangerous to all of us if ideas and models are not challenged.

Sure, the medical profession was bewildered by this thing called "diabetes" How do we make sense of it? How will we control it? A flurry of thought processes arose, but so did the confusion that resulted in fake glucose cut-off points, fake labels, and theories (guesses) like glucose-related damage when glucose was just only one part of a vastly bigger picture.

Are the complications of diabetes due only to glucose toxicity (glucotoxicity)? This glucose guess (***Glucose Hypothesis***) has been proven false through the lens of time. No one factor, such as glucose, can cause all the biological damage or biological rot we see in "diabetes". So now, the medical field has shifted focus to lipid fractions like LDL. This shift to lipids as the enemy is called the ***Lipid Hypothesis*** – another guess. We will look at the LDL myth in detail later.

Remember, a hypothesis is an educated guess, plain and simple. Look at how chaotic this classification system is. Insulin resistance is a period in this continuum until blood glucose levels rise to a particular threshold, which then becomes "prediabetes". At an even higher glucose level, it then becomes "diabetes". How do we arrive at this "prediabetes" glucose cut-off? It is when someone has Impaired Fasting Glucose (IFG) or Impaired Glucose Tolerance (IGT) where glucose levels are high. IGT is discovered using a glucose tolerance test (GTT), which checks blood glucose levels after a glucose load.

However, to truly complicate matters, 75% of those with "prediabetes" will have MetS, and 86% of those with frank Type-2 Diabetes Mellitus will have MetS (Grundy 2006). Go figure.

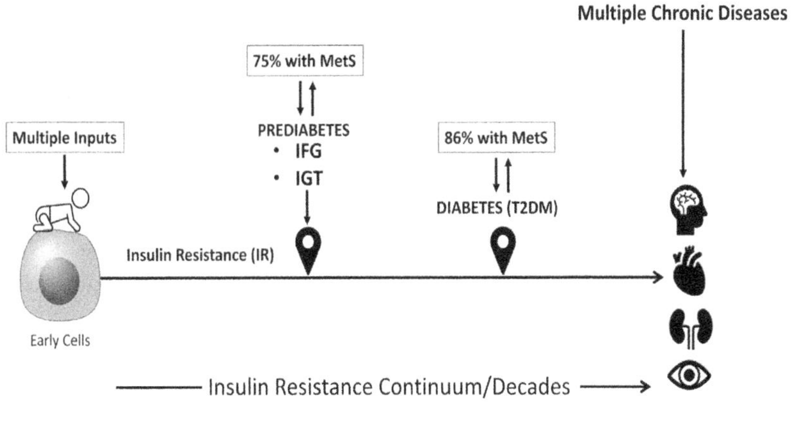

Oh, what a complicated mess. If this confuses you, then be reassured; doctors are also confused. Doctors don't question this highly arbitrary and fragmented way we use glucose cut-offs along an insulin resistance continuum. We are caught in a rut that the medical profession can't back out of now as they will have to be on their knees in a mea culpa moment, saying we have stuffed up.

Grassroots doctors, Endocrinologists who specialise in diabetes and dietitians think, who are they to question this "wisdom" being imparted by revered gurus of medicine? Wow, they have the title of Professor, so what they say can't be questioned. These gurus that strut stages spruiking drugs should be interrogated about what they say and why they say it. They should all have a forensic examination of their income to see who is being influenced by Big-Pharma.

If you look at the chapter "***Revolution Time***", I discuss the "Speaker Programs" that landed Pharma conspirators in prison. Watch the movie "*Pain Hustlers*" to see how corrupt those who strut medical stages can be, and you will get a deeper idea of how sickening this corruption is and why this chronic metabolic disease disaster is ongoing. However, most medical or dietetic gurus are not corrupt, just confused and conned to accept false constructs and feel powerless to change the system they have inherited and twisted to comply with. Many gurus do challenge this system, and kudos to them. Medical mavericks are the ones who will change the system and "keep the bastards honest".

The fact that all these terms overlap, such as "prediabetes", "MetS", and "diabetes", further reinforces that we have a common pathway – our insulin resistance continuum. As Professor John S Yudkin states, the cut-offs for diabetes are based on the risk of developing microcirculation damage such as retinopathy (small blood vessel disease of the eye's retina) or large vessel disease that will lead to heart attacks or strokes. The retina is our "window" to viewing our microcirculation health directly, as our small vessels are easily seen. Others will define these very high glucose cut-off points as a risk for developing "diabetes", but to cause even more confusion, cut-offs also vary in different laboratories and countries.

Blood glucose cut-offs are irrelevant as they do nothing to halt, reverse or cure any related metabolic disease. No drug treatment exists that will stop in its tracks insulin resistance and the **S**low,

*I*ncremental and *C*umulative (*SIC*) progression of biological damage (biological rot) that increases cellular entropy. No drug stops our microcirculation networks from imploding before or after any glucose cut-off point. Professor Yudkin states:

> *"Lesser degrees of hyperglycaemia increase the risk of developing diabetes and maybe arterial disease. But in both cases, the risk is graded, making any choice of cut-off point purely arbitrary." (Yudkin and Montori 2014)*

In this chapter, I will discuss the focus on developing T2DM as highly irrelevant and a medical disaster. Diabetes, as discussed, is only a mere point on a risk continuum and not a destination we need to obsess about. Our absolute focus should be on a continuum of risk that totally damages our critical microcirculation networks, leading our organ systems to deteriorate and crumble.

Lower blood glucose levels are a micro and macrovascular risk long before any glucose cut-off point. A sobering thought is that individuals classed as having "prediabetes" with glucose levels far lower than that used to diagnose "diabetes" have a 50% increased risk of coronary heart disease, where damage and blockages occur to the arteries of the heart. Studies show around 60% of those with Impaired Glucose Tolerance (IGT) as a cut-off for prediabetes will develop a fake "diabetes" level (Yudkin and Montori 2014). Remember, "diabetes" is a hop, step and jump away from all our healthcare-crushing chronic metabolic diseases. So, "prediabetes" is far from a benign problem that can be considered "mild" and then ignored.

Professor Edwin Gale's take on fake glucose cut-off points

> *"The difficulty they all faced was that blood glucose, as measured within a population, forms a continuous gradient between health and disease. Any cut-off between the two will, therefore, be somewhat arbitrary." (Gale 2005)*

This astute statement recognises that this damaging insulin resistance process, leading to many chronic diseases now crushing healthcare systems, is a continuum (continuous change or gradient). This continuum of metabolic change proceeds down a predetermined and highly predictable path to an inevitable end – our challenging and chronic diseases highly resistant to drugs and current dietary dogma.

A linear path with incremental and cumulative adverse effects over its course should tell you that every point on a continuum is highly significant and that choosing a particular point on this path is arbitrary and grossly underestimates future negative health impacts of ANY point on that continuum no matter how early that point is in this course and no matter whether that signal of metabolic dysfunction is a flicker or a blinding cut-off biomarker point.

Professor Edwin Gale expanded on the fairytale of arbitrary (fake) blood glucose cut-off points and stated:

> *"And so the wise men decided that the important thing you need to know about blood glucose is how high it has to be before it harms your blood vessels. Here, they came up with an answer: if your blood glucose goes up a little, this is bad for your arteries, but if it goes up a lot, your small blood vessels will suffer as well." (Gale 2005)*

What Professor Gale is saying above is essentially true with one very important qualification. A wealth of research now shows that it is the other way around to what was stated in the quote above. ***It is our small blood vessels, i.e. our microcirculation, when damaged, that becomes the "motor" that drives large vessel disease, not the other way around*** (Stokes and Granger 2005). This small vessel or microcirculation damage occurs, as we have discussed, long before glucose rises beyond the upper limit of a normal range. Microcirculation damage is the major driver of the biological rot I mentioned and the reason we are getting nowhere in metabolic disease management.

Damaged microcirculation networks are our ultimate nemesis in this metabolic dysfunction process, as these damaged small vessel networks are a crucial point of our vascular systems responsible for distributing oxygen and nutrients and removing cellular waste. These damaged small blood vessel networks thus become the small blood vessel "assassins" of organ systems.

All roads lead to microcirculation damage. We have insulin resistance, metabolic dysfunction, and frequent postprandial (after-eating) hits on a daily basis to ensure ongoing damage to these small microcirculation blood vessels over our lifetime. We must start to pay a lot more attention to the smaller things that have gigantic biological impacts.

The glucose hypothesis (glucose guess) has backfired on us.

We focus intensely on glucose when it is just one factor out of many, as I have mentioned, that damages our health and drives the metabolically induced biological rot that causes chronic organ failure. Glucose can cause much damage directly through the glycation of proteins to the point of creating Advanced Glycation Endproducts (AGEs). Glucose can also latch onto LDL, the so-called "bad" cholesterol, to create glycated LDL (gLDL), a far more pathogenic form of LDL that becomes "sticky" and is one trigger towards plaque formation in arteries, leading to heart disease or strokes. It is important to remember that with all these biomarkers, we allowed them to reach a point where they become damaging due to neglect! Biomarkers like glucose initially offer an energy (fuel) advantage to cells struggling with those acute insults that rob them of energy. We have allowed glucose to show its other damaging face through neglect in not preventing ongoing glucose damage.

Once this LDL becomes sticky, it can grab hold of and fasten onto the lining of arteries (the endothelium) and, at this point, can become oxidised-LDL (ox-LDL) equally as pathogenic or more in creating vascular damage. This modified LDL leads to plaque formation that could rupture to cause a heart attack or stroke.

We must remember all the changes in insulin resistance from hypertension, high glucose levels, inflammation, oxidative stress, increased Reactive Oxygen Species (ROS), and lipid changes also damage the blood vessel lining of our endothelium, making the lining sticky like "***Molecular Velcro***". This "velcro" enables modified LDL to latch on much easier to initiate plaque formation. It is not just glucose but a range of IR changes that lead to vascular disease.

When have we ever stopped the surges in glucose after eating by modifying food composition inputs on a meal-by-meal basis, which makes the high glucose level of advanced insulin resistance and diabetes worse? Still, as you see from the effects of insulin resistance listed above, glucose is only one part of a long line of risk factors. Inflammation itself damages and modifies LDL to cause oxidised LDL (ox-LDL). Knowing this, you can see that our focus on glucose is incredibly naïve and simplistic. Inflammatory damage to proteins or LDL can also occur in the postprandial (after-eating) period, meal by meal, and snack by snack.

The fact that glucose can't get into cells because insulin doesn't work and that we need higher glucose levels for fuel to enter cells doesn't stop us from hammering glucose lower and lower in the blood as enemy number 1 with drugs that make glucose less available than it already is to cells. Remember, in the early stages of insulin resistance, high glucose is an adaptation and an advantage. If glucose can't get into cells, we need to bypass insulin resistance and offer cells a different energy substrate. We bypass glucose as fuel by using ketones. More on this when we look at dietary modification. Ketones will give glucose-starved cells a fighting chance to reverse internal cellular structural damage, ramp up enzyme production, and create ATP to fight off all the entropy (decay) that has accumulated. How unbelievably silly that we do not adopt this nutritional strategy in the very early stages of metabolic disease to stop this process in its tracks.

"Metabolic Memory" and not Type-2 Diabetes Mellitus (T2DM) should be our focus

"***Metabolic memory***", also known as the "***legacy effect***", is a powerful consideration when we don't take steps very early in the

Insulin Resistance Continuum to protect our endothelial glycocalyx and prevent small vessel damage. Remember, it is this small vessel (microcirculation) network that is the driver of all the biological rot we see as organ failure (chronic diseases). This irreversible damage by poorly controlled glucose levels to the smallest blood vessels that make up our microcirculation networks is a major reason we have not won this medical war against chronic metabolic diseases. This persisting damage to small blood vessels highlights our outdated thinking, where awareness and management start way too late.

Metabolic memory is where structural microcirculation damage has occurred to the point of no return (Jax 2010). It is hard to reverse anything when vessels become so incredibly stiff, scarred and obstructed out of neglect to do something meaningful. Medicine never seems to learn the lesson of preventing damage in the first place and starting management early. Management is always after the fact. Please keep in mind that our only hope to reverse this metabolic memory is to use nutrition-based management. Drugs have proven to be incompetent in reversing this glucose legacy effect.

It is well known that if you begin intensive (drug) treatment **soon after** a diagnosis of diabetes is made, then there is a significant decrease in cardiovascular events. However, a delay in treatment after just eight (8) years of persisting diabetes will mean no reduction in cardiovascular events (López-Jaramillo, Velandia-Carrillo et al. 2014). Imagine how brilliant the results would be if we acted in a nutritional sense long before diabetes developed, as we could have halted and reversed microvascular damage before it had a chance to become a threat and long before this metabolic memory issue. It is Sad, then, that nutritional modalities of treatment are "sacrilege" to doctors who worship at the altar of Pharma and are blinded by drug-centric approaches only.

The problem is that "prediabetes" and "diabetes" go unnoticed in a huge number of people in populations worldwide. Globally, almost 50% of all diabetes cases go undiagnosed, ranging up to 80% in many countries (Beagley, Guariguata et al. 2014).

Leaving diabetes untreated for just eight (8) years seals the fate of an individual in terms of cardiovascular events.

If we had changed the composition of food to stop postprandial hits to our blood vessels with each meal, creating high glucose/insulin levels, we would have slashed the risk of metabolic memory and organ damage. Drugs, even if used early to decrease cardiovascular risk, will ultimately have no effect if all the inputs discussed in this book are not managed well.

Imagine all the 100s of millions of individuals with no idea they have "prediabetes" or "diabetes" consuming masses of grain-based foods, other carb-rich foods and dairy, sealing their fates. How sad then that many of those individuals will reach a point of no return in microcirculation damage without even knowing the damage that is occurring by stealth in their bodies and small blood vessels.

Concerning "metabolic memory", we recognise persisting damage to microvascular beds irrespective of glucose control. (Orasanu and Plutzky 2009). In other words, if we reach this early threshold of significant microcirculation damage, then glucose control will do nothing to reverse it. By not focusing on preventing microcirculation damage, we have screwed things up.

Small vessel damage worsens glucose control, and this worsened glucose control then damages our microcirculation networks even further. If our blocked small vessels can't deliver glucose to their target cells, tissues, and organs, it is obvious then that the unused fuel (glucose) will rise higher and higher in our systems. What's the use of targeting glucose when the "pipelines" are getting more and more damaged, blocking the delivery of fuel to where it is needed? Thus, it is no wonder that drugs can't reverse this memory effect of glucose damage. It was such a dreadful blunder of logic and neglect.

This result of metabolic memory is what we get by our laser-like focus on one biomarker – glucose. We allowed this to happen. Is it just bad luck or incredible negligence? Targeting glucose won't work, as it is a simplistic notion that one biomarker causes all the biological damage (biological rot) in our insulin resistance-metabolic dysfunction continuum. Once again, this metabolic memory phenomenon is another nail in the casket of glucose cut-off points.

Gestational Diabetes Mellitus (GDM). The "mother" of future-generation insulin resistance continuums

The womb seems more important than the home (nurture) as it determines an individual's long-term health outcomes and longevity. We need to remember that diabetes in pregnancy (gestational diabetes mellitus or GDM) has tripled in only recent months (Mnatzaganian, Woodward et al. 2022). GDM is the factor that condemns our children, grandchildren and great-grandchildren. We Program future generations for metabolic disease, and as I have discussed, we are epigenetically programming future generations for earlier and earlier onset of multiple cancers. How sickening that our generation is responsible for so many future health problems, misery and death.

Professor David Barker of 'The Barker Hypothesis' fame discussed below, wrote a paper published in the British Medical Journal (BMJ) titled:

"The fetal and infant origin of adult disease. The womb may be more important than the home" (Barker 1990)

The Barker Hypothesis states that epigenetic programming can hardwire fetal changes in the womb, which is more important than nurture (our immediate environment/home after birth). Such epigenetic programming is, in essence, how one generation passes on information to another about the state of the environment around the mother. See Appendix-6.

Pregnancy is a turbocharged generator of insulin risk for four (x4) generations, one being the mother. Pregnancy is an incubator for future metabolic diseases and a massive generator of future insulin resistance prevalence in populations as a result of affected individuals born to mothers with gestational diabetes mellitus (GDM). Babies born to a mum with GDM can have significantly impaired mitochondrial function (a huge mitochondrial handicap), which means a significant reduction in cell energy (ATP). The level of this epigenetically inherited mitochondrial dysfunction handicap is expanded upon in the dedicated chapter on cell starvation. A study from Yale University and published in the journal Diabetologia found that children born to mothers who had GDM:

> *"...had at least a 5x greater risk of developing IGT than those not exposed to gestational diabetes." (Holder, Giannini et al. 2014)*

Remember, IGT is Impaired Glucose Tolerance, a glucose cut-off point we discussed as a marker for "prediabetes". This huge 5x risk of IGT is a sign that these children have been programmed for chronic diseases early in life. It is truly irresponsible that we don't move heaven and earth to ensure this epigenetic programming never happens during pregnancy, as it is catapulting numbers in populations with the IRC ⇄ MetDc ⇄ MVDc risk that progresses to chronic metabolic diseases.

Sadly, a mother who suffers from GDM will be at a very high risk herself for future Type-2 Diabetes Mellitus (T2DM) and cardiovascular risk. This risk for T2DM is a huge 10-fold (10x) increased risk of that affected mum developing diabetes within 15 years (Egeland and Meltzer 2010). To put this into perspective, let's say a mother is a 25-year-old woman who develops GDM. She then runs the risk of having diabetes by the ripe old age of 40 or younger.

On top of this 10x increased risk of diabetes, a woman with gestational diabetes (GDM) has a 65% increased risk of stroke and a 2x increased risk of heart attack, heart failure and peripheral vascular disease (Yu, Soohoo et al. 2022).

What kind of society are we to allow young women in the prime of their lives to suffer early life-threatening diseases by not pulling out all stops to prevent this GDM problem from manifesting in pregnancy, where risk should be looked at long before pregnancy? Where are the dedicated prepregnancy and pregnancy clinics run by nutritionally savvy practitioners who won't sacrifice the life of a mother and future generations for economic imperatives? And why do we allow children to be born to suffer early chronic disorders?

Hardly a healthy human is left, as Aldous Huxley stated, all because we have become a dysfunctional group of humans on this planet numbed by the misery and death surrounding us by preventable diseases, even when our own lives are at stake. Why are we allowing corporations to get away with this carnage? Why are we enabling exponential growth of epigenetically programmed disease as gestational diabetes skyrockets when all of this could be prevented?

The Oral Glucose Tolerance Test (OGTT) has the subtlety of a sledgehammer to test for Gestational Diabetes Mellitus (GDM)

With such a huge risk of GDM to the mother and future generations, what do we do? We use an absolutely blunt tool in the form of an Oral Glucose Tolerance Test (OGTT) to look for an advanced glucose signal late in the pregnancy when epigenetic programming of the child (and mother) may have already occurred long before this pregnancy test result shows a positive outcome, condemning both child and mother to biological damage (rot).

The OGTT is a primitive tool akin to a hammer and chisel rather than using early markers before pregnancy or developing early signals in pregnancy. But no, we wait for that blinding glucose signal during a late-stage OGTT in pregnancy, and like glucose cut-off points, the damage has already been allowed to occur in the mother and child, including the generational damage that occurs due to epigenetic programming. Late glucose signals in pregnancy are setting the mother and baby up for the deadly consequences mentioned above.

We should never be looking for a problem late in pregnancy when the stakes are so high. What we should be doing, if we have any sense of decency at all, is to look for trouble long before pregnancy starts through testing for early biomarkers or the use of wearable technology to warn us this woman is at risk. I have mentioned actively looking for and finding trouble ahead of pregnancy, and this could be done in dedicated pre-pregnancy clinics through highly trained nurses who have a sound and deep knowledge of uncorrupted nutritional modalities of management and not the drug-addled, nutrition naïve way we do things currently. I discuss this in the chapter ***Revolution Time***.

Most women with gestational diabetes mellitus (GDM) already have beta cell dysfunction and chronic insulin resistance lurking in the background long before falling pregnant. Pregnancy becomes a "stress test" for bringing out diabetes during foetal development (Kaaja and Rönnemaa 2008). An oral glucose tolerance test (OGTT) at 24-28 weeks of pregnancy is the sledgehammer approach for diagnosing gestational diabetes. A "gold standard" it is not.

"The oral glucose tolerance test (OGTT) has been the mainstay for diagnosing gestational diabetes for decades. However, this test is deeply flawed" (Bogdanet, O'Shea et al. 2020)

We ignore many early biomarkers to warn that a woman is at high risk of GDM long before falling pregnant and long before that OGTT late in pregnancy that looks for the fake high glucose cut-off signal. See Appendix-31. Do GPs and obstetricians look at the fasting insulin level as a highly predictive indicator for future diabetes or Quintile Climbs in various biomarkers? What about the woman's weight, waist circumference, and history of fatty liver? Are there inflammatory markers in this woman's blood work? Does she have a high risk for diabetes based on her family history? Our assessment of the risk for gestational diabetes long before a woman falls pregnant is pathetic.

The advanced glucose cut-offs have proven useless in preventing skyrocketing acquired chronic metabolic diseases, and yet we are using this "deeply flawed" OGTT test to guide "management". Suppose a woman has the OGTT and develops a high glucose level or hypertension. In that case, all we do is try to control glucose or hypertension in pregnancy, which will do nothing to stop epigenetic programming. Once again, we have neglected to prevent these problems from arising in the first place or put in place an intensive nutrient-dense program before or during pregnancy. It is no wonder that population health is decreasing while the prevalence of metabolic diseases is skyrocketing as we always do things back to front.

Governments need to wake up to all of this and stop wasting our money on futile models that will see all of us sick before we should be and will see our lives crushed by inaction and mindless policies. We jeopardise the health of the mother, the child, and individuals not yet born in future generations because of inaction. Simply deplorable.

Metabolic markers are not enemies but highly predictable adaptations to cells in an energy crisis

Declaring anything as an enemy will require an army to engage in a war against this "enemy". Big Pharma sends out its soldiers, their drugs, to fight this pointless battle. It is senseless because this war continues with no victory in sight despite a plethora of weak medications.

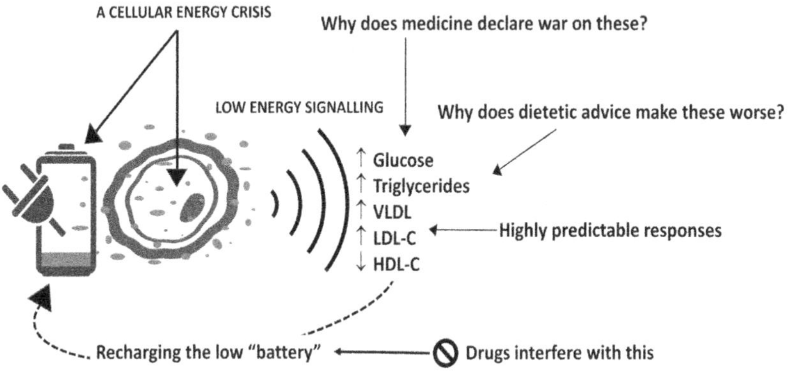

Highly predictable metabolic marker behaviour is not a freakish aberration. The pharmaceutical industry was given an absolute gift when the medical profession and Pharma decided to target these biomarkers as enemies. Seeing these metabolic markers as adaptations responding to cells in an energy crisis is far more intelligent. The ***Cell Starvation Model (CSM)*** views these biomarkers in the light of adaptations to cells in distress. They didn't just pop up to be labelled as enemies only to prop up the bottom line of Pharma.

Why do we ignore evolution in all of this, where a cellular bioenergetic decline is considered an existential threat for those cells caused by cellular starvation pressures? More on this in the dedicated cell starvation chapter. We have lost the war on chronic metabolic diseases due to our complete ignorance of what these biomarker adaptations mean to a cell in an energy crisis and where structural deterioration mandates cellular nutrients and building supplies to fix this increasing decay.

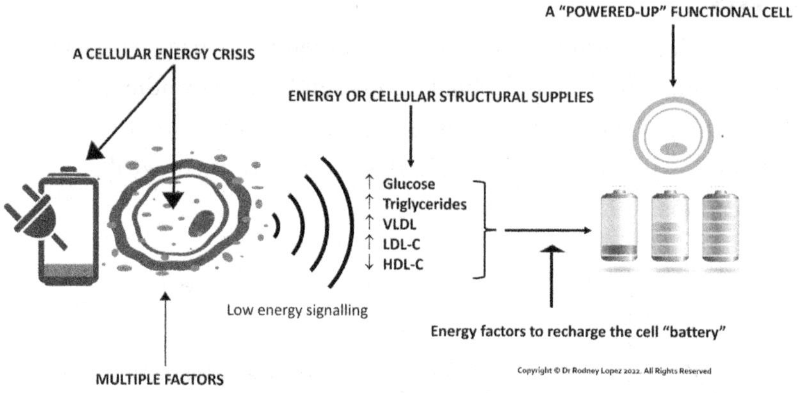

Multiple every day and highly common cell shocks or insults are discussed in the BIG-10 Womb-to-Tomb list. These ultra-common factors can easily pull the rug from under cell energy (ATP) production. In the graphic, we have cells with a diminishing ATP supply, represented by a battery demanding to be recharged and reenergized. This process of bioenergetic decline (our cell "batteries" losing energy) occurs gradually from birth and may also exist in the womb. Multiple and incredibly common factors I discuss in the BIG-10 Womb-to-Tomb list that will shortly follow can easily hammer cell energy pathways. Diminished cellular energy is an existential crisis for cells. Thus, they signal they are running out of power and "cry out for help" by biomarkers and other energy-depletion signals. This "cry" for help is that they need glucose, amino acids, and lipids (fats) as fuel to generate energy (ATP) to top up the cell "battery" and that they need supplies for structural repair – amino acids, cholesterol, and lipids.

If cells have low energy levels, then how can they power the repair or construction of proteins, enzymes, receptors, signalling molecules, organelles and other cellular components or reverse entropy? Our failure to recognise these blood biomarkers for what they are as supportive adaptations has propelled this metabolic dysfunction problem into the stratosphere and helped us lose this medical war. Many have lost their lives from aggressive drug management of these biomarkers, and this adverse pharmaceutical effect occurs for a good reason. Drugs work counter to these evolutionary adaptations. For example, if we view glucose as fuel to top up cellular energy, then trying to hammer glucose lower and lower will create an energy crisis in cells. If triglycerides or LDL are energy or structural supplies for cells undergoing structural decay, then what are we doing by lowering these critical supportive biomarker changes? Gurus wanting to defend drugs then take note that these biomarkers were allowed to become enemies by the irresponsible delay in managing metabolic disease very early on using non-drug nutritional approaches. Horrific complications have occurred with drug treatments, which is easily understood if we view drugs trying to inhibit biomarker adaptations that have cell survival implications.

This premise of blood biomarkers as enemies has become questionable and murky as medicine and dietetics have become increasingly embedded in the pharmaceutical and food industries.

Blood biomarker changes are highly predictable. This amazing biomarker predictability is shaped by evolution because if the medical profession actually opened their eyes, they would have seen that all these metabolic biomarkers are either an energy source or a cellular building component or both. You can bet with great chances of winning that someone with cell energy starvation and insulin resistance will have the following biomarker characteristics:

- A raised glucose level,
- Raised triglycerides
- Raised LDL
- Raised VLDL (a hallmark of chronic metabolic disease),

- Low HDL (raising HDL can be dangerous)
- Elevated Uric Acid level
- Raised inflammatory markers.

Drugs have been developed to target all of these blood biomarkers. There is a huge sum of money to be made in seeing biomarkers as enemies. Has this war caused chronic diseases to plummet? Quite the contrary, it seems as if medications have served as 'fertilisers' for these conditions. Dietetic advice makes all of this far worse.

Any drug has to be cautiously used in a Goldilocks Zone of dosing. Nothing happens if the drug dose is too low, and if it is too high, cells cannot cope due to reduced energy and structural supplies. Even if used in this Goldilocks Zone, drugs come nowhere near the benefits of food-based, nutrient-based approaches.

Glucose to Fructose in the brain: High carb madness damaging our brains

More and more, we are finding how dangerous the high-carb intake madness is. An incredible finding by Yale researchers has shown that 30% of blood glucose levels can be shunted to fructose in our brains. High-carb intakes easily achieve high blood glucose levels.

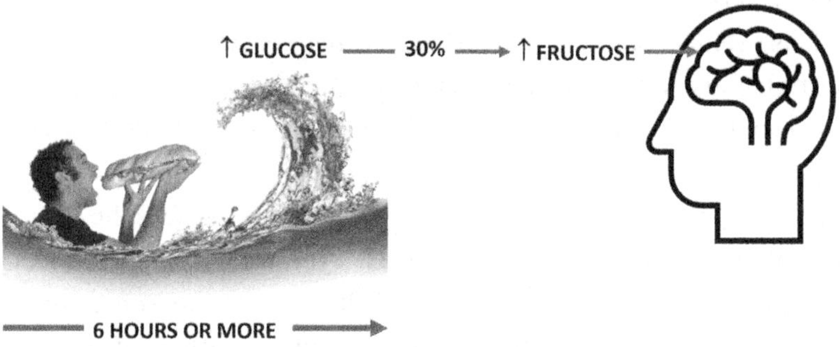

Fructose is a rapid robber of cell energy. Finally, we are waking up to the fact that neurodegeneration and mental health disorders are caused by bioenergetic decline. Fructose is discussed in a dedicated chapter as fructose is ubiquitous in foods consumed and a colossal factor in the bioenergetic decline in cells.

With vested interests gaslighting about carbs and fructose to protect their industries and with dietetics too embedded in politics wanting to please the government's interests in agriculture and then please food corporations, we continue to consume huge carb loads.

The Yale study reveals that chronically elevated glucose, or even spikes in glucose levels after eating, can be diverted to fructose, which in turn may lead to a decline in brain energy and an increased risk of dementia. Glucose spikes after eating can linger for 6 hours or more or never come down due to insulin resistance. This blood glucose to brain fructose conversion and bioenergetic decline makes sense as to why people with diabetes are so prone to dementia. This increase in brain fructose from blood glucose is one factor, out of many others, that adds to dementia risk for everyone. It is a factor that an individual can greatly control through dietary management.

We will look at this blood glucose to brain fructose conversion in more detail in the next chapter under "***Brain glucose to fructose conversion***". This striking level of fructose in brain fluid is a disaster for brain cells due to the rapid depletion of energy (ATP) triggered by fructose. How fructose depletes cells of ATP so rapidly is discussed in the "***Fiendish Fructose***" chapter.

Imagine those with mental health disorders or neurodegenerative diseases that are made worse by fructose acquired through sugar (50% fructose) and these elevations in blood glucose caused by twisted dietary guidelines. Who warns these people?

We now have a mechanism of how brain cell armageddon can occur as cells are rapidly depleted of energy by fructose. This brain fructose conversion worsens matters where insulin resistance (IR) turbocharges this effect by ensuring glucose is blocked from entering cells; this glucose-blocking effect leads to a further increase in blood glucose that can then be converted to fructose in the brain. What a beautiful synergy, and yet we seem so incredibly confused as to why we are seeing an "explosion" in dementia or mental health disorders. We bide our time until these problems become tsunamis that drown us. Why are we looking for drug targets for diseases like Alzheimer's that have proven useless? Why do we continue with pointless biomarker drug wars rather than declaring war on something so damaging as fructose?

We love looking for simple solutions like Beta-Amyloid or single targets for neurodegeneration with a view to making mega dollars from a drug silver bullet solution. We have yet another example of simplistic thinking regarding diseases of the brain.

BIG-10 Womb-to-Tomb allostatic factors, cell starvation and microcirculation impacts.

I have no doubt whatsoever that our so-called "healthy" staple foods are propelling this chronic disease pandemic to greater and greater heights. From ancient times to our modern era, staple foods have driven diseases, as I will discuss below.

Although the following graphic is based on fake glucose cut-off points and labels, let's use this flawed medical construct and all the flawed labels in our discussion, knowing in our minds we are dealing with a continuum of risk. The evidence strongly points to the Insulin Resistance Continuum (IRC) forming a progressively worsening bidirectional relationship with metabolic dysfunction (MetD), with both these powerful factors progressing in our lives as continuums.

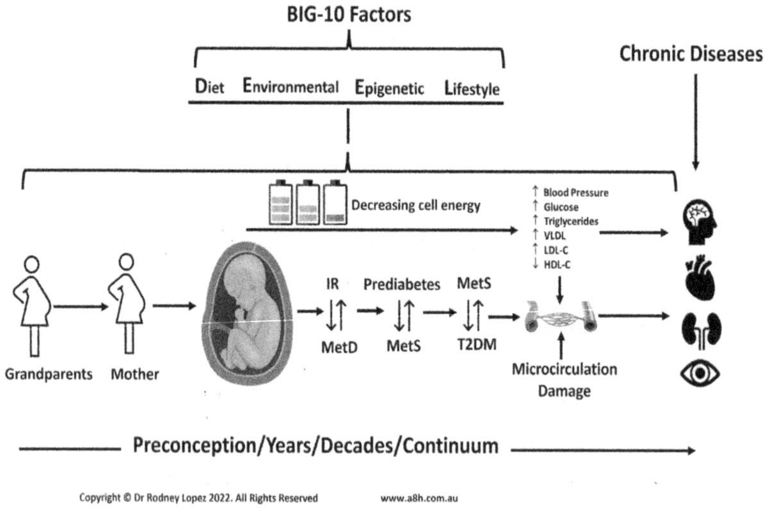

IR = Insulin Resistance; MetD = Metabolic Dysfunction; MetS = Metabolic Syndrome; T2DM = Type-2 Diabetes Mellitus.

This link between IR, MetD, and microvascular disease (MVD) is the engine that drives chronic metabolic disease, as we have discussed. The *BIG-10 Womb-to-Tomb List* that follows gets the ball rolling with the sequence of events shown in the illustration. Suppose the IRC ⇄ MetDc ⇄ MVDc combo is in action. In that case, we will have ongoing biological damage (rot) through the ***S***low, ***I***ncremental and ***C***umulative (SIC) progression. As we move along this continuum, we will then see blood biomarkers start to rise.

Our vascular risk begins when this continuum is left to run its course uninterrupted. All roads from this combination of factors acting simultaneously eventually lead to microcirculation damage, and our microcirculation networks are critical for the delivery of oxygen, fuel, and cellular building supplies. ***Insulin resistance plus microvascular damage reducing blood supply to cells and organs is a deadly duo one-two punch in this metabolic disease crisis.*** This combination is a massive threat to cell energy systems. We allow the microvascular system to assassinate our organ systems. It is always important to keep in mind the enormity of this insulin resistance and metabolic dysfunction problem that we have been clueless about.

What follows are the top 10 ultra-common reasons that impact our ability to produce energy in cells, leading to cell structural and ultrastructural damage and ongoing damage to our small blood vessels (microcirculation). All of this starts early in our lives. Insulin resistance magnifies any dietary shortcomings, of which there are plenty, worsening the intracellular chaos produced by the BIG-10 list. Insulin's actions are expanded upon in the dedicated chapter on cell starvation.

Many factors act simultaneously to make us ill, with processes adversely impacting our lives from the womb to the tomb, shaping our health destiny.

(1) Postprandial (after-eating) glucose and triglyceride surges: This is a colossal problem throughout our lives. Food is a double-edged sword. On the one hand, food keeps us alive while slowly killing us at the same time. We damage our bodies by consuming food maybe three times a day, maybe more and let's not forget those snacks. The sooner we can view the components of each meal on our plates and then visualize how that food or the elements within it affect our blood and bodies soon after eating and for hours more, the more we will appreciate how we are being damaged with each meal and snack driving biological rot.

For example, suppose we can look beyond the expected taste of the food we are about to eat and can see how the mound of rice as a risotto or pasta or potato mash in front of us will dramatically increase our blood glucose level for hours on end, damage the lining of our all our blood vessels, drive up inflammation and increasing small dense LDL (sdLDL), oxidized LDL (oxLDL) and triglycerides all factors damaging to large and small blood vessels and where high blood glucose will result in glycation (glucose damage) of proteins.

In that case, we may then think twice about a huge serving of such starchy carbs. All starch in carbs will be converted to glucose in our bodies. Let's not forget that spike of blood glucose after a starchy carb load like grains, bread, or potatoes, etc, where 30% will be converted to fructose in our brains, shutting off brain energy (ever feel the need to sleep after a large carb meal?). What about a huge slab of animal flesh full of fat and calories helping shut off ATP production (nutri-stress) and increasing our waist circumference and also increasing triglycerides and TMAO in our gut, a heart risk, driving up inflammation and adding to bowel cancer risk? This is a short list of the damaging things that can happen after eating. Every time we eat to live, we take ourselves close to disease and death, and all these food impacts are incremental and cumulative.

The other important factor regarding food is the timing of our meals, i.e. when we eat, that can make food intake even more dangerous. This ***chrononutrition effect*** is discussed in the final chapter. In the final chapter, I expand on this concept of the best time to eat to reduce cardiovascular risk. This after-eating damage to our bodies is nothing new. We have known about the damaging effects of food after eating for decades. So, why don't most people know about such an important effect caused by food? Could this knowledge put a dent in food sales? Could this knowledge damage the status quo of government tax incomes from food production and consumption? Are dietitians even aware of how dangerous after-eating effects can be, especially when they greatly impact those with insulin resistance and metabolic disease where these individuals are now the norm in populations? See Appendix-18 to get an idea of the unbelievable changes in our blood after eating food.

Highly damaging changes occur in our blood after eating that can last 6 hours or more in ***healthy people*** (Ceriello 2003). These glucose elevations or elevations in triglycerides or insulin may never come down in those with insulin resistance. These are not mild or benign changes that can occur in our blood after a meal. These changes can be deadly acutely and in the long term. Insulin resistance makes these postprandial surges far more dangerous and fatal over our lifetimes. All these after-eating effects can cause slow, incremental and cumulative damage over our lifetimes.

High triglyceride levels after consuming a large carbohydrate meal can increase appetite and decrease cognition. It is interesting a paper published in the prestigious journal Nature stated that:

> *"Triglycerides cross the blood-brain barrier rapidly, are found in human cerebrospinal fluid, and induce central leptin and insulin receptor resistance, decreasing satiety and cognition." (Banks, Farr et al. 2018)*

Grains and starchy carbs are not exactly benign and cause harm in many ways, and yet carbs are constantly being pushed onto people seeking dietary help. Legumes can be up to 45% starch (carbs), and the more you consume, the higher blood glucose will need insulin to control it. The problem is that those with insulin resistance and diabetes are already struggling to produce enough insulin to meet demand. These postprandial effects will age you as proteins and all blood vessels slowly but surely become damaged by glycation caused by glucose spikes after consuming starchy carbs.

The medical and dietetic professions unbelievably ignore this highly damaging process happening 2, 3 or more times a day with every meal and snack consumed (O'Keefe and Bell 2007).

Colossal numbers of individuals within populations worldwide are at risk of these postprandial effects due to the increasing prevalence of insulin resistance and chronic metabolic diseases. But it is important to remember that even if you don't have insulin resistance, these after-eating damaging effects will take you out meal-by-meal and snack-by-snack. It is the lifelong damage caused by food that all humans suffer from. The food itself can not only cause insulin resistance but worsen it over time to diabetes and beyond. Our microcirculation is particularly vulnerable to these postprandial effects, and lipid molecules like LDL can be modified by glycation after these blood surges from eating. High carb loads make matters worse by glycating LDL and proteins. This glycated LDL (gLDL) is far more dangerous.

Interestingly, our blood plasma, after we separate the blood cells from the plasma, looks milky after a meal due to the fat being transported to our tissues and organs. This milkiness is due to the fat levels (triglycerides) in the bloodstream after digestion. This after-eating triglyceride or fat level in the blood causes a "soaring" inflammatory response in the body (Margioris 2009). This episodic inflammation with each meal damages our whole body and can oxidize LDL (oxLDL), making this form of LDL highly damaging to our entire vascular networks. Each meal is seen as a threat that is stressful enough to mobilize homeostatic (balance) mechanisms (Margioris 2009).

What do our kids eat? These postprandial impacts harm our microcirculation early on in our lives and set the scene for progressive vascular damage and organ destruction (Ceriello 2000). Tight biomarker control will never account for the high level of heart and vascular disease seen (Ceriello 2000). We must take into consideration multiple factors all acting at once, and these after-eating daily effects are powerful biological impacts we ignore that lead to vascular and organ failure.

Microcirculation damage is the greatest threat to us. It is often the small blood vessels that take the brunt first, such as the penile artery in men with erectile dysfunction (ED), but these small blood vessel effects causing ED provide an early warning signal that other vascular beds are affected. ED warns that microvascular networks are damaged all over the body and not just in the penile blood vessels. Dietetics fails to understand that their recommendations are damaging to the masses of insulin-resistant individuals in populations as this mass of individuals seems to be forgotten in their recommendations. High energy inputs with each meal can hammer energy production – as discussed in the next point.

(2) Nutrient overload (nutri-stress) shuts off cell energy production—high-energy food intake in the context of sedentary lifestyles.

Pointless consumption of carbohydrates, fats, and protein can impact and overwhelm energy-extracting systems and impair mitochondrial function. In the chapter on cell starvation, we will look at a critical redox system, the NAD^+/NADH redox couple, as the regulator of cell energy. Mitochondria, as an "engine", can be overwhelmed and "overheated" by too much food energy. The overwhelming amount of excess food energy intake is particularly relevant to fat intake and mitochondrial impairment (Ruegsegger, Creo et al. 2018).

Lower NAD^+/NADH also deactivates Sitruins. Sirtuins are NAD+-dependent metabolic signalling proteins involved in metabolic regulation and mitochondrial biogenesis (creating more mitochondria). Chronic nutrient overload can permanently damage mitochondria and the endoplasmic reticulum (ER) (Qiu and Schlegel 2018). When do people stop consuming unnecessary calories? Importantly, the ER regulates protein and lipid synthesis, transport, and protein folding into their 3D shapes to make them functional. Our cells rely on the ER for structure and function. Once the ER becomes permanently damaged, there will be a downward spiral of structural cell decline. So, those with high-carb, high-protein, and high-fat diets and those who consume ultra-processed foods (UPFs) are warned of the worsening bioenergetic crisis ahead of them.

Chronic food energy overload is a problem throughout the lives of those in the West, and it is increasingly becoming prevalent in developing countries consuming Western food. However, those in developing countries consume high-carb loads of rice, legumes, and other grains. Countries with soaring levels of diabetes also have high intakes of sugar and sugar-sweetened beverages. See below. The consumption of ultra-processed, high-energy, micronutrient-poor foods in pregnancy is particularly concerning, with around 50% consuming energy-rich, nutrient-poor ultra-processed foods (UPFs) (Cummings, Lipsky et al. 2022).

A great concern is that 98% - 99% of pregnant women are not getting anywhere near their fruit and vegetable intake (Slater, Rollo et al. 2020). Intrauterine epigenetic signalling is a primal and evolutionary hardwired mechanism to pass information about the environment from mother to child. The commonly encountered overfed yet undernourished mother creates fetal malnutrition, which is an epigenetic signalling disaster that programs the child for insulin resistance, obesity, diabetes and a predisposition to mental health problems. We see disastrous epigenetic outcomes when babies born to malnutrition pressures in pregnancy are primed for insulin resistance (IR). These IR babies have a 30% reduction in ATP production (Petersen, Dufour et al. 2005). This mitochondrial handicap means their cell energy output is 1/3 lower than that of others not born with this handicap. More about this is in the chapter on cell starvation. Just think about what we feed babies after birth that can drive insulin resistance. From high dairy intakes to high carb loads to high fructose loads, we prime children for a life of disease—all in the name of Big Ag, staple food sales and food corporations.

(3) High fructose intake: Fructose rapidly pulls the rug from under cellular ATP production. This rapid cell ATP depletion with fructose happens despite fully functional mitochondria. The chapter *Fiendish Fructose* shows how this fruit sugar hijacks our energy pathways and incapacitates the Krebs Cycle and mitochondria, thus dramatically lowering cell ATP production. Sugar is 50% fructose, and sugar contaminates so many foods. See Appendix-8 for high fructose foods. Giving large amounts of fruit, processed fruit-based foods, and fruit-based snacks, plus a high fruit juice intake, is irresponsible in childhood. All our diseases begin in childhood. Increasing fructose loads from a young age is not a good idea. Fructose can set the scene for hypertension and metabolic diseases.

One glass of orange juice can raise central arterial (aortic) pressure (Pase, Grima et al. 2015). High fructose intake can elevate blood triglyceride (fat) levels and increase uric acid levels. Uric acid can decrease Nitric Oxide (NO) formation, thus decreasing NOs' potent effect on blood vessel dilation (diameter widening). It is NO that has a powerful impact on blood flow in the microcirculation, and if not enough NO is available, the situation is made worse by other damaging chemicals that worsen vascular flow (Gutterman, Chabowski et al. 2016).

A lack of Nitric Oxide (NO) will make small or large blood vessels stiff. If blood vessels can't dilate effectively, blood delivery to cells, tissues, and organs will be reduced. Insulin's ability to increase glucose uptake depends on the NO vasodilation effect. This NO effect worsens insulin resistance (IR) (Jia, Aroor et al. 2014).

Fructose is 7 – 10x more damaging than glucose in terms of glycation, thus far more dangerous to our cells, tissues, organs and blood vessels (McPherson, Shilton et al. 1988). Fructose can induce hypertension, MetS and Non-Alcoholic Fatty Liver Disease (NAFLD), and this fatty liver worsens insulin resistance (IR), where IR is an almost universal finding in fatty liver (Utzschneider and Kahn 2006). We prime children for a life of chronic disease, and we allow adults to damage themselves by not knowing the dangers of fructose and sugar, which, as mentioned above, is 50% fructose.

Foods full of sugar and sugar-sweetened beverages create sugar-rich foods, making people sicker, while pharmaceutical companies benefit from disease care and not health care. Gaslighting about sugar and fructose is not only ignorant but highly dangerous. It is not as if nutritionists with frivolous knowledge are not creating unnecessary confusion by saying things they shouldn't in the public arena to promote foods that harm. This confusion kills millions yearly!

(4) High sugar (sucrose) intake: The composition of table sugar or sucrose is 50% glucose and 50% fructose. Sugar is a main source of fructose in diets. So, high intakes of sugar will boost glucose and fructose simultaneously, which is highly damaging to our ATP-generating systems, which I will discuss in depth in this book. Furthermore, it is important to remember that glucose can be converted to sorbitol through aldose reductase, which is then converted to fructose. Glucose thus boosts fructose effects even further. This sorbitol pathway is expanded further in point 5. Fructose is, therefore, hidden in many foods with a high fructose or sugar content. In chapter one, we discussed how we can damage our brains through the glucose to fructose shunt, creating bioenergetic havoc in our brains.

It is thus wise to consider the sugar content of foods consumed, like the hidden sugar in hamburger buns and pizza bases and high sugar levels in condiments or sauces. Sweets, sweetened beverages, and desserts provide huge hits of sugar. Sugar is another highly modifiable component in food composition that we ignore to allow the food and beverage industry to survive while its customers slowly become sick and die prematurely. It is foolish when you consider that society has to pick up the tab in dealing with chronic diseases and early loss of productivity and let's not forget the premature loss of life.

(5) High starchy carbohydrate intake: When you think of starchy carbs from potato and pasta, bread to rice and other grains, you should believe that all of these are just pure glucose. Starchy carbs are ultimately broken into glucose! It is important to remember our vegetables are also carbs, but not the glucose-spiking starchy type. Veggies and low-fructose fruits are desirable non-starchy carbs. Don't let any dietitian or nutritionist convince you carbs are essential because they are not. They are not the only sources of glucose. Our bodies can produce glucose when needed, even from our triglyceride (fat) glycerol backbone.

So, a high starchy carb intake is equivalent to high blood glucose levels after eating, especially if an insulin-resistant individual is consuming this high-carb diet. Carb intakes need to take into consideration if someone has insulin resistance or metabolic dysfunction or if they are elite athletes needing to restore glycogen stores. It is not as if a dietitian or GP sees elite athletes as their bread-and-butter clientele; far from it. Their clientele is made up predominantly of the sedentary, disease-riddled, insulin-resistant, overweight or obese types on multiple medications. We seem to discard the enormous prevalence of insulin resistance in such individuals, yet we promote grains and other starchy foods to keep up the sales of agricultural products.

High-carb intakes will demand more insulin from a struggling pancreas and increase insulin/IgF-1 levels. You will see how important this hormone shift is when reading *Lessons Learnt from the Laron Syndrome* in Appendix-33. It is mind-numbing that medicine and dietetics have ignored high carbohydrate intakes for so long, disregarding the colossal numbers of people now suffering from insulin resistance and metabolic dysfunction.

Glucose is toxic to these insulin-resistant individuals, so what do dietitians do? Provide foods that increase blood glucose even more. Grains are yet another staple damaging us. Shame on dietetics to be so confused about the 101 principles of starchy carbohydrate intakes. In the next chapter, you will see the overwhelming evidence for the use of low-carb diets and the amazing impact it has on metabolically ill people.

Grains could be modified for lower carb contents, yet we stick to a limited number of grains like wheat, maize or rice. Dietetic advice seems to be given in a vacuum to what is happening in populations. As Professor Marion Nestle, a renowned molecular biologist, public health advocate and nutritionist, has stated, it was the food revolutions of the 1960s and 70s, the Green and Farming revolutions that produced a glut of cheap cereals that set us on this path to a metabolic disease disaster (Nestle 2022). Dietetics and the dietitians they generate that guide us on all things diet were manipulated into becoming the sales force for grains. Throw in advertisements showing that elite athletes get to that level by pouring cereals out of a box along with copious amounts of milk and fructose-rich honey, and voila, you now have grains taking a central position in our diets.

We have seen what these food revolutions have done to population health, and because we have a dietetic profession either too self-interested or too embedded with vested interests, they don't challenge the grains are good dogma. And so this chronic disease disaster continues to soar in populations globally.

The farmers producing these grains would vote sympathetic politicians into government, and these politicians would then become powerful lobbyists to promote grain consumption. Food corporations would ensure their interests were embedded in undergraduate and postgraduate education. In 1992, the USDA released its first food pyramid, and you may have guessed that the base of this pyramid recommended 6-11 servings of carbs (cereals, pasta, bread, rice) (Willett and Stampfer 2003) – how absurd. You only have to glance at Appendix-38 and look at the base of this food pyramid to see the influence of farmers and politicians on how populations become pawns in the political and food production game. So the message was carbs are good, and fat is bad. Dietitians still seem caught up in a time warp, recommending huge amounts of carbs without question, as suggested by this vested interest food pyramid—agricultural leverage impacting dietetic recommendations.

Insulin resistance means that insulin doesn't work well, so those with insulin resistance (almost everyone now) cannot deal with the high glucose levels after eating high starchy carbs – See Appendix-13 and Appendix-14. The resultant glucotoxicity in the postprandial (after-eating) state is a disaster. We fail to understand the dangers of glucose spikes or excursions after eating, which are damaging us with every meal and every snack. However, these glucose spikes are also nutrient overloads, as discussed in point-2, which hammer our energy-extracting systems. Our cells and mitochondria cannot cope with the high energy inputs of overconsumption. These acute high food energy disruptions to cellular ATP production and diminished structural integrity can produce irreversible defects in energy production systems (Qiu and Schlegel 2018).

> *"A major deficiency in our understanding of the role of hyperglycemia in the pathogenesis of chronic diabetic complications is the contribution made by exaggerated postprandial glycemic excursions, in contrast to that made by chronic fasting hyperglycemia." (Toya, Sara et al. 2020)*

You can switch the term "glycemic excursions" to "glucose spikes". So, high glucose levels after eating are more damaging than chronic glucose elevations, where the term chronic means that glucose is constantly elevated. Imagine that. How many millions of lives have been lost due to clueless and dangerous dietary guidelines? Yet, it is ironically the medical profession and not dietetics pushing for low-carb diets. The masters of medicine, I suppose, are Pharma and not food corporations, unlike dietetics, entrenched with food corporations and food sales imperatives.

We forget when giving high-carb intake recommendations that glucose is converted to fructose through the sorbitol-aldose reductase pathway, as mentioned above—high carb intakes → ↑ glucose after eating → ↑ sorbitol → ↑ fructose → ↓ cellular ATP energy → ↑ Insulin resistance → ↑ oxidative stress and ↑ inflammation and ↑metabolic markers → ↑ modified LDL and other lipids → damage to blood vessels, microcirculation networks and organ systems.

The conversion of glucose to sorbitol is a way of bypassing the inability of the cell to cope with the glucose volume (hexokinase saturation); thus, this sorbitol or polyol pathway is a defence mechanism to protect cells from glucose toxicity. So much for high-carb intakes! Shunting glucose to sorbitol occurs in many tissues and is the main reason for diabetes cataracts and peripheral nerve damage. In the next chapter, we look at a profoundly important finding of high blood glucose levels, whether from after-eating surges or those with established insulin resistance and diabetes, found by Yale University researchers. This finding involves the shunting of this blood glucose to fructose in the brain we have touched upon. We know fructose rapidly deletes body and brain cells of energy (ATP).

Is it any wonder why people with diabetes have dementia and Alzheimer's Disease at far higher rates than someone without high glucose levels? However, the type of food you have, in particular high starchy carb intakes with those glucose spikes, can put you at risk as well over your lifetime, irrespective of whether you have overt insulin resistance or diabetes.

The glucose spikes after eating are like mini diabetic episodes.

So much for high-carb recommendations to sell more grains. More on this in the "prediabetes" chapter. Why don't we learn from research over decades about the postprandial (after-eating) dangers of food impacts? It is as if these findings have been forgotten or totally ignored for commercial reasons, even though the weight of postprandial research could crush us -Appendix-18.

(6) Staple food intake: The end of staples, as we know, is coming to a fast end. As discussed above, we regard staples as benign, but this is far from the case. The effects on our bodies created by staple food impacts add to the burden of disease. Staples like eggs, dairy, meat, cereals, honey, and high fructose fruit juices and fruits have all been used for millennia in populations and, indeed, throughout our evolutionary history. Thus, staple foods are well-known and loved. But just because we have used these foods throughout evolutionary history and that we love them doesn't mean they are benign by any means. Can you imagine a breakfast that is not heavy on eggs and bacon or the huge carb loads from some breakfast cereal poured out of a box? Pancakes with maple syrup, etc. We seem to think they are fine. However, we will see how staple foods can cause harm in many ways.

Eggs, dairy, cereal-based foods, fruit juice and horrific breakfasts out of the box, including oats and porridge, are made even more toxic by adding milk (see GI-Insulin Dissociation below) and then adding honey (40% fructose 30% glucose) or agave (70% fructose). A combination like this to start the day is incredibly highly toxic, producing a huge glucose spike and a large food energy overload with a postprandial effect that will linger on for 6 hours or more (Ceriello 2003). Imagine all that damage to our trillions of cells, blood vessels and organs lasting 6 hours or more or 24/7 in insulin-resistant individuals. Energy overload is not the only problem. All that glucose that floats around in our bloodstream also causes harm. It glycates our proteins, damages the glycocalyx and endothelium (lining) of blood vessels, and contributes to the fructose load from sugary foods. Even the glucose spikes from starchy carbs are converted to fructose, damaging our body and brain cells. Fructose, I have pointed out, is 7 – 10 times more damaging to proteins than glucose. Let's not forget that the shunting of glucose to fructose in our brains after a high carb load increases our risk for dementia.

Our dreadful population prevalence figures tell us insulin resistance and metabolic dysfunction are becoming the norm, so don't you think dietetics is incredibly negligent not recognizing that times have changed since the food revolutions? It is a disgrace. Insulin resistance magnifies this after eating glucose elevation from starchy carbs. These persistent elevations in glucose after eating can potentially cause long-term damage to cells, especially in those with advanced insulin resistance such as "prediabetes, "MetS" or "T2DM". The fact that cells can develop persistent damage and impairment from poorly planned food intakes is something we will look at later. We discuss the amazing ATP-depleting effect of fructose in the "Fiendish Fructose" chapter.

Many dietitians recommend damaging breakfasts out of the box plus honey or agave in the false belief that these are safe, natural, and are not artificial sweeteners and thus must be OK. I don't think oats steel-cut or not is safe. Oats have a high carb load. Vested interests will market these boxed cereals to the hilt to convince us these nutrient-poor, glucose-spiking grains are good for us. Staples damage us in many ways, and Big-Ag and Big-Food will gaslight us about this danger. Dietitians continue to promote grain products due to their training and indoctrination. Unfortunately, dietetics is highly influenced by food boards and the food industry. Sponsored research will just muddy the water. Let's look at some staples and how they can damage us:

Staple Food Concern - Eggs: Eggs can increase oxidized LDL (ox-LDL). This modified LDL is a pathogenic form of this lipid carrier and leads to vascular diseases. The Heart Foundation of Australia limits recommendations to seven (x7) eggs a week if cholesterol is elevated. Why would a heart foundation do this? It is stated in research that an egg yolk will raise low-density lipoprotein (LDL) by 10% and yet, at the same time, increase highly damaging oxidized LDL (ox-LDL) by a whopping 34% (Spence 2002) (Levy, Maor et al. 1996). Egg composition is vital to its effect on oxidized LDL (ox-LDL) (Shapira and Pinchasov 2008).

So, are eggs essential to human life? The answer is a resounding NO. Only nutrients are crucial, not a particular food. So, in a world of unbelievable risk of dying of a cardiovascular event, making heart and vascular disease the number one killer on this planet, who do we believe? Gaslighting nutritional gurus?

In a study involving 4439 women and followed up for six (6) years, it was shown that there was weight gain in postmenopausal women (Greenberg, Cheung et al. 2024). Is weight gain acceptable in this age group at risk for cardiovascular disease and, in particular, Alzheimer's dementia when eggs are not essential for health? There are many plant-based egg substitutes now available in most supermarkets, and the supplement regimen I suggest will mean you will not suffer from a nutrient deficiency if you don't eat any eggs.

Perhaps we must build better eggs rather than gaslighting or muddying the waters about eggs, putting people at risk! You will see comments about this LDL oxidation effect caused by eggs depending on an individual's diet or antioxidant intake. So if 7 in 10 individuals are overweight or obese and metabolic disease is so high in populations all eating a Standard American Diet (SAD), this means that the norm is a poor diet and increasing LDL oxidation is the result of poor diets and after-eating impacts. Thus, eggs are adding to this existing burden of oxidized LDL, and increasing oxidized LDL is a risk with such a dominant diet and adverse postprandial impacts. We will look at the risk of modified LDL in the chapter "*That's no way to treat a metabolic biomarker.*"

Another cause for concern in men is that we also have papers pointing out that men who consume 2.5 eggs a week have an 81% higher risk of lethal prostate cancer than men who consume less than 0.5 eggs a week (Richman, Kenfield et al. 2011).

Professor Artemis Simonopoulos, an expert on omega-3s, studied the composition of a supermarket egg versus wild Greek eggs as would be found in Greek islands of the Mediterranean. The comparison was astounding, with the supermarket eggs having 19 times (19x) the ratio of omega-6s to omega-3s, whereas the wild Greek egg had an omega-6 to omega-3 ratio of 1.3 (Simopoulos and Sidossis 2000).

Omega-6s promote inflammation through the omega-6 eicosanoid pathway. See Appendix-23. Omega-6s compete with omega-3s, as both paths use the same enzymes to produce either inflammatory or anti-inflammatory eicosanoids. We have competition for the same enzymes by Omega-6s and Omega-3s. If we consume more omega-6s, that pathway will hog those shared enzymes, forcing the production of inflammatory compounds. We get a huge intake of omega-6s from cheap vegetable oils or processed and ultra-processed foods, so consuming many eggs will add to this inflammatory Omega-6 burden, already stoking the fires of inflammation where inflammation drives so many cancers, chronic diseases and mental health disorders.

Factors driving inflammation will mean our immune super-system will be constantly activated, and as a super-system, it hogs energy and nutrient resources, making matters worse for already struggling insulin-resistant cells starving of fuel, nutrients and building supplies. We have never heard this kind of depth of knowledge from those who work in the egg industry. They only want you to continue eating eggs, irrespective of the damage caused.

Staple Food Concern - Dairy: Dairy intake can cause spikes in insulin-IgF1 due to GI-insulin dissociation, as discussed above. Dairy is designed for baby animals, not humans. Dairy may have helped save early humans from starvation, but this does not mean there is no risk. We need to view these staple food risks through the lens of "The Laron Syndrome" – see Appendix-33.

The insulin effect of dairy is 3x to 6x that expected from the glycaemic index (GI) (Östman, Liljeberg Elmståhl et al. 2001)

> *"Milk and dairy products have been identified as potent insulin secretagogues, as their consumption stimulates acute hyperinsulinemia" (Tucker, Erickson et al. 2015)*

So, "***potent insulin secretagogues***" mean a powerful insulin production effect. Is this something smart to do with a massive number of individuals in populations suffering from the Insulin Resistance Continuum (IRC)? Beta cells in the pancreas of these individuals are already under stress to supply insulin. The IRC is now the norm in societies, and yet we practice medicine or provide dietetic guidelines as if this insulin resistance and metabolic disease disaster don't exist. "Experts," write articles in lay media without acknowledging that those with insulin resistance are now a dominant force in global populations, let alone the mass of chronic metabolic disorders that have insulin resistance as the basis.

We demand more and more insulin from this struggling pancreatic organ through high carb loads or sugar or even high protein and fat loads, and then on top of these loads, we consume a lot of dairy that has a disproportionate demand on insulin production relative to its carbohydrate level. This dairy consumption helps the dairy industry make a dollar, but it is unethical when dairy is ***NOT*** an essential food item. You can get every nutrient in dairy from other food sources. Dairy boards and the dietetic industry will have you believe you can consume as much dairy as you like without repercussions. We do this for kids, don't we? We give them a lot of dairy, often from birth when mothers can't breastfeed. After weaning, we provide these children with copious amounts of dairy, such as milk, yoghurt, flavoured milk, and custards. Add to this dairy intake all the other insulin-spiking grain foods that are constantly driving up insulin levels in children as well as adults.

The prevalence of Eosinophilic Oesophagitis (EoE), according to trends seen in the Netherlands, has multiplied 316-fold. Like our metabolic disease disaster, we downplay dietary impacts. An article published in the Australian Doctor in June 2024, however, does implicate dairy and gluten in this terrible disease of the oesophagus that can cause difficulties swallowing and a choking hazard that can shorten one's life after a long period of misery (Skardoon 2024). Australian Doctor is distributed to all Australian doctors free of charge and is well respected in the medical profession as a reliable source of information. Thus, with dietetics pushing staple foods and where dairy and gluten-rich cereals are the icons of our staples, then is it any wonder diseases like EoE are surging worldwide?

As discussed in this book, we now know that high blood insulin levels can trigger insulin resistance. So, what are we doing for our kids? Do we set kids up for insulin resistance and prediabetes later in life? What about the children born to mothers with Gestational Diabetes Mellitus (GDM) with a 5x increased risk of prediabetes? We set them up for a lifetime of misery and ill health. We see this happening so widely in populations. What are we doing for those born with insulin resistance with already struggling beta cells? Are we pushing individuals with IR towards beta-cell burnout? This burnout happens when the beta cells in the pancreas pack it in because of the constant insulin demand from our foods. To me, this is a logical conclusion that we create all these problems by the very food we are made to believe is essential in our lives. But, if certain foods are not crucial to life, it becomes unethical to push those damaging foods when they could be detrimental to our health.

Do those who drive dairy consumption do it out of ignorance of concepts such as the GI-Insulin Dissociation? Or are they embedded in the commercial interests of the food and dairy industry by research grants, food board funds, or scholarships? But remember, undergraduate degrees are riddled with vested interests. So budding dietitians know no better but are programmed at universities to push these foods and prop up these industries. Many dietitians are clueless as to their indoctrination but accept what they were taught as fact. See the chapter "*Revolution Time,*" where this is exposed.

Staple Food Concern - Animal Flesh: The WHO and other watchdogs have been sounding the alarm about red meat and cancer, including bowel cancer, for decades. All cancers are increasing dramatically globally, with bowel cancer in the under 50s rapidly growing, as we have discussed. The meat industry and some dietetic groups would love you to believe that meat is essential. No food is vital, as I have mentioned, as we only need critical nutrients within food to sustain life. If one food lacks certain nutrients, or if we avoid that food, we can always get those nutrients from another food or supplements.

Women who reported a high heme iron intake from animal flesh had a threefold (3x) increase in gestational diabetes (Shah and Fonseca 2011). I will discuss how gestational diabetes is rising rapidly and acting as an "***epigenetic engine***" to affect three (3) future generations. So we love to promote animal flesh as a staple food and yet ruin the lives of future generations. Truly sad.

Protein is a nutrient from multiple food sources, but minerals like iron are rich in animal flesh. But other foods also have iron; let's not forget we can supplement iron, which is often needed in those with iron deficiency anaemia, an ultra-common problem worldwide. If specific foods are not crucial, why take the risk? We now have plenty of plant-based protein options rather than consuming fat-rich, energy-rich animal flesh. Our only guiding principle is to ensure nutrient sufficiency, which we can do from supplementation if we avoid conceited and arrogant statements by professionals with huge vested interests in the food and drug industry who would prefer you harm yourself with unnecessary non-essential foods.

Bowel cancer is exploding in populations, and this deadly cancer occurs in younger and younger individuals. Red meat has always been a suspect in the cause of bowel cancer. The WHO has classified pork, beef and lamb as Group-2A – probable carcinogens. Processed meats (bacon, ham, salami, frankfurts) are classified as Group-1 carcinogens. Group-1 carcinogens include the highly dangerous asbestos or benzene compounds. These processed meats act as strong promoters of bowel and stomach cancer. In addition, the Nurses' Health Study showed a strong association between beef, lamb and pork consumption and bowel cancer risk (Aykan 2015).

Gestational Diabetes Mellitus (GDM) is a mega-engine that can drive future metabolic disease, as we have discussed. We need to put the brakes on GDM as soon as possible before GDM drives us rapidly to the Metabolic Singularity point and over that healthcare cliff. It is irresponsible not to warn women who have a high intake of heme iron from animal flesh that there is a three times (3x) increased risk of gestational diabetes (Shah and Fonseca 2011). Should we warn women or protect Meat and Livestock?

Dietetics encourages people to cook chunks of animal flesh to provide amino acids. This meat has a high energy and fat content but may not be digested completely (think powerful proton pump inhibitor antacids) or for older people with decreased hydrochloric acid production that impairs digestion of meat. Undoubtedly, future generations will see us as primitive beings who went down a path of staple food consumption voluntarily, forgetting we were forced to consume these staples in our evolutionary history. But not now.

We are already seeing revolutionary changes in food. Appendix-33 shows the use of staples in the context of the Laron Syndrome and why we need to care about high dairy intakes, meat, eggs, processed foods, and increased glucose loads. Cancers don't just happen without help, and foods are a huge driver of many cancers by many mechanisms. Only those who benefit from misery and disease due to self-interest and vested interests are confused by the need now to abandon staples.

(7) Common micronutrient insufficiencies and deficiencies, Essential Amino Acids (EAAs), Omega-3s, Choline and L-Citrulline (Nitric Oxide generator)

Micronutrient deficiencies are extremely common, considering the high intakes of processed and ultra-processed foods and the pitiful intakes of fresh vegetables and fruit. It is downright foolish and dangerous now to make witless comments about "an optimal diet" as no such thing exists. Dietetics love to downplay these population deficits in micronutrients as this makes them appear to be doing a stellar job guiding all of us to consume staple foods.

Populations are riddled with micronutrient deficiencies. It is simple gaslighting and deceit. An optimal diet only exists in the minds of dietetic practitioners whose main aim is to increase the sales of whole foods and support Big Ag. Critical nutrients often fall far below the intake for optimal cellular function, and any micronutrient insufficiency or deficiency of even one vitamin, mineral or trace element can incapacitate energy-extracting systems from the glycolytic pathway and Krebs Cycle to the Electron Transport Chain (ETC) protein complexes in mitochondria that require copious amounts of cofactors (minerals) or coenzymes (vitamins) to keep the cellular machinery fully functional.

Energy-rich, nutrient-poor foods are incredibly common—these are the overfed yet undernourished individuals. Think fast-food outlets, drive-throughs, food malls, packaged meals or meals delivered to the door. Energy-generating systems in metabolism cannot work without vitamins, minerals and trace elements acting as cofactors or coenzymes in these pathways. ATP formation cannot occur without magnesium (rich in dark green leafy veggies, sadly lacking in diets).

Iron, too, can severely decrease ATP production. We will look at iron deficiency in the chapter on cell starvation, which affects 1 in 3 people worldwide (Kumar, Sharma et al. 2022). Iron deficiency is common before pregnancy and accelerates in severity during pregnancy. Any impact on cellular energy will also impact cell structural integrity and trigger insulin resistance. This impact on cell structure and ATP production may never recover.

Insulin signalling declines without magnesium. Likewise, without Nitric Oxide (NO), insulin's ability to clear glucose is limited (Jia,

Aroor et al. 2014). Our microcirculation beds play a huge role in delivering oxygen and nutrient supplies to our tissues and organs. We need our microcirculation to provide enough L-Arginine or nitrate from food to produce Nitric Oxide and even to deliver the hormone insulin to cells.

We consume far more Omega-6s in comparison to Omega-3s, and this is a driver of inflammatory eicosanoids, as we have discussed, thus adding to the background inflammatory processes as noted above. Inflammation drives virtually all diseases known and can increase the risk of malignant spread. See Appendix-23.

Essential amino Acid (EAA) supplementation could provide highly bioavailable amino acids for children and adults, needing little to no digestive power from hydrochloric acid in the stomach to be absorbed with none of the dangers of high energy from animal protein sources. These EAAs have very few calories and could meet our protein needs without the risks posed by staples. These essential amino acids will decrease the ***protein leverage*** drive, which can increase the risk of obesity. Protein leverage will be discussed in the final chapter. We either eat to satisfy a primal urge or eat nutrient-dense foods for health. We must remember that many medications can cause micronutrient deficiencies and that we need far more nutrient resources during illness and recovery. Proton Pump Inhibitors (PPIs) are commonly used in the population for GORD and heartburn, and these can greatly impair protein digestion and mineral and vitamin absorption. Medicine itself adds to the misery in populations with iatrogenic (medicine-induced) disease. Research articles on the "safety" of PPIs are blatant lies funded by Pharma.

(8) Low intake of dietary antioxidants, phytochemicals and dietary fibre diversity: My final chapter will discuss a diet that shows our way out of this metabolic mess is to ensure a diet rich in micronutrients, phytochemicals (beneficial plant compounds) and dietary fibre diversity. We forget that our gut microbiomes exert a powerful effect on our immune system. We risk systemic inflammation that needs to be controlled by free radical quenching compounds from plant phytochemicals in food and food-based antioxidants.

Insulin resistance (IR) is associated with oxidative stress and inflammation. We need to offset this side-effect of IR by consuming a wealth of anti-inflammatory dietary components. Many of these phytochemicals are prebiotics that can enhance gut microbiome health. Lacking these valuable food components will only increase or drive disease states.

(9) Epigenetic mitochondrial programming: Offspring born to diabetic parents are 40% to 70% more likely to develop diabetes early in life, depending on whether one or both parents have diabetes (Ali 2013). This high prevalence of programmed risk is made worse by postprandial surges of glucose, all due to the impaired capacity of mitochondria at birth to deal with glucose spikes due to epigenetic programming in the womb and the mitochondrial handicap that ensues.

The "ticking clock" of small and large blood vessel damage tells us that cardiovascular and microvascular disease exists long before diabetes manifests and predates diabetes by decades. This vascular risk is determined in the womb and accelerated from birth onwards. We need to tackle this problem of epigenetic programming; otherwise, the fate of humanity is set in stone. That we don't look for early markers for gestational diabetes mellitus (GDM) before pregnancy is an absolute disgrace as we condemn the mother (and baby) to a very high cardiovascular risk and condemn future generations for ill health. We condemn those born with mitochondrial defects due to gestational programming to a life of early disease and death.

(10) Environmental toxic impacts, including common medication toxicities: PFAS, the "forever chemicals", fragrances made up of 100s of chemical compounds, herbicides, pesticides, VOCs, POPs, etc., surround us in our daily lives. We are exposed to toxicities on the roads we drive down, in our homes and offices, and in our food, air and water. These compounds can hammer cell energy-extracting systems. It is important to remember the vulnerability of pregnant mothers to these toxic influences and the susceptibility of the developing fetus to poisonous exposures. These harmful exposures can add to epigenetic programming in the womb with long-term consequences. Many of these compounds are hormone-disrupting chemicals, either blocking or enhancing the effects of estrogen and testosterone.

We look at this shocking state of affairs regarding 350,000 chemicals released out there. Appendix-32 is a sobering story about AETT, a fragrance used without testing for 20 years. It is shocking.

Common medications can be incredibly damaging to cellular energy-extracting systems, from Proton Pump Inhibitors (PPIs) to toxic antipsychotics directly impairing components of the Electron Transport Chains (ETCs) in our trillions of mitochondria. It is no wonder that PPIs or antipsychotics can trigger Type-2 Diabetes Mellitus. And as you will see, we use powerful PPIs in babies and children – go figure.

BIG-10 influences on cellular bioenergetic impairment are tremendously common. It is disappointing that medical research and the medical and dietetic professions seem to move forward with their eyes closed to these damaging influences.

CHAPTER 2

"Prediabetes": A huge missed opportunity

"Prediabetes": A vast, silent, and ever-expanding "balloon" of individuals with insulin resistance predisposed to Type-2 Diabetes Mellitus, vascular, heart, dementia, mental health illness and chronic disease

Time and again, you see in research papers or repeated by medical experts that "prediabetes" increases the risk of "diabetes", and so we have one fake label increasing the risk of another fake label. Somehow, this seems to make sense to the medical establishment rather than a continuum of risk from one to the other that has nothing to do with a glucose level. However, it is important to recognise that the longer blood glucose levels stay elevated and poorly managed, the higher the risk of biological damage (our biological rot).

We have been utterly irresponsible by not dealing with glucose levels as early as possible in this process, but it is not just glucose levels that we love to focus on, but all the other factors that drive biological rot that I discuss throughout this book not the least of which are all the after-eating impacts of so-called "healthy" staple foods.

A meaningless high glucose level that sounds a very loud alarm bell states the blatantly obvious observations that at this high glucose diabetes cut-off point, we will have a higher level of risk of vascular and organ damage – not exactly an earth-shattering revelation. We allowed that risk to reach a dangerous level. The glucose levels that define "prediabetes" are short of the very high glucose levels used to define Type-2 Diabetes Mellitus (T2DM or just diabetes); hence, the term "prediabetes" is used. Whether this fake glucose cut-off for a label of "prediabetes" proceeds to the just as fake high "diabetes" glucose cut-off point is highly irrelevant. Both fake labels are on the same path to chronic diseases, and only the presence or absence of biological rot (cells decaying, metabolic markers worsening, vascular systems crumbling, and organ systems failing) matters. Nothing else matters.

Suppose we use the poster child of metabolic diseases, the USA, as a guide for the prevalence of "prediabetes' in many other countries. In that case, the CDC has calculated that 1/3rd of Americans have "prediabetes" (34.5%). This prevalence may seem alarming, but it would pale in comparison if figures derived from very early biomarker signals were used to define metabolic health.

As a sobering thought, just changing the cut-off points used from lower levels of waist circumference to blood pressure or blood glucose levels revealed that 88% of Americans were not metabolically healthy (Araújo, Cai et al. 2019). Wow! Staggering findings. So, what about you and your chances of not having an abnormal metabolic marker of some kind? It is incredibly low that you are "normal" in this 21st-century era.

Using cutting-edge ways to find early biomarker changes or early microvascular disease would show that we are already at or are frighteningly close to the ***Metabolic Singularity*** – our universal metabolic disease prevalence. It is shocking then to know that all these individuals with early signs of metabolic disease are sitting ducks and time bombs waiting for large blood vessel disease (macrovascular disease) and small vessel disease (microvascular disease) to manifest clinically or, worse still, take their lives suddenly with a heart attack or stroke. Surprisingly, prediabetes carries an "essentially identical" risk for cardiovascular disease as diabetes (Gottwald-Hostalek and Gwilt 2022).

Should this surprise us? Well, it shouldn't because large or small vessel vascular risk is created by many factors acting simultaneously, not just by glucose, which we seem to have elevated to the status of chief villain in metabolic disease for no brilliant reason that relegates many other risks lurking in the background as having minor or no significance but are just as damaging. As I have mentioned, microvascular disease is the "motor" that drives large vessel disease. Allow our small microvascular networks to be damaged, and you hammer not only all our large blood vessels that depend on their very own microvascular blood supply (the vasa vasorum) but also put every organ in the body at huge risk of eventually deteriorating and failing.

So why are we so fixated on "prediabetes" transitioning to "diabetes" as a pivotal point in a continuum of risk and biological damage where all points have the potential to reach a state of vast microvascular damage to ongoing biological injury that then devastates all organ systems, driving them to failure? In my mind, the problem in all of this is:

1. All roads in this metabolic process lead to microcirculation network failure. This means less glucose can be delivered to cells, tissues, skeletal muscle, and organs, and less glucose is burnt off as energy. This lowered glucose utilisation allows a buildup of unused glucose to rise in the blood. This increased level of blood glucose, in turn, causes more microcirculation damage, leading to even higher blood glucose levels, and so it goes on and on – a vicious bidirectional loop.
2. There is a failure to understand the significant postprandial effects of recommended 'healthy' staple foods that elevate various biomarkers such as glucose, triglycerides, and inflammation in this after-eating period, adding to the already abnormal biomarker changes caused by our insulin resistant –

metabolic dysfunction "mother" and all these after-eating impacts damage our microcirculation networks meal-by-meal.

3. Glucose cut-offs and fake labels do have a political purpose as they become barriers. Let's say we go on a campaign to find early metabolic disease, and we indeed find vast numbers that fit the bill for early disease. Governments and healthcare systems will shake in their boots as they feel compelled or pressured to do something for them. However, by having high biomarker cut-offs, we are drastically limiting this needy group as high biomarker cut-offs will drastically cull the numbers affected. We can thus ignore this group of individuals with early disease. So, it is shortsighted because doing something for this massive cohort with early metabolic disease will ultimately have profound beneficial effects for populations and nations.

This so-called "prediabetes" period has been dreadfully handled. We have made an absolute mess of trying to understand this insulin resistance-metabolic dysfunction continuum, which is our "mother" of chronic diseases, and why is this the case? For such a long time, we have seen insulin resistance as separate from "prediabetes", which was then separated from "MetS" and "Type-2 Diabetes Mellitus (T2DM)". Only now are we seeing that this is one long metabolic dysfunction continuum of change (the "mother") creating havoc in all our cells, depriving them of energy and decreasing structural integrity. I describe this fictitious "prediabetic" state as this has been the case historically in medicine.

In medicine, as professionals, going about their business earning a dollar yet knowing that they are not winning at all is unforgivable. How can they not know when every major watchdog is screaming out loud that we have metabolic disease armageddon out there in populations? It is what professional lemmings do, which is to protect their turf and income regardless of outcomes.

This herd mentality doesn't occur just in the medical or dietetic professions but is a universal human problem. This human frailty is why the book ***Hippocrasy: How Doctors Are Betraying Their Oath*** is so important, as it shows the true hypocrisy in medicine and the cult of lemmings that never question anything. However, many mavericks in medicine or dietetics put their professional status on the line to buck the trend. This has always been the case in medical history. Those whose names are esteemed in medical history were often broken people who called out what they saw as wrong thinking or practices at the time. Buck the trend and dare to threaten income streams, and you pay the price.

Could the resolution of chronic metabolic diseases, which constitute the vast majority of problems doctors see and treat in their clinics, pose a significant threat to their livelihoods? Of course, it does, but what do we do? Can we protect professional incomes and lifestyles while population health deteriorates globally?

Yet, in life, there are no threats, only opportunities. Doctors and dietitians can become relevant again by reskilling and re-tooling to deal with 21st-century diseases that have not responded to their current skills or current drug-based tools. Regulatory bodies need to wake up and change the system; otherwise, this disaster will simply roll forward to our ***Metabolic Singularity*** and tsunamis of disease.

Diabetes glucose cut-off points are the Mount Everest of glucose levels. Why?

We must now get past this huge hurdle of seeing this insulin resistance, metabolic dysfunction continuum, our "mother" of chronic illness as having significance ***ONLY*** if it reaches that massive increase in blood glucose level we term Type-2 Diabetes Mellitus (T2DM).

As I have stated, there is no such thing as "prediabetes" or "diabetes" or "MetS"; hence, these terms are put in inverted commas to denote a fake label, but what we do have is a ***Pre-disease continuum*** made up of an uninterrupted process of cell energy decline followed by cell structural damage (increasing entropy) followed by insulin resistance and metabolic dysfunction that culminates in all our chronic metabolic diseases. We have one "mother" of a problem leading to chronic disease.

Trying to divide and conquer this continuum of risk and damage is a pointless exercise and a huge laugh because, as mentioned above, we have no drug cure at ***any*** point along this continuum of risk.

We now need to get this straight: we have one continuum that is the cause of all these deadly chronic diseases (our "mother") that is a linear and continuous process from birth to our tombs.

Glucose cut-off points are absolutely irrelevant on a continuum of glucose change. These glucose cut-off points are an abomination now and a relic of the past that should be discarded as Dark Age thinking.

We must now choose either a linear path or a convoluted one to guide us in metabolic disease management

Occam's Razor, as I have mentioned, is a philosophical principle that states that the least complicated path to solving a problem will be the right one. If we accept the principle of simplicity as the correct solution, we should then choose Path (1), as shown in the graphic below, hands down, that blocks the development of chronic diseases.

However, Path (2) is the one the medical profession has chosen, and in doing so, it has truly destroyed our chances for a healthy life and chosen the worst path possible for population health.

Path (2) is a crazy, tangled path that has either been designed to maximize pharmaceutical profits or is a twisted path created by monumental medical blunders. In fact, Path (2) is an amalgamation of corrupt behaviour, self-interest, and vested interests that drove this convoluted path. We have allowed Pharma and food corporations and governments with conflicts of interest to call the shots, and we have permitted unbelievable autonomy for the medical and dietetic professions to stumble along and create this metabolic disease nightmare. Shouldn't these professions be accountable for this disaster?

If you have been given this diagnosis of "prediabetes", "MetS", or "diabetes" (T2DM), then understand you may already have advanced vascular or organ disease and that you need to be investigated.

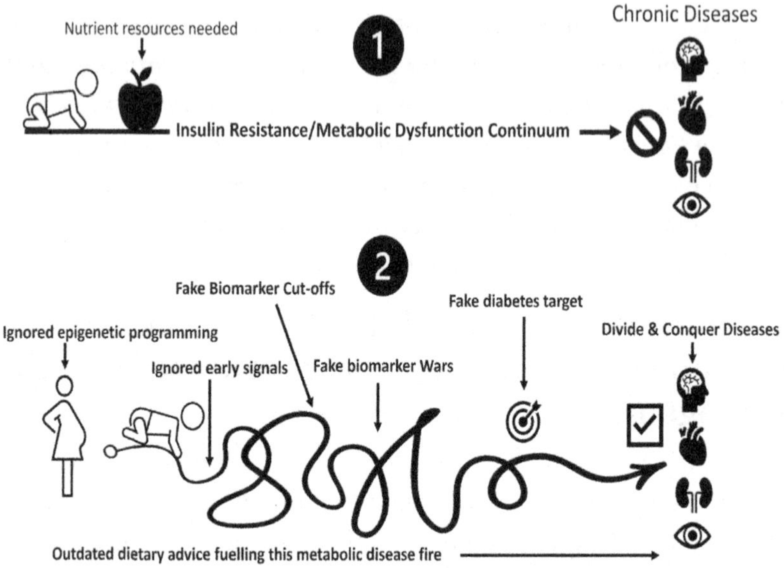

The dietary protocol and supplements I suggest are all designed to boost vascular health, but critically, we need to stop insulting our vascular system. Medicine and Pharma will, in future, concentrate on our microvascular beds, but as usual, it will be a drug approach that totally discards all the other harmful inputs that demand modification and if what's past is prologue, then the medical profession will discard the vital need for nutrient support in the future. Drugs without comprehensive big-picture nutritional support that addresses the cellular defects in insulin resistance is a pointless and deadly exercise.

A pandemic of fatty liver

Insulin resistance is an "almost universal finding" in non-alcoholic fatty liver disease (Utzschneider and Kahn 2006). Fatty liver in this day and age is considered the liver manifestation of Metabolic Syndrome (MetS) (Flisiak-Jackiewicz, Bobrus-Chociej et al. 2021).

With up to 1 in 3 people in Australia having fatty liver, and this is up to 5.5 million people affected, this problem is not exactly rare (Roberts, Majeed et al. 2021). Fatty liver is a global problem affecting an average of 25% of the world population, and this pandemic of fatty liver runs in parallel with the ever-increasing prevalence rates of overfat, obesity and Metabolic Syndrome (MetS). It is something I have regularly seen mentioned in CT scans and ultrasound reports of abdominal imaging.

In the ***Fiendish Fructose*** chapter, we will look at cheap nutrient management that is jaw-droppingly effective yet ignored by the medical profession. Why? Because Pharma can't put a registered trademark on natural compounds. It is sad when so many lives have been destroyed by the arrogance and conceit shown against food-based, nutrient-based treatments, giving a false impression that a drug-based solution is our only hope. It is absolutely not!

We have an explosion of fatty liver (NAFLD) associated with metabolic dysfunction that is now a pandemic of liver disease. Most people don't know they are suffering from this problem, which can have dire consequences even in childhood. There has been a 3-fold increase in fatty liver since the 1990s, and it is expected that by 2040, 55.7% of the world's population will have fatty liver (Le, Yeo et al. 2022).

Fatty liver is the consequence of a "prediabetic" state that we have messed up through our desire to use drugs instead of what is required to stop this madness. If you have been diagnosed with fatty liver, then read the ***Fiendish Fructose*** chapter. A simple abdominal ultrasound can reveal this deadly problem in an individual, especially if you have other features of MetS such as a big belly, hypertension, raised uric acid or glucose or raised triglycerides, all powerful indicators that you are well on your way along this metabolic dysfunction continuum.

A pre-disease continuum should be our concern

The CDC would much rather we change the term "Prediabetes" to "**Prevent**diabetes" (CDC 2022). As mentioned above, we could regard the whole course of the insulin-resistant-metabolic dysfunction continuum as a "***Pre-Disease Continuum***". The CDC would like everyone, including doctors and the lay public, to understand that what we term "prediabetes" can be prevented.

Historically, in medicine, we have used artificial blood glucose cut-off points termed *Impaired Fasting Glucose (IFG)* and *Impaired Glucose Tolerance (IGT)* to arrive at the label of "prediabetes", which are points way too far along the continuum that has allowed biological damage (biological rot) to have occurred long before these fake glucose cut-off points are discovered. This early biological damage then snowballs throughout our lives because, as I have mentioned, it robs us of our health and puts us at risk of early death.

It is estimated that close to 4 million people in Australia are "prediabetic" (Deed, Barlow et al. 2015), as are nearly 100 million Americans (CDC 2019)(CDC 2019) – this is a staggering 1 in 3 Americans with advanced glucose cut off points. As frightening as these statistics are, it is important to remember that they are derived from advanced glucose cut-off points, as mentioned above, and thus miss the massive numbers with early metabolic markers long before those later glucose signals manifest.

Advanced glucose cut-off points vastly underestimate disease prevalence. This underestimate makes medicine and dietetics feel good about themselves that they are doing a "great job" when, in fact, they are doing a lousy job of keeping us all healthy. They have failed. We need to move beyond the hocus pocus of prevalence figures based on shonky glucose cut-off points.

Our only focus should now be to prevent biological damage that occurs long before any glucose cut-off point and long before any fake metabolic label.

The Centers for Disease Control (CDC) USA states:

"Don't let the "pre" fool you. Prediabetes is a serious health condition...Prediabetes puts you at increased risk of developing type 2 diabetes, heart disease, and stroke."(CDC 2022)

By ignoring early signals for metabolic disease, we allow our metaphorical "prediabetes" balloon to keep on expanding, and we put our healthcare system at huge risk of collapsing.

Ditch the glucose cut-offs and fake labels

Labels given to glucose cut-off points are anachronistic and a huge embarrassment now. Insulin resistance and beta-cell dysfunction may exist for years and even decades before the "prediabetes" glucose cut-off signals manifest (Khan, Chua et al. 2019). To think that once the insulin resistance and metabolic dysfunction continuum starts with even a barely measurable flicker, we will have set into motion the inevitable, ***S***low, ***I***ncremental and ***C***umulative (SIC) biological damage (biological rot). Our absolute focus should be halting and reversing biological rot through well-established, evidence-based nutritional principles.

The term "prediabetes" would have to be the worst construct in medical history. Some interesting quotes follow:

> *"In conclusion, prediabetes, far from being benign, is a toxic environment that is associated with the development of microvascular and macrovascular complications." (Brannick, Wynn et al. 2016)*

Professor John Yudkin once stated:

> *"Professor John S Yudkin of University College London, UK, wrote in 2014 that "Prediabetes is an artificial category with virtually zero clinical relevance." (Gottwald-Hostalek and Gwilt 2022)*

At first glance, I thought that "*virtually zero clinical relevance*" meant that this "prediabetic" state doesn't matter. Nothing could be further from the truth. However, the clever professor may have also meant that as an "*artificial category*", it is meaningless in the context of a continuum of risk and dangerous outcomes. However, the dominating sentiment in the medical and dietetic professions is that this "prediabetic" state can be ignored as "mild" and insignificant. If we ignore this metabolic phase, we are then condemned to early chronic disease and early death. Imagine then that 100s of millions of lives were destroyed by this fake diagnosis of "prediabetes' that was left untreated, allowing all these souls to perish. We are still doing the same today because we wait and wait for that easy solution – a drug rather than implementing established and highly effective dietary principles we know can stop the biological rot in its tracks.

"Prediabetes": The nemesis of healthcare systems globally

We are caught up in a time warp. Acute diseases, such as infections, now comprise only a small fraction of the disease burden in this century. Infectious diseases made up only 1.7% of the total disease burden in Australia in 2018 (AIHW 2022). Yet we think we can fix these chronic conditions as if they are acute problems like infections using a silver-bullet mentality from the last century. This silver-bullet thinking is so last century using antibiotics, which were indeed wonderful silver bullets at that time, but this silver-bullet era has long gone. We now have a world of chronic diseases that silver bullets can't fix:

> *"The emerging burden of chronic disease over the past half-century fell upon a medical profession that was born in an era of acute disease predominance, had become imbued with cure as the goal, assumed individual physician authority with patient passivity, and was structured to treat disease as a passing episode in the patient's life...*
>
> *Despite the change in the major problem confronting it, the profession has remained largely locked in those attitudes and practices designed for acute disease. When applied to chronic disease, the attitudes and practices are neither effective nor efficient. The development of appropriate healthcare practices for chronic disease is central to solving the healthcare crisis." (Holman 2005)*

The balloon and conveyor belt analogy explains why "prediabetes" is unstoppable.

So why is this problem of metabolic disease getting bigger and bigger? Insulin resistance (our real "prediabetes") has been doubling or tripling over the last two decades, so there is nowhere to hide from this disaster now. We need to deal with insulin resistance head-on. Please refresh your memory of the metabolic dysfunction balloon discussed in chapter one. Trapped in that metaphorical "prediabetes" balloon are affected individuals, all with insulin resistance, who wait silently to become acutely and seriously ill. Crammed in that metabolic dysfunction balloon, they all undergo the ***S***low, ***I***ncremental and ***C***umulative ***(SIC)*** progression of biological damage (increasing biological rot), leading to more and more wicked complications. We have no hope of halting this progression with drugs or halting the massively increasing numbers of those with insulin resistance being crammed into this ever-expanding balloon.

Once patched up by drugs or maybe a stent in a blocked artery that cures nothing, affected individuals are thrown back into that balloon to suffer more biological damage (rot), which is inevitable as this continuum of metabolic damage will power on regardless of these band-aid approaches. No patch-up job with pharmaceuticals or a stent will stop this metabolic process from driving on relentlessly in the background of an affected individual.

These sick individuals are then discharged continuously from that balloon onto a metaphorical disease conveyor belt that will then dump them at GP clinics or hospital settings in a never-ending but ever-increasing cycle of more and more complicated disease outcomes that we have no answer for. The huge problem is that the numbers of those discharged from that balloon have dramatically increased decade after decade. The conveyor belt is not fast enough now to deliver these diseased individuals to medical facilities where GP clinics and hospitals become the choke points at the end of the conveyor belt as GPs and hospitals simply can't cope with the flood of complex (wicked) chronic diseases and the outcomes. Hospitals find it hard to discharge severely sick individuals who languish in those hospital beds for long periods, blocking others just as seriously ill from getting a hospital bed.

No drug in over 60 years has been able to stop this sheer volume of diseases flooding our healthcare systems. No drug has stopped the numbers with insulin resistance continually filling that metaphorical balloon, and no drug has stopped the biological rot that will result in horrific medical complications that are never fixed. How can this be sustainable when prevalence rates are accelerating and where we now wait for tsunamis of these diseases to overwhelm us in the coming two decades? We wait and wait for medical reductionism to provide an answer, with the medical profession begging for an answer from Pharma to find that blockbuster drug to resolve this embarrassment of skyrocketing disease prevalence. It is not as if the dietetic industry is shouting for change in dietary inputs.

We allow distorted food-based inputs to keep putting us at risk. Our true saviour is to ensure absolute nutrient adequacy to generate cellular energy that then powers cells to reverse entropy (decay) over time. You don't stop biological rot if you cannot reverse entropy (cellular chaos, decay) through the investment of ATP energy. The ongoing implementation of a dietary approach that minimizes the post-meal impacts of food while ensuring the continuous supply of nutritional resources is the only way forward. How easy is this concept to understand compared to the medical and dietetic model management mess? Pharma and food corporations won't like this approach. Should we care?

Microvascular disease (MVD). Chaotic, asymmetric organ damage that leads to the many clinical presentations ("faces") of disease

Microcirculation network damage is the powerful link that ties together seemingly unrelated medical disorders of the body and brain. It is microcirculation damage that affects multiple organs simultaneously to produce the many clinical "faces" of metabolic disease we see and the cause of multimorbidity. So, one abnormal metabolic process that links multiple organs at any given moment in time. Many current diseases remain poorly understood, yet we can explain many of these conditions by considering insulin resistance, metabolic dysfunction, bioenergetic decline, and cellular decay (entropy) at the heart of those clinical problems, all exacerbated by disruptions and blockages in microcirculatory networks.

All that cellular energy decline and structural decay and all those increasing blood biomarkers made even worse by after-eating surges in glucose, triglycerides, and inflammation can lead to damaged and dysfunctional small blood vessel networks. Once this happens, our cells, tissues and organ systems have no hope as the "pipeline" for everything they need, from fuel, oxygen, nutrient supply and waste removal, becomes more and more choked off.

All tissues and organs have their specific microcirculation network. Our skin, for example, has a rich network of small blood vessels, and our bones and skeletal health depend on a healthy microcirculation to stay healthy. We can age rapidly due to small vessel damage, and we ignore this impact to our peril. All our mental health problems can be viewed as cellular bioenergetic and structural decline made massively worse by microcirculation network obstruction. The fact we allow this microcirculation damage to occur due to cell starvation, the neglected changes in blood biomarkers, and the neverending postprandial (after-eating) meal-by-meal hits to our vascular system many times a day is sheer negligence—such a huge missed opportunity.

What we need to get our heads around is that microcirculation damage to our organs will never be symmetric, and it will always be chaotic as inputs will vary from day to day, which means some organs are affected to a lesser or greater extent than others at any point in time. Our microvascular networks will be damaged chaotically and never uniformly and never symmetrically in any organ as this chaotic asymmetry of organ damage depends on genetics, epigenetics and personal allostatic loads or congenital and acquired structural and vascular defects. All of these will vary from individual to individual.

Thus, asymmetric microvascular damage, even within organ systems, along with chaotic acute and chronic inputs, are the hallmarks of chronic disease, and these factors will determine how these disorders present to medical practitioners, i.e. the clinical "faces" of these diseases, whether the crushing chest pain of angina or the slow and inevitable memory loss of vascular dementia. We must grasp this concept now that a singular process with multiple inputs can produce variable clinical presentations.

As the text "Fundamentals of Chaos Theory" states:

> *"Almost all natural, physical, and socio-economic systems are inherently nonlinear." (Sivakumar and Sivakumar 2017)*

So, chaos is a nonlinear system where small differences in inputs can result in drastically different outcomes over time. Thus, regarding metabolic disease, we have variability, uncertainty, and unpredictability that impact organ systems. This variability is the hallmark of metabolic and microvascular disease, leading to biological deterioration. These chaotic features lead to the complexity of medical presentations that are so hard to cope with in a medical sense. It is this complexity of presentations that is poorly understood in medicine, and as a result, these complex (wicked) presentations are crushing healthcare systems globally. All of these variables will determine which organ makes the most "noise" first, but this doesn't mean that other organs are not affected as well simultaneously but are making less "noise" at that time. Less "noisy" organs will make much more noise later on. Remember, this is a progressive ***multisystem*** disaster of a problem.

Microvascular disease worsens hyperglycaemia (high blood glucose) and vice versa in a bidirectional vicious loop. Large blood vessels have their specific microcirculation, the Vasa Vasorum (vessels of vessels)

Of concern is that microcirculation damage can occur early in the glucose continuum. Microvascular disease (MVD) can precede hyperglycaemia (high glucose levels) long before glucose cut-off points, which, as mentioned, we put way too much emphasis on. In fact, microvascular disease can occur with glucose levels well within the normal range (Emanuelsson, Marott et al. 2020). It is a scary thought that we have a small vessel problem, the silent "assassin of organs," happening in the so-called normal biomarker range, making glucose cut-off points a redundant and dangerous concept.

As mentioned above, when small blood vessels are affected, we have less glucose being delivered to our huge skeletal muscle bed to dispose of (burn off as energy). It is well documented that skeletal muscle is responsible for around 85% of blood glucose disposal to be used as an energy source (de Wendt, Espelage et al. 2021). Our skeletal muscle has a vast microvascular network. So when we lose muscle mass (sarcopenia) or if our skeletal muscle microvascular network is affected, then huge amounts of glucose are not being burnt off as energy. Blood glucose then increases as a result. This skeletal muscle disposal of 85% of glucose also depends on insulin working normally.

MVD and hyperglycaemia are bidirectional, where MVD can drive hyperglycaemia, and hyperglycaemia can worsen MVD in a vicious loop. This loop worsens insulin resistance and metabolic dysfunction. This microvascular-glucose loop is firmly documented (Stehouwer 2018).

The retina of the eye is our window to cardiovascular health. Retinal vessels also act as a proxy for the microcirculation health of the brain. These two vascular beds are also tightly linked (van Dinther, Voorter et al. 2022).

> *"The retinal microvascular network offers a powerful tool to study the role of the microcirculation in cardiovascular disease."* (Struijker-Boudier 2023)

It has been known since 1876 and described by W. Koester how the vasa vasorum are the small blood vessels of larger coronary arteries, i.e. the vasa vasorum is the microcirculation of larger arteries and contributes to plaque formation, inflammation and plaque rupture in our larger conduit arteries (Xu, Lu et al. 2015). So, our larger arteries need their specific microcirculation to survive. Vasa Vasorum means the "vessels of vessels".

We ignore small vessels to our peril. As mentioned, microcirculation damage is now seen as the "motor" that drives large vessel disease (Stokes and Granger 2005) and a motor that also drives inflammation.

> *"The microcirculation is recognised as the site where the earliest manifestations of cardiovascular disease, especially inflammatory responses, occur that may play a pivotal role in driving the atherosclerotic process in conduit vessels ... By the time symptoms develop or clinical signs of atherosclerosis can be detected in conduit vessels, the disease process is already at an advanced stage." (Lockhart, Hamilton et al. 2009)*

Conduits are the large artery "pipelines" that deliver blood to organs through the smaller blood vessel networks that branch off these larger vessels. As usual, medicine waits and waits for something to go wrong, like angina, a heart attack, heart failure, vascular dementia or stroke, but as you see in the quote above, all of these problems are very advanced points of damage to large vessels.

We have totally missed the opportunity to avoid these problems by not dealing with microvascular disease in the very early stages This microvascular protection can be achieved through nutritional means, and we should never depend on drugs, thinking they will stop the ongoing damage from all the harmful factors I mention in this book as they won't. However, the delivery of oxygen, micronutrients, and waste removal occurs in our small vessel networks - our microcirculation networks.

Impaired Fasting Glucose (IFG) or Impaired Glucose Tolerance (IGT), as mentioned, are glucose cut-off points we use to declare someone has "prediabetes". But the International Expert Committee states:

> *"Moreover, the categorical classification of individuals as high risk (e.g., IFG or IGT) or low risk, based on any measure of*

glycemia, is less than ideal because the risk for progression to diabetes appears to be a continuum." (IEC 2009)

As mentioned previously, statements like this litter the medical literature where they state there is the likelihood or not of "***progression to diabetes***". It would be far more accurate to state, "***progression to chronic metabolic disease appears to be a continuum***" instead. However, this absurd focus on "diabetes" makes no sense unless we see it as a Mt Everest of glucose cut-offs that are designed to cull numbers who will need public funds for intervention.

It is incredibly important to know that microvascular density is 50% less in diabetic animals and thought to be far worse in humans with Type-2 Diabetes Mellitus (T2DM) due to the added burden of hypertension culling these fragile small vessels even further (Wiernsperger and Bouskela 2003).

These factors will make hypertension worse, thus culling even more small blood vessels in a vicious cycle. This lack of microvascular density puts people with diabetes at huge risk for all the complications we see, hastening organ damage and failure, and this microcirculation damage will worsen the postprandial surges in glucose. Carbs anyone? We have been naïve and very foolish by promoting blood glucose-spiking high-starchy grains and foods to vulnerable people simply to sell agricultural products.

Let's not forget that glucose to fructose shunting in the brain will be powered by this culling of small blood vessels spiking blood glucose further and increasing hypertension, making dementia risk even greater. You can see how simplistically we think about these diseases and manage them.

Tik-Tock: Poiseuille's Law, microcirculation armageddon: Small decreases in capillary diameter produce dramatic reductions in blood flow and dramatic increases in blood vessel resistance

"It has long been an axiom of mine that the little things are infinitely the most important." Sir Arthur Conan Doyle

A 20% reduction in small vessel diameter can result in a 100% increase in resistance and a 50% reduction in blood flow
(Gutterman, Chabowski et al. 2016)

Wow! This fact is staggering, as small decreases in small vessel diameter can result in a huge 100% increase in blood vessel resistance. Imagine blood flow being slashed by half in organ systems. It is known that preterm babies have microcirculation dysfunction that can lead to long-term cardiovascular complications (Puchwein-Schwepcke, Grzybowski et al. 2019). We need to put in far more research on early microvascular damage and long-term outcomes. However, you as an individual can truly protect your small blood vessels just by dietary means and stop the incessant harmful insults to your small vessels. Imagine what we can achieve by just ensuring nutrient adequacy or thinking about food composition before we eat anything to protect against postprandial (after-eating) vascular damage.

Conventional wisdom states that microcirculation damage occurs at the onset of diabetes and that large vessel disease occurs decades before (Haffner, Stern et al. 1990). But this has to be challenged now, and this thinking has to be "turned on its head" as microvascular disease predates "by a mile" large vessel disease driving atherosclerosis. Microvascular beds are the tick-tock ticking clock of adverse cardiovascular events (Lockhart, Hamilton et al. 2009).

Microvascular damage and, indeed, all vascular diseases are part of a continuum, as I have discussed. We can extrapolate from the figures above that even a 5% reduction in small vessel diameter would produce a 25% increase in blood vessel resistance and a 12.5%

reduction in blood flow. A micronutrient deficiency in pregnancy may program a child for chronic vascular diseases.

Hypertension, a hallmark of this insulin resistance continuum, is itself a continuum (Duprez and Toleuova 2013). The likelihood of having hypertension without metabolic dysfunction or diabetes without hypertension is slim (Cheung 2010). If we didn't have blood pressure increasing trying to "push" blood through blocked (resistant) small vessels, we would not survive as we deprive cells, tissues and organ systems of this critical blood pipeline, thus depriving all our cells of essential factors such as oxygen, fuel (glucose) and micronutrients and getting rid of cellular waste. It is said that 2 billion people suffer from at least one micronutrient deficiency (Christian and Stewart 2010). Imagine then the vast number of people with microcirculation damage restricting the delivery of micronutrients even further to our biological tissues.

Without nutrients and oxygen, oxidative phosphorylation (OXPHOS) cannot proceed effectively in mitochondria, and as a result, ATP production in mitochondria diminishes greatly. ATP production worsens as blood vessel resistance increases and blood flow decreases disproportionately. This progression of microcirculation damage and ongoing cell structural destruction is a major reason patch-up drug treatments will never work. Poor dietary advice that adds to this synergy of adverse effects needs to be condemned. Blood vessel resistance continues to grow incrementally despite ad hoc treatments. Hypertension is now seen as a continuum of damage leading to horrendous consequences long-term.

The brain is a selfish super-system that demands a lot of glucose to function. Imagine early and relentless microcirculation damage impacts on the brain far earlier than our research gurus consider, leading to a decline in bioenergetic and structural decline over decades. The Yale University finding of glucose-to-fructose conversion in brains is groundbreaking, worsening bioenergetic decline in brain cells. Fructose pulls the rug from ATP production.

We waste billions on beta-amyloid treatments for Alzheimer's that have proven almost useless or wonder why mental health problems are skyrocketing and forget that the brain not only needs an immense amount of glucose for energy to survive and function, but it also needs a wealth of nutrients and oxygen to function and repair normally. It is a pity that we have been so backward in recognizing the importance of the microcirculation networks in chronic disease and have allowed this microvessel damage to assassinate our organ systems over time when we could have halted this destruction long before it happened. All we do is aim for drug treatments with a view to driving financial gain for Pharma and lazy medical practices that never deal with the heart of the problem, and that is to consider what cells need to function and survive.

The endothelium (the cells lining blood vessels) is a huge endocrine (hormone-producing) organ. This lining becomes"Molecular Velcro" to latch onto damaged (modified) lipids

> *"Dysfunction of the vascular endothelium is thus a hallmark of human diseases." (Rajendran, Rengarajan et al. 2013)*

Insulin resistance has a range of damaging impacts on our blood vessels, heightened by postprandial (after-eating) consequences, which occur daily and many times during the day. You are familiar with Appendix-18, which shows the detrimental effects of this postprandial state, and yet we ignore these cumulative after-eating effects over our lifetimes to our detriment health-wise.

Meal-by-meal, snack-by-snack, we hammer our endothelium, and because food inputs don't change for the better, the vulnerable endothelium becomes more and more damaged over time. The damaging postprandial (after eating) effects occur on top of the metabolic markers, oxidative stress and inflammation created by our insulin resistance metabolic dysfunction continuum.

This "prediabetes" period will increase the expression of an adhesion molecule called VCAM-1, described as "Molecular Velcro" mentioned previously. We are all familiar with Velcro, which has tiny hooks to attach things. Normal blood vessels have very little VCAM-

1, but damaged blood vessels have a lot. This molecular VCAM-1 “Velcro” then grabs onto passing inflammatory white blood cells or modified LDL, like hooks in normal velcro, to begin the atherosclerosis process (Libby, Aikawa et al. 2000).

Let's now throw into the mix modified lipids such as glycated LDL (gLDL) or oxidised LDL (ox-LDL), which can increase in the after-eating state (Lechleitner, Hoppichler et al. 1994). Modified LDL can trigger a cascade of events that can harm the endothelium, activating white blood cells like monocytes, which then stimulate the production of VCAM-1 (Toma, Sanda et al. 2016) and start the plaque-building process in the larger arteries and increase endothelial dysfunction and stiffness along with obstruction in the microcirculation. We must wake up to this issue and shift from decreasing total LDL to preventing LDL from being modified by an ignored insulin resistance process magnified by after-eating (postprandial) effects that leads to LDL damaging blood biomarkers, oxidative stress, inflammation and postprandial hits.

The endothelium is the largest organ in the body. The 1.2 trillion endothelial cells lining our blood vessels comprise the largest endocrine organ (one that produces hormones and biologically active compounds). The vast array of biologically active compounds produced by endothelial cells includes but is not limited to - vasoactive peptide hormones, coagulation factors, growth factors and adhesion molecules (Baumgartner-Parzer and Waldhausl 2001).

Thus, when these endothelial cells are damaged and activated from all the factors mentioned in this book, we trigger a highly significant inflammatory response that affects our entire bodies and all the larger conduit blood vessels. Our brains can become inflamed locally from the damaged endothelium of these small blood vessels deep within the brain and indirectly from the systemic inflammation created by the inflamed endothelium of large and small vessels elsewhere in our bodies.

> *“Furthermore, the inflammatory response, characterized by endothelial activation initiated in the microcirculation, plays an*

important role in driving the atherosclerotic process in large vessels." (Lockhart, Hamilton et al. 2009)

The surface area of the endothelium lining is a whopping 400 square metres (Änggård 1990). It is five times (5x) the size of our hearts in mass and six (x6) times the size of a tennis court (Hassan 2006). The endothelium is the largest endocrine organ in the body.

"Recent evidence clearly establishes the endothelium as the body's largest endocrine organ." (Glasser, Selwyn et al. 1996)

It is important to note that most of this huge endothelium surface area is from the smallest blood vessels in the microcirculation beds called the ***capillaries***. This large endothelial surface area nourishes our cells, tissues and organ systems. Nutrients, oxygen, fuel supply and waste removal all occur through these endothelial cells lining our smallest blood vessels. The fact that the endothelium is not only the biggest organ in the body but the biggest endocrine (hormone-producing) organ makes it easy to see how microcirculation damage drives not only disease of large blood vessels (vasa vasorum damage) but is also the engine that drives organ failure, e.g., cardiovascular disease, neurodegeneration such as Alzheimer's and virtually all the chronic diseases related to insulin resistance.

The UKPDS demonstrated that intensive glucose control significantly reduces the risk of microvascular complications (such as retinopathy, nephropathy (kidney), and neuropathy (nerves)) but has a less pronounced effect on macrovascular complications (such as heart attacks and strokes). But this will only happen if diabetes is treated early and does not linger to severely damage small blood vessels. It only takes eight (8) years for metabolic memory to kick in, as I have discussed, where we have irreversible microcirculation damage (López-Jaramillo, Velandia-Carrillo et al. 2014).

We will look at the aggressive lowering of blood glucose and the consequences later in the chapter titled "*That's no way to treat a metabolic biomarker*." We discussed microcirculation damage and "metabolic memory" previously. No amount of glucose-lowering will wipe away this metabolic memory of microcirculation damage, which marches on irrespective of our drug-centric treatments that try to control blood glucose and will thus lead to more and more complicated future clinical presentations. The key is early nutrient management to prevent, halt and reverse microcirculation damage.

Studies other than the UKPDS showed no improvement in cardiovascular mortality with glucose control, and strict glucose control does not decrease cardiovascular risk or mortality. The Action to Control Cardiovascular Risk in Diabetes (the ACCORD study) showed intensive glucose lowering increased mortality after 3.5 years and did not reduce cardiovascular events (Chawla, Chawla et al. 2016) so much for focusing on glucose and applying intensive glucose-lowering treatments that punish cells already lacking glucose fuel in a cellular energy crisis. Gurus will continue to gaslight these findings and move on to any crumb of information that helps their agenda of drug sales.

As the microcirculation beds worsen, we reach a point where drugs become less and less effective, and the risk of using drugs increases as it becomes more risky to decrease cell energy supplies as cellular energy and structural integrity deteriorate even more. Cutting off the energy and structural supplies using drugs is not clever. We never see biomarkers such as glucose as a positive for cells in terms of fuel supply. This microcirculation damage and metabolic memory will persist long after blood glucose has been normalised (Orasanu and Plutzky 2009). All these studies show how highly flawed this glucose-centric way of thinking is. We need to deal with metabolic disease on many fronts, not just focus on glucose or any other single biomarker.

Vascular disease is a continuum! For example, microvascular diseases like retinopathy (small vessel damage in the retina) increase with increasing glucose levels (IEC 2009). So, the moral of the story is to stop this glucose damage early and not to forget that multiple other factors are involved in this damage.

That diabetic microvascular (small vessels) and macrovascular (large vessel) disease are continuums is not in doubt (Dzau, Antman et al. 2006). However, we must treat all factors and recognise that microvascular disease can drive large vessel disease. This flip in focus from large vessels to the smallest vessels now needs to be firmly entrenched in the minds of medical practitioners. But who is educating medical practitioners about this switched way of thinking?

It is important to recognise that 20%-25% of all those with an initial adverse cardiovascular event have only one (x1) risk factor, and only 50% have elevated LDL (Dzau, Antman et al. 2006). It is also a sobering thought that around 50% of individuals presenting with a heart attack or sudden cardiac death had these life-threatening medical presentations as the first sign of underlying (hidden/silent) vascular disease (Lockhart, Hamilton et al. 2009).

How negligent and immoral have we been knowing that the principles behind the Lyon Diet Heart Study on the Mediterranean Diet could have stopped all of this in its tracks, but we worship at the altar of failed drug approaches and food economic imperatives. A whopping 73% reduction in new cardiovascular events was seen in the Lyon Diet Heart Study (De Lorgeril, Salen et al. 1997), and yet we flog the dead horse of drug management. Money from drug and food sales does indeed matter!

Inflammation: The role of the endothelium

The size of the lining of all our blood vessels, the endothelium, is staggering. One important component of the endothelium that lines the internal blood flow facing cells is the glycocalyx, as I have mentioned. Many nutrients can support the carbohydrate-rich components of the glycocalyx and strengthen this important part of the endothelium. In our rush to use a pointless drug that will do nothing for someone who has vascular dementia or heart failure due predominantly to microcirculation damage, we then do absolutely nothing to support the glycocalyx with readily available nutrient resources that could make a world of difference to outcomes.

I mentioned some statistics above, but here is another one.

> *"...the endothelium actively maintains approximately 60,000 miles of blood vessels in the human body." (Rajendran, Rengarajan et al. 2013)*

Imagine that 60,000 miles or 96,560 kilometres of blood vessels are maintained by cells lining our blood vessels. We are constantly "poking the bear" with the BIG-10 Womb to Tomb factors which damage our vast and highly active endothelium in an astronomical network of blood vessels where most of the endothelium is found in our small blood vessels (microcirculation networks).

There is no mystery as to why we will all suffer from heart disease or dementia in our lifetimes. If we don't watch every meal and snack we consume, and if we don't take measures to minimise our BIG-10 Womb-to-Tomb hits every day, damaging cell energy and function, then our health destiny is set.

It is a fact that artificial, cherry-picked antioxidants and anti-inflammatories fail to produce a positive effect in most studies. It would be tempting to think that if we can diminish inflammatory processes, we can make some positive strides. Declaring war on inflammation backfired on researchers studying this and found that anti-inflammatory drug approaches actually caused harm, which is unsurprising if we see inflammation as an adaptation and not an enemy. We discuss this inflammation treatment "paradox" in the chapter "***That's no way to treat a metabolic biomarker.***"

In a nutshell, though, by targeting inflammatory processes downstream of cells (beyond and after cells) rather than dealing with the upstream factors (factors that impact cells and the cells themselves), then attacking inflammatory processes (a result of our distressed energy and nutrient-deprived cells) becomes counterproductive as inflammation is an adaptation.

Cellular complexity is far too great to use a brute of a drug to fine-tune balance. Antioxidants through food and nutrient resources should be a part of a far bigger cell rescue and maintenance picture that can dampen down inflammation. Food-based approaches can be rich in phytochemicals and antioxidants if that diet is well structured. Let's not forget the anti-inflammatory effect of a diet rich in Omega-3s and a well-balanced gut microbiome if that microbiome is well nourished by a diversity of prebiotics (food fibre). We get these anti-inflammatory compounds from a range of multicoloured low-fructose fruits and vegetables.

Our only job to get cells back on track and become well-balanced is to provide food and nutrient inputs that don't cause harm. In medicine, we do things in a lopsided way. We must offer a wide range of nutrient resources to cells and then leave our miraculous cells to work their magic to restore cell function and resolve metabolic dysfunction.

A damning paper in the journal *Inflammopharmacology* was titled "*COX-2 inhibitors: a story of Greed, deception and death.*" COX-2 inhibitors are selective anti-inflammatories, but these drugs block a prostaglandin called prostacyclin. Doing this stops the vasodilating (blood vessel widening) effect of prostacyclin, diminishing blood supply to cells, tissues, organs and larger blood vessels. Remember that most people already have a defective microcirculation, and we then throw in a COX-2 anti-inflammatory "grenade" that worsens things dramatically by diminishing the ability of blood vessels to widen. Heart attacks, strokes and deaths were all well documented within three years of release of certain anti-inflammatories (Halpern 2005). Halpern's paper stated: *"The manufacturers faced a possibly complicit, toothless and bloodless FDA, and used every maneuvering to fleece the patients."*

It is not just the COX-2 anti-inflammatories but also general anti-inflammatories that can lead to dangerous cardiovascular outcomes (Howes 2007). If we consider diminished microcirculation a major contributor to cardiovascular outcomes, how irresponsible are we to pull the rug from under the critical blood and nutrient supply to our cells by using mindless anti-inflammatory approaches that decrease vasodilation (preventing the opening up of blood vessels)? By preventing vasodilation, we block the delivery of fuel (glucose), oxygen and nutrient resources to cells and organs. That we allow Pharma to get away with these deaths is unforgivable, and yet we do.

As the Halpern paper stated: "*Who cares about the cost of innocent lives when Pfizer and Merck have hired some of the best and brightest* *lawyers as hired guns, and when Celebrex had sales of US$ 3.3 billion last year?*" Celebrex was created as a COX-2 inhibitor.

Inflammation, in reality, is an adaptation that benefits energy-struggling cells by widening (vasodilating) blood vessels, thus increasing blood, oxygen, fuel, and nutrient supplies to struggling cells (Ramanlal and Gupta 2020). Inflammation can be a friend, but the medical model only sees it as an enemy.

So instead of providing the body with Nitric Oxide (NO) generating compounds such as L-Citrulline (See Appendix-12) or providing a wealth of phytochemicals, nitrate-rich foods and food-based antioxidants that can have tremendous positive benefits on a failing microcirculation, or ensuring a diversity of fibre (prebiotics) to our gut microbiome, we continue with drug-obsessed thought processes: money, money, money to be made I guess.

We know that antioxidants can improve endothelium-dependent relaxation and they can reverse oxidised-LDL (Ox-LDL) and prevent the inhibition of eNOS, the enzyme that converts L-Arginine to Nitric Oxide (Rajendran, Rengarajan et al. 2013). L-citrulline is a far better oral source of L-arginine than taking L-arginine by itself. Adding food nitrates found in beetroot and other foods also helps boost nitric oxide (NO) over time, thus boosting blood flow.

Alzheimer's Disease (AD): A microcirculation problem with cell bioenergetic decline

The story of Alzheimer's disease is the story of insulin resistance and the crucial role impaired insulin signalling plays in AD, thus linking insulin resistance, metabolic dysfunction, MetS, mental health disorders and AD. It is no wonder, then, that, like all our body organ damage that occurs over years and decades, the same is true of AD, where we have a slow progression over years to decades prior to memory loss and physical decline. As you will learn, Alzheimer's is a vascular problem, and once again, our very small vessel network (the brain microcirculation network) is at the crossroads of functional and structural damage to the brain in AD.

Instead of seeing AD as the result of ***one*** pathological metabolic process, we want to find the specific biochemical, molecular or environmental factor (target) that is the killer problem in AD. So, we drill deeper and deeper into the molecular effects that result in AD rather than the cause of AD. This drilling down confuses everyone and delays life-saving prevention and treatment. We must recognise that, like all our other chronic metabolic diseases, this problem begins early, with bioenergetic and vascular decline playing a central role, along with subsequent cellular structural decay in brain cells driven by increasing microvascular damage.

Alzheimer's is one disease that sends a shiver up the spine of many people as they age. AD has robbed ageing parents of the ability even to remember their children. There is no heavy-hitting genetic variant that causes AD, yet we treat it as something that results in a vacuum separated from all the dietary and environmental factors I describe in the BIG-10 Womb-to-Tomb list that impact the brain cells metabolically and depleting them of energy. Our brain glucose-to-fructose shunt, as discussed in Chapter 1 and below in more detail, is a big hit to brain energy.

Like all diseases, the Holy Grail is to find a money-making biomarker to target, like beta-amyloid, which has proven next to useless in reversing AD if we target this abnormal protein. As this quote rightly points out, AD is a vascular disease and, more specifically, a microvascular disorder.

> *"The collective data presented in this review strongly indicate that the present classification of AD is incorrect and should be changed to that of a vascular disorder." (de la Torre 2002)*

All of the risk factors known to be associated with AD, from diabetes to hypertension, hyperhomocysteinaemia (high homocysteine level), atherosclerosis, apoE4, and menopause – all have a vascular component and are all associated with decreased brain perfusion (blood flow) (de la Rocha, Sanchez-Muniz et al. 2009).

A 2023 paper stated:

> *"...almost all AD brains display evidence of endothelial and capillary degeneration even in the absence of other forms of macrovascular pathology." (Tarawneh 2023)*

Capillary degeneration is microvascular degeneration. The "*almost all*" statement can be replaced with 100%, as researchers don't like using absolutes. This small vessel disease can be seen in the absence of large vessel disease (macrovascular pathology). Finally, we have a true sense prevailing in AD, recognizing microvascular disease as the final nail in the coffin to nerve cells causing so much biological and brain damage. This brain cell damage is increasing entropy (decay, chaos, degeneration) as a result of decreasing brain cell energy to the point it cannot reverse this decay or entropy. Once the blood supply is severely restricted through microvascular disease, the rest is history, as structural and ultrastructural damage will then accelerate along with complex molecular impacts caused by neuronal degeneration long before the tau and amyloid aggregates manifest (Tarawneh 2023).

Like all our chronic metabolic diseases, we have focused our attention on the wrong end of this problem. We have been focusing on the effects of this process rather than the metabolic process, which results in cellular energy and structural decline. In other words, these aggregates are not the cause of AD but simply reflect the damage caused by bioenergetic and structural insults along with decreased waste removal, such as amyloid, as the brain microcirculation becomes increasingly damaged and blocked and not functionally effective for waste removal.

We have two forces colliding to sap cells of energy, thus hastening structural decline:

1. Our BIG-10 Womb-to-Tomb impacts robbing cells of energy
2. Our small blood vessel "pipelines" become obstructed, further robbing cells of the supply of oxygen, fuel, and nutrients, therefore worsening ATP production and increasing structural decline. Points (1) and (2) act synergistically to damage cells and our brains. You often

hear that depression and hearing loss are big factors for dementia. What you never hear is that microcirculation damage can lead to both these modifiable issues.

These two points above are fundamental to the damage caused in all cells, tissues, and organ systems in the body, not just the brain.

The single most important genetic risk for Alzheimer's Disease, apoE4, reduces the efficiency of mitochondria to produce ATP (energy)

If anyone has this apoE4 genetic variant, and we then throw in what I have described in points (1) and (2) above, we add to this genetically decreased mitochondrial efficiency.

With a tsunami of Alzheimer's disease expected in the coming decades, do we have time to wait for this drug-targeted solution, which, in my mind, will never come? Like all other drugs dealing with metabolic disease, these drugs for Alzheimer's will be stop-gap solutions that act like bandaids that barely hold back the inevitable.

Now, let's get back to our apoE4 gene. You inherit one apoE4 gene from the mother and one from the father. Having one apoE4 gene doubles or triples the risk for Alzheimer's, but having two genes (x2) increases your risk by 8x to 12x (Mayo-Clinic 2023). However, the ApoE4 gene is insufficient and is not necessary for Alzheimer's to develop (Kamboh 2004). AD needs far more than a gene and involves all the factors discussed in this book to generate such brain damage. Points (1) and (2) above are constantly in the background acting synergistically and are the major forces leading to organ damage, including our brains, through cellular bioenergetic and structural decline. Just add that glucose → fructose shunt in the brain, as I have discussed previously, to create a sledgehammer bioenergetic decline effect in the brain and then let's add microcirculation network failure to hammer our brains truly.

Animal studies have linked this apoE4 genetic variant to decreased ATP production, as discussed, but apoE4 also adversely affects the critical NAD^+/NADH levels that are vital in OXPHOS and

ATP production (Yin, Nielsen et al. 2019). High food energy consumption (nutri-stress) also decreases NAD^+/NADH, and this lower redox couple action then acts to decrease ATP production, where energy is required to prevent or repair damage to mitochondria. Thus, the only susceptible genetic marker we know is the ApoE4 gene, which has everything to do with cell bioenergetics and ATP production.

The "***grand unified theory***" of neurodegeneration focuses on mitochondria, which are the energy powerhouses of ATP production. Still, in my mind, we are focusing on one aspect of cell ATP production. We seemingly disregard the huge contribution to cell energy production by the optimal delivery of blood, oxygen, fuel (glucose) and micronutrient supply via our microcirculation networks, which are all critical factors in cell energy-producing pathways. Without micronutrients, all our energy-producing pathways, including the Electron Transport Chain (ETC) in mitochondria, come to a crashing halt. It is amazing how little we think of nutrients in the causation of disease, and when we do use nutrients in management, we love to forget the effects of high-energy whole foods causing nutri-stress and scrambling the ability of cells to produce energy or repair and rebuild themselves. We also need to consider fully functional biochemical pathways like the glycolytic pathway or Krebs Cycle, which are vital before energy production in mitochondria kicks in. These biochemistry cycles are micronutrient hogs. A failing microcirculation, and hence micronutrient delivery, greatly affects all these components needed for energy production to occur.

Multiple enzymes exist in both the glycolytic and Krebs cycle, each susceptible to micronutrient deficiencies or environmental or medication toxicities. This focus on mitochondria is reminiscent of the medical professions focusing on single biomarkers as the bad guys. We now know how focusing on one factor and not the whole picture can create a disaster. To see how the Glycolytic Pathway, Krebs Cycle and Mitochondria all link up, see Appendix-29.

Interestingly, a medication for prostate enlargement called Terazosin can bind onto and boost the enzyme phosphoglycerate kinase 1 (PGK1) to stimulate ATP production in the glycolysis pathway. Men taking this medication had a 37% decreased risk of developing Parkinson's Disease (Cai, Zhang et al. 2019). This effect once again reinforces the importance of an adequate cellular energy supply in neurodegeneration. We don't need a drug like Terazosin to improve brain energy; all we need to do is reverse microcirculation damage and provide cells with all the oxygen and micronutrients they need to boost ATP production.

Those who think microcirculation damage cannot be reversed have not read research on diets like the Lyon Diet Heart Study or have read research showing *glycocalyx* supplements can improve microvascular health (van der Velden, IJpelaar et al. 2024). The glycocalyx is a micro-thin gel layer made up of carbohydrate components (glycoproteins, glycolipids) lining the endothelium. In animal studies, it has been shown that:

> *Reduction of weight via calorie-based diet and exercise in animal models of obesity results in significant improvement of endothelial function both in large vessels and in the microcirculation, primarily due to attenuation of oxidative stress and inflammation. (Csipo, Fulop et al. 2018)*

Imagine then using a supplement like ***Endocalyx***™ or support nutrients that help strengthen the glycocalyx, along with a well-structured diet like the one in the last chapter, which generates ketones assisting cells to bypass the insulin-blocking effect on glucose (fuel) getting into cells with this alternative fuel.

Microvessel disease is thus a progressively worsening problem that adds even more misery to bioenergetic impacts. Here's another quote about the prevalence of microcirculation damage - "***Practically all***" individuals with AD have microvascular degeneration (de la Rocha, Sanchez-Muniz et al. 2009). These studies scream that AD is part of a vascular and bioenergetic decline continuum. So, how does the brain repair itself and create neurotransmitters or myelin sheaths if it lacks the energy to do so or suffers nutrient supply shortages all because of damaged and blocked small vessels?

We need to dump now our flawed thinking of organ failure like the brain. This drain on oxygen, fuel, and nutrient resources should be our obvious target. We will discuss nutrient vasodilators such as L-Citrulline later that boost Nitric Oxide (NO), nitrate-rich foods that do the same and flavonoids that support vascular health.

Alzheimer's has long been suspected as a prion-related disease. Prions are toxic proteins that have an alteration in their 3D shape. In other words, they are misfolded. However, prions can pass on this protein folding abnormality to normal proteins to cause a chain reaction of proteins damaging proteins. Proteins can only work if they have the right 3D configuration. Beta-amyloid (Alzheimer's) and alpha-synuclein (Parkinson's) act like prions to spread protein misfolding in the brain (Frost and Diamond 2010). 3D protein folding and activation occurs in the cells' Endoplasmic Reticulum (ER). Nutrient limitation and insulin resistance affect the creation and repair of ER systems.

An emerging area of interest is the ***brain microbiome in Alzheimer's Disease***. Many pathological organisms can contribute to dementia, where antibiotics may be able to reverse the dementia completely. More research will emerge, but just like bad foods can cause havoc with the gut microbiome that then affects the whole body, such diets can affect the brain microbiome, making this collection of brain microbes sick and adding to disease risk.

How many other brain disorders are affected by a dysfunctional brain microbiome? We need vast amounts of energy to keep microorganisms in check as we need to feed the immune system to deal with abnormal changes in microbiome makeup. Our mental health problems could be at the mercy of pathological organisms. We have discovered now that even our renal tract has its specific microbiome. Just targeting organisms without targeting the metabolic process that can hammer brain immune system function and brain energy will be a mistake. It is all or nothing and not piecemeal simplistic approaches that never work.

More on the brain glucose to fructose conversion: This Yale University finding explains brain bioenergetic decline, neuroinflammation and dementia risk

Yale University researchers, for the first time, have shown the extent of blood glucose to fructose conversion in our brains that can occur after eating glucose-spiking foods, as discussed previously. Remember, with insulin resistance, glucose can't get into cells as it should, resulting in higher blood glucose levels after eating starchy carbs, where these high glucose levels hang around for 6 hours or more.

We now know that within 20 minutes of blood glucose elevation, 30% of that glucose can be converted to fructose in the brain through the polyol pathway. It does not matter whether an infusion of glucose causes elevated blood glucose, as used in the Yale study, or whether we raise glucose by consuming starchy carbohydrate consumption. Elevated glucose is elevated glucose, plain and simple. In fact, if we infused fructose rather than glucose, even if it was a large amount of fructose, it increased brain fructose by only a small amount in comparison to high blood glucose levels being converted to high fructose levels in the brain. This finding led the authors to state that brain fructose levels are a:

"*...highly sensitive neuronal signal for carbohydrate ingestion.*" (Hwang, Jiang et al. 2017)

Imagine that, with all this damage being caused by high carb recommendations. There can be a 50% reduction in brain ATP production in Alzheimer's Disease (Johnson, Gomez-Pinilla et al. 2020), and such a reduction in ATP levels shows the extent of the bioenergetic decline in this neurodegenerative disorder.

This fructose production from glucose in the brain is an unbelievably important finding from Yale University researchers (Hwang, Jiang et al. 2017). These same researchers showed a 20-fold (20x) increase of fructose in the brain fluid as a consequence of high blood glucose levels. High blood glucose levels are seen after any meal with a high-carb load that can lead to glucose to fructose shunting (Johnson, Gomez-Pinilla et al. 2020).

All starchy carbs are glucose molecules linked together and broken apart in digestion. After the digestion of starchy carbs, blood glucose levels rise rapidly and can stay elevated after a high-carb meal. In fact, these levels may never come down in those with significant insulin resistance. This high carb and sugar consumption means a never-ending supply of glucose to be converted to fructose in the brain. A very good reason not to buy into the generalized mantra of grains or carbs are always good, irrespective of the clinical circumstance and that you can have as much as you like with no consequences. Is this what dietetics is saying? Why haven't they qualified their recommendations for those with insulin resistance, established Alzheimer's dementia or women undergoing the glucose transition in menopause, where brains don't use glucose effectively once oestrogen declines?

Shouldn't dietetics recognise that these clinical problems don't tolerate high-carb loads? What about the glucose-to-fructose conversion that will make matters much worse for women undergoing the "menopausal switch" (glucose transition) away from using glucose as a fuel, putting them at unnecessary risk? Do we need the next century to conclude that we need to cut down on carbs? Brain bioenergetic decline should not be argued anymore. A bioenergetic decline in all cells should now be seen as the ultimate cause of metabolic disease. Any impact on brain energy levels is amplified by microcirculation decline in the brain.

A low-carb approach is far more effective than potentially harmful medications that never deal with the dominant forces that drive metabolic and brain diseases.

Low-starchy carb diets: Let's look at the huge evidence-based benefit: Mini diabetic episodes

It is well established that sugars and processed carbs can cause Type-2 Diabetes Mellitus even in the absence of other risk factors (Bhardwaj, O'Keefe et al. 2016). As indicated, each high starchy carb meal can produce a "***mini diabetic event***" as blood glucose levels will soar after such a meal. To think that episodic glucose surges won't cause harm is akin to believing in the tooth fairy, so why aren't individuals in populations warned about these damaging meal-based impacts?

> *"Lifestyle modifications should be the primary focus when treating insulin resistance. Nutritional intervention with calorie reduction and avoidance of carbohydrates that stimulate excessive insulin demand is a cornerstone of treatment." (Freeman and Pennings 2018)*

Having a glucose-spiking high carbohydrate load is the most powerful insulin-generating effect (Bonsembiante, Targher et al. 2021). We need to imagine what each meal will do with regard to elevated blood glucose and insulin demand if we are to have any hope of preventing chronic metabolic diseases. Think about that huge mound of risotto or pasta you are about to eat, the pile of potato mash, the bread or pastries or a dessert and the mini-diabetic event that follows. Consider potato fries (French fries). Will you dip them into a sugar and fructose-soaked tomato sauce or condiment? Do you really need that dessert that will push your blood glucose level sky-high? Consuming these foods at the wrong time of the day (chrononutrition) will have a big impact on your long-term health. I discuss this in the final chapter. All these food impacts should be seen as nails in your coffin meal-by-meal or snack-by-snack.

A UK study has shown how a Low Carbohydrate Diet (LCD) can help individuals lose weight, and after 23 months on an LCD, 46% of people with diabetes were drug-free through deprescribing as drugs were not needed anymore (Cucuzzella, Riley et al. 2021). This positive finding through a food-based change must surely be every pharmaceutical CEO's nightmare scenario, where they imagine diminishing drug sales. Are the medical and dietetic professionals listening, or is it the game to keep supporting corporations at the expense of lives? A low-carb diet is ***a low-starchy-carb diet*** that does not restrict a huge range of non-starchy vegetables and low-fructose fruits.

Lay nutritionists writing in a Sunday paper wellness pullout never seem to grasp the complexities of nutrition and never seem to consider how generalized statements can cause tremendous harm, especially when vast numbers within populations they are talking to are already at significant metabolic risk.

However, the same UK study above also showed that HbA1c (a biomarker for diabetes control) was decreased to a non-diabetic level in 93% of individuals using a low-carb strategy (Cucuzzella, Riley et al. 2021). A staggering result! A normal HbA1c means that our proteins are not being glycated (damaged by glucose), which also means that our blood glucose levels are good overall. Thus, as a result, this finding also implies that there will be less glucose to be shunted to fructose in our brains. Do we need 1000 years of useless reductionist research to tell us this when dementia levels are poised to skyrocket?

Drugs, rather than dietary guidelines, fail to stop the destructive march of insulin-resistant chronic diseases. Unbiased dietetic guidelines can make a massive positive impact.

Only 48 hours of persistently high glucose levels are needed to produce significant insulin resistance – high-carb diets, anyone?

Just look at the following research findings in relation to a carb-mad world that constantly spikes blood glucose and insulin levels. It is easy enough to achieve persistently elevated blood glucose and insulin levels with the wrong type of foods we consume. See Appendix-18.

The research was carried out on 15 young individuals, all healthy and all having normal Glucose Tolerance Tests (GTTs). The normal GTT excluded any existing prediabetic or diabetic state. These young individuals had no family history of diabetes, and none were on medications that could have interfered with glucose metabolism. Nevertheless, these healthy young individuals underwent testing for insulin responses by exposing them to artificially **induced persistently high blood glucose levels** through a glucose infusion.

The worrying result of persistently high blood glucose levels was that:

> *"Significant insulin resistance" was noted in as little as 48 hours of testing (Del Prato, Leonetti et al. 1994).*

Moreover, after eating in normal, non-diabetic individuals, each meal's effects on glucose can linger for 6 hours or more (Ceriello 2003). Do people eat non-stop or continue to have large carb-rich meals late at night with elevated blood glucose levels persisting throughout their sleep? If the dietetic world denies this carb-mad eating, they must be walking around with a blindfold on.

> *If we can't change the quantity of food consumed, we better change the composition of food consumed by populations and do this quickly.*

We discussed how the insulin-spiking effects of dairy can put us all at risk for insulin resistance.

The Framingham Offspring Cohort Study shows that increasing carbohydrate intake can trigger insulin resistance, MetS and diabetes (McKeown, Meigs et al. 2004). With worsening carbohydrate (glucose) intakes, we worsen fasting glucose and fasting insulin levels that may never return to normal as insulin signalling is dampened, which may, in turn, trigger persistent insulin resistance. Remember, there are two types of research: 1. The type that is real and produced by dedicated researchers who want the truth known or 2. Financial incentives drive many industry-funded researchers to do anything for a dollar. They are bought by industry to muddy the waters as far as food impacts are concerned or if they want to gaslight drug benefits.

Here is a statement by the researchers about the dangers of persistently high blood insulin levels (hyperinsulinaemia):

> *"These findings indicate that hyperinsulinaemia should be considered, not only as a compensatory response to insulin resistance but also as a self-perpetuating cause of the defect in insulin action." (Del Prato, Leonetti et al. 1994)*

There is no essential carb. Our bodies can create all the glucose they need from amino acids or the glycerol backbone of triglycerides – found in our body fat. With 60% -70% of many populations overfat, overweight and obese, do you think there won't be a wealth of triglycerides from excess body fat to produce glucose as required? If insulin resistance can be created in 48 hours of high glucose levels, why are we pushing grains and insulin-spiking dairy? Foolish. Grains or dairy are not essential for life and yet pushed due to vested interests. Deplorable! Governments are to blame as they demand support for the agricultural economy from dietetic recommendations and fake food pyramids. Foods such as cereals, oats, sugar, fructose, dairy products, honey, and agave can lead to high glucose and insulin levels, which can be highly detrimental to your health. Keeping blood glucose (and insulin) levels high 24/7 is not hard in the 21st century.

Adenosine Triphosphate (ATP) is a hydrotrope

A low ATP level doesn't just affect energy levels. ATP can help decrease brain aggregates common in many neurodegenerative disorders. It is now becoming difficult not to recognise brain disorders as one of bioenergetic decline. Beta-amyloid in Alzheimer's and Alpha-Synuclein in Parkinson's Disease are misfolded dysfunctional proteins that form aggregates like neurofibrillary tangles in Alzheimer's Disease.

Interestingly, ATP is seen as a hydrotrope, i.e. it can solubilize (dissolve) protein aggregates (Cai, Zhang et al. 2019). So, lower cellular energy means less ATP available to decrease protein aggregate formation. As you can see, Alzheimer's management is far more complex than just trying to remove beta-amyloid from the brain. Beta-amyloid is yet another simplistic approach. It is far smarter to help cells boost ATP production by supplying them with all the nutrient resources they need to do so.

We must keep in mind that insulin resistance is a huge problem in brain disorders and that to bring cells back from the brink of disaster, we need to supply them with an alternative form of fuel. This strategy to shift to ketones as an alternative fuel is a no-brainer to me (pun intended). We delve into this in the final chapter.

Glial Cells, Astrocytes and Neuron Bioenergetics

Glial cells are the brain's resident immune cells that support and protect brain nerve cells (neurons). Cross-talk exists between the glial cells and the peripheral immune system (Greenhalgh, David et al. 2020). As you can see, we can't separate the body from the mind. Astrocytes are said to make up around 40% of the glial cells. Astrocytes provide critical metabolic support to neurons through lactate supply, which can be converted to pyruvate to enter the Krebs Cycle for conversion to ATP in neuron mitochondria.

Astrocytes use anaerobic glycolysis to produce lactate from glucose. This lactate is metabolic fuel for neurons and, thus, another fuel for neurons (Qi, Mi et al. 2020). Therefore, if nerve cells are highly active and need a rapid energy supply, anaerobic glycolysis (ATP produced without oxygen) in Astrocytes can convert glucose to lactate to provide fast energy to the neurons they support.

This glucose-to-lactate conversion to supply nerve cells is called the "***Astrocyte-Neuron Lactate Shuttle***" (Chih and Roberts Jr 2003). Anaerobic glycolysis is thus the go-to for this very fast nerve cell energy supply. This anaerobic glycolysis process is 100 times faster than oxidative phosphorylation (OXPHOS) in the mitochondria to create ATP (Stojan and Christopher-Stine 2015). OXPHOS is the usual way mitochondria produce ATP in the presence of oxygen. Anaerobic glycolysis, as the name suggests, occurs in the absence of oxygen. The downside to anaerobic glycolysis is that it is a glucose guzzler, taking 16 glucose molecules to create 32 ATP. On the other hand, we only need x1 glucose molecule to create 32 ATP via OXPHOS in the mitochondria using oxygen.

So, anaerobic glycolysis chews up a large amount of glucose to meet its energy needs. It is a pity if our microcirculation is damaged and the glucose supply needed for this glucose-guzzling anaerobic glycolysis process is not delivered. If we now add insulin resistance to this mix, we will have an impairment of glucose getting into cells for lactate production. Throw in fructose, as mentioned, created by the glucose (fructose shunt), and now we have a real cellular disaster for brain cell energy production.

Astrocytes are thus critical for providing highly active nerve cells with an energy resource in lactate. The factors mentioned above will sabotage the high glucose needs of Astrocytes, therefore debilitating neurons in the process. Remember, our glucose to fructose shunt in the brain due to high glucose levels in insulin resistance, diabetes or after eating high carb loads doesn't help by rapidly depleting brain cells of ATP. So, one bioenergetic impact after another to sap brain cells of energy to function.

Just from viewing the complexity of astrocyte metabolism, you can see why the simplistic beta-amyloid hypothesis has been a disaster. We need to restore cell energy through nutrient support, not simplistic drug approaches, with a view to making a huge amount of money.

The MIND diet has firmly established that memory can be wound back 7.5 years (Morris, Tangney et al. 2015). Yet we want to use nation-crushing expensive drugs that have proven almost worthless compared to food-based, nutrient-based approaches for brain health.

It is medicine and Pharma trying to present a far more complex picture than is necessary to intellectually bludgeon the lay public, politicians and public health advocates into submission to do things their way or the highway. Don't be conned!

Metabolic Psychiatry: Mental health disorders and bidirectionality - all for one and one for all. Truly sad we don't focus on brain bioenergetics?

Professor S Sethi from Stanford University coined the term ***Metabolic Psychiatry*** after noticing the tight relationship between metabolic disease and psychiatric presentations. Professor Sethi recognised that to treat mental health disorders, she needed to address two problems at the same time. By using psychiatric drugs exclusively, we are ignoring the profound impacts of metabolic disease driven predominantly by dietary factors but other modifiable inputs as well.

Professor Sethi recognised that Schizophrenic patients presenting for the first time had existing insulin resistance and a disorder of glucose metabolism in the brain. (Sethi 2022). We are dealing with a bioenergetic crisis in all cells, but with such an energy-intensive organ as the brain that devours glucose to function and where the brain is an organ that is always switched on, even a minor disruption of blood, oxygen, fuel, and micronutrient supply will be devastating.

When do we learn our lesson and stop inflicting harm by not recognizing this fundamental fact and stop harming millions of people with mental health diseases? Professor Sethi from Stanford University knows the potential benefit provided by ketones to minds struggling with mental health problems. This simple tactic of switching from glucose to ketone body fuel can result in huge benefits, but how we arrive at ketosis is critical for long-term health. It is not just about ketosis, though, but a ***gentle ketosis*** diet that also provides the wealth of nutrients needed for all organs to function normally. It is this enlightened approach that we all need now.

We must recognise now that with insulin resistance, glucose entry into cells, whether in the brain or body, is severely restricted. So if glucose can't get into cells to act as fuel for ATP production, then why the heck aren't we switching from glucose to ketones, which can easily get into body and brain cells without the help of insulin?

The link between insulin resistance and mental health problems is massive and undeniable, and yet we use primitive drugs to deal with a problem that can be significantly improved by diets rich in nutrients and where we shift from ridiculous carb-based glucose-raising dietary inputs when glucose is actually banned from getting into cells due to insulin resistance to a far more clever ketone body-producing dietary approach as a glucose alternative.

We allow this pandemic of mental health disorders all through the way we deal with this so-called "prediabetes" state and the fact we do nothing to prevent worsening insulin resistance and bioenergetic decline in cells. In fact, we are programmed for mental health disorders in the womb. Shouldn't we be focusing on the pre-pregnancy stage and the health of children? Seems logical, right? But we in medicine are interventionists, and we wait for a medical disaster to manifest before we act, and then we act using drug tools that have proven to be a disaster for metabolic diseases and mental health problems. This medical model is stunningly inadequate, but governments need to wake up to this failure of intervention versus prevention and take action instead of being misled by the profession.

Mentally impaired individuals are often unaware of this link between cell bioenergetics and brain health. Instead of addressing this through diet, most turn to drugs, risking metabolic dysfunction and shortened lives. Many studies have shown an undeniable link between sugar consumption and a higher risk for mental health disorders (Knüppel, Shipley et al. 2017). No one knew why this was the case, but the Yale University finding of the glucose-to-fructose conversion in the brain, which I have mentioned many times now because of its importance in brain health, shows that with sugar, the glucose component is just as important as the hugely impactful fructose component in causing biological damage or driving a bioenergetic decline in brain cells.

Ordinary sugar, composed of 50% glucose and 50% fructose, triggers brain energy decline. Individuals with mental health disorders often self-medicate with high-energy drinks containing sugar, caffeine, or guarana, exacerbating their condition. Let's heed Yale's critical finding and prioritize dietary changes over sluggish medical and dietetic models.

The drug-centric model for mental health disorders harms patients. It affects brain energy, causes sluggishness, and impacts the Electron Transport Chain in brain mitochondria. Drug approaches can lead to weight gain and diabetes. Prioritizing nutrient support over drugs is essential.

Mental health disorders are all linked. One process with many mental health presentations

Multiple mental health disorders—ADHD, bipolar disorder, schizophrenia, depression, anxiety, delirium, and eating disorders—actually stem from a single metabolic process. This process depletes cell energy and leads to structural impairment in brain cells. Our declining microcirculation is the root cause of body and brain diseases. No single gene or structural defect can account for mental health disorders.

A Danish study has shown that if you have one mental health disorder, you are likely to have a high risk of developing any other mental health disorder (Plana-Ripoll, Pedersen et al. 2019). These mental health issues are thus ***bidirectional***, but how can one mental disorder so strongly be associated with another unless there is a common pathway?

This bi-directionality is explored in the book "Brain Energy" by Harvard Professor of Psychiatry Christopher Palmer (Palmer 2022). It seems absolutely absurd to think that one specific impact will cause Schizophrenia or another specific impact will cause Manic Depressive Disorder. It is far more intelligent to see this as one process that, because of individual minor genetic variants, anomalies in brain vasculature, micronutrient insufficiencies or deficiencies, epigenetic programming in the womb and ongoing microstructural damage by processes we allow to continue that we have the many "faces" of mental health all driven by one metabolic process designed to rob the brain of energy and function.

Insulin resistance is a process that links all our acquired metabolic illnesses to Alzheimer's Disease (AD) and mental health disorders.

Insulin resistance is closely tied to microvascular disease (MVD), which worsens over time. Alzheimer's disease (AD) is even called ***Type-3 Diabetes*** due to this link to insulin resistance. Recognizing this connection can help combat mental health issues.

Neurodegeneration and mental health are influenced by modifiable factors—the BIG-10 Womb-to-Tomb list. These include insulin resistance, metabolic dysfunction, brain fructose, microvascular decline, neuroinflammation, oxidative stress, and impaired cell repair. Mental health research must consider these factors so we can finally manage mental health effectively and save these poor souls from a life of misery.

As mentioned, the brain is an organ with a voracious appetite for energy. It is one of three selfish super-systems that hog energy and nutrients. The brain consumes 20% of our energy intake in the form of glucose but makes up only around 2% of body weight. Glucose fuels 95% of ATP generation in the brain (Cunnane, Trushina et al. 2020). So, anything that disrupts the energy supply, particularly the glucose supply, will create profound changes in the brain. The huge need for glucose to drive brain function makes it the most energy-intensive organ of the human body (Chandra, Li et al. 2017).

It is incredibly important to know that 60%-70% of oxygen exchange to cells in organ systems occurs through the microcirculation networks (Munoz, Lucas et al. 2020). The implications are staggering if you look at the section in this chapter titled ***Tik-Tock: Poiseuille's Law, Microcirculation Armageddon***, how small decreases in diameter could cause a devastating effect on brain oxygen delivery. Imagine then the impacts this would have on mental health disorders or neurodegenerative disorders.

This disruption to glucose supply is easily achieved through microcirculation deterioration and insulin resistance, and for women undergoing menopausal change, we have estrogen as a factor that will deprive brain cells of energy, turning the ***metabolic switch*** away from glucose being used as a primary fuel source after menopause by around 30% less glucose being utilized by the brain in post-menopausal women– ouch! A 1/3rd reduction of primary glucose fuel supply. How idiotic we don't warn women that the brain loves ketones as a fuel source. We keep women ignorant, waiting for a drug solution to arrive for a quick-fix script solution that will never come. And so we allow the brains of women to deteriorate to an

Alzheimer's dementia state instead. We will look at gentle ketosis strategies in the final chapter that have every chance of helping women dodge a dementia bullet, mental health disorders or Alzheimer's as a result of this menopausal glucose transition.

So imagine astrocyte armageddon post-menopause when astrocytes are denied the vast amounts of glucose these glial cells need to supply lactate for nerve cell energy production. Astrocytes, as specialised brain glial cells, are said to outnumber neurons (nerve cells) fivefold (5x) (Sofroniew and Vinters 2010). So, as the key regulators of brain energy, astrocytes exist in vast numbers in the brain, all needing huge amounts of glucose to support neurons. Even slight reductions in fuel supply will create havoc in the brain, leading to neurodegeneration and mental health decline. Our focus should be nutrient-based approaches for neuroprotection, not ridiculous inaction and drug worship that destroys lives.

So why does it seem that we have one dominant mental health disorder?

Minor genetic variants have a role, and variations in microcirculation supply to various parts of the brain parts will determine brain-related symptoms and signs. Some parts of the brain are affected more than others asymmetrically, as we have discussed. This asymmetry is no different from universal vascular disease, which involves some vessels like the heart arteries or carotid arteries more than others. But the great mistake we make is that when we have one organ making the most "noise", we forget we still have widespread but silent (for now) vascular disease in other organs that will sooner or later also start to "scream".

The medical profession's downfall lies in overlooking widespread microvascular damage. Specialists often focus on their narrow field—like a cardiologist (heart specialist) treating heart disease—while ignoring related issues (such as carotid involvement leading to stroke or kidney failure). Specialization with a narrow focus harms our approach to metabolic diseases. Only adopting a big-picture approach will do. We need a specialist who has a Master of Metabolic Disease instead of fragmented medical care.

The "pull" and "push" of brain blood supply activity

Different parts of the brain fire at various times, and the demand for blood, oxygen, glucose and nutrient supply is a "***pull***" effect and not a "***push***" effect (Cunnane, Trushina et al. 2020). So, increased focal brain activity will "pull" blood to it as the brain does not directly (push) blood to highly active brain parts. So, brain tissue activity is the determinant of where blood is directed. This "pull" effect has the potential for a "***vascular steal syndrome***" that I alluded to previously, where highly active brain parts steal (pull) blood supply away from adjacent less active parts due to their energy and nutrient demands at any given moment.

So, some parts of the brain may be inhibited just by other parts being active, drawing in glucose and nutrient resources to support this activity. Just this fact alone tells you how we can have various mental health presentations due to these local vascular effects determining which parts of the brain are firing and supported and which parts of the brain are inhibited by vascular pull factors.

"Stealing" of fuel and nutrient resources from other adjacent brain areas is a factor for our various mental health presentations or "faces", which, on the surface, seem chaotic but are easily understood. It is the triage mechanism I have spoken about at a focal level in the brain where active parts rob Peter to pay Paul. Poor fuel and nutrient supply will also create micro and macro-structural brain damage, and this damage will then also determine the clinical "face/s" shown in terms of a mental health presentation.

Brain degeneration is complex and influenced by nutrient sufficiency or insufficiency. We then have the pull and push of blood supply, as well as factors that determine asymmetric blood supply, along with structural and ultrastructural defects that determine mental health presentations. Rather than labelling disorders separately, we must recognise that all of this is an interconnected process.

80% of ATP consumption in the brain is used for brain signalling, neurotransmitter release, synaptic transmission, and ion exchanges (Balasubramanian 2021). So, imagine a microcirculation-induced energy supply crisis, with brain cells misfiring or firing erratically (hyperexcitable cells) or are inhibited from firing due to the blood supply steal syndrome described above or where there are errors in neurotransmitter synthesis or ion exchanges due to ATP decline.

Low fuel and energy will mean synapses are ill-prepared for a barrage of rapid-fire signals such as pain signals. How can you create neurotransmitters, repair synapses, or fuel synaptic transmission with diminishing microvascular function, delivering inadequate fuel, oxygen and nutrient resources when a barrage of signals arrives at various brain locations not prepared or fully resourced for this assault in signals?

So, if glucose entry into brain cells is impaired by all the factors described above, is ketosis then feasible in mental health disorders?

> *"The administration of a ketogenic diet in this semi-controlled setting to patients with treatment-refractory mental illness was feasible, well-tolerated, and associated with significant and substantial improvements in depression and psychosis symptoms and multiple markers of metabolic health." (Danan, Westman et al. 2022)*

When brain cells lack glucose, switching to ketones is essential. We must provide all necessary nutrients—not just cherry-picked ones—without mega doses of any nutrient being used. Nutrients are not drugs. The final chapter delves into this nutrient strategy alongside a gentle ketosis diet that provides great hope for all metabolic diseases of the body and brain.

An epidemic of back pain: Once again, we see the destructive impact of our damaged microcirculation at work

We now have a staggering prevalence of lower back pain. According to the Sydney Alumni Magazine (SAM) from Sydney University, it is estimated that 800 million will be affected by back pain by 2050 - a huge jump of 36% from 2020 (USyd 2023).

To think this growing pandemic of back pain has nothing to do with the insulin resistance pandemic is truly ludicrous. Pain is a function of both peripheral nerve impulses and brain processing that requires fully functional brain cells with an unimpeded supply of all the nutrient resources necessary for operational and anabolic purposes and repair. What connects all these inputs is a bioenergetic decline and progressive microcirculation damage.

Incoming pain signals from damaged peripheral tissues or joints won't be processed as they should in the region of the brain receiving these pain signals as the brain becomes less and less resilient to deal with a barrage of signals coming from damaged tissues. The neurons in these regions are already struggling with energy and structural defects. These cells can't cope, and so they will deteriorate further. With problems like back pain, the perceived pain is often no longer from damaged peripheral tissues; instead, chronic pain now resides in the central nervous system (CNS) and is a brain problem, not a peripheral one (Yang and Chang 2019).

The Insulin Resistance Continuum (IRC) and progressive microcirculation damage set the brain up as a fertile breeding ground for chronic pain syndromes. All of the factors described above set the brain up to not cope with constant pain signals. These pain-related overstimulated brain cells need more resources due to persistent pain signalling, but these nutrient resources are compromised.

Diminished microcirculation perfusion (blood supply) to the vertebrae and discs occurs from age 35 onwards. This poor microcirculation supply initially affects the bone marrow and is followed by bone loss and intervertebral disc deterioration (Ou-Yang and Lu 2015). Is it any wonder that so many surgical approaches to back pain fail? Remember that microcirculation perfusion defects are common in the brain or spinal cord, limiting oxygen and nutrient resources to brain tissue. Perfusion defects must be addressed.

Uric acid levels – A potent early marker for ATP depletion, insulin resistance and NAFLD. Look for a uric acid quintile-climb

Many people have a history of gout, an acutely painful condition of a joint that becomes swollen, red, hot, inflamed and extremely painful. The affected joint is usually in a big toe and seems to have come on as if a switch had been flicked on. If someone develops this condition, they will get a spiel from a doctor or nutritionist that eating too much of this or that will trigger gout and that they need to avoid those triggers. After all, how much time does a doctor have in a 6-minute consultation to get across what is necessary?

The other issue is that, as we have discussed, we live in a world riddled with fatty liver, insulin resistance and metabolic dysfunction, and so what practitioners need to be aware of is that a high uric acid level, even if in the upper quintile of a normal range, will predict you will die early from a chronic metabolic disease or if you don't die early in life then you will be riddled with a debilitating disease where you may as well be dead.

Uric acid has a pivotal role in creating an energy crisis in cells. Uric Acid (UA) is an independent marker for cardiovascular disease (CVD) and a sensitive identifier for ATP depletion in liver cells. The liver is one of the major sites for uric acid production, and the liver, along with skeletal muscle, are the two major sites that significantly impact the level of insulin resistance seen in metabolic dysfunction.

> *"Uric acid production by hepatocytes is a very sensitive index of ATP depletion" (Petrie, Patman et al. 2013)*

A high blood uric acid level is not all about gout. Check for the uric acid quintile climb if you have serial blood results.

Fructose rapidly and significantly depletes cellular ATP and causes an increase in uric acid levels. We consistently give children large amounts of fruit juice, tinned fruit, dried fruit, fruit bars with added sugar, etc., thus setting them up for ongoing cellular ATP depletion and insulin resistance. The message is that cell starvation leads to energy, and structural decline begins early in life. We need to reconsider our staple food addiction with regard to what we feed our kids.

We thus have uric acid levels as a sensitive marker for ATP depletion in an organ (the liver) that is a major player in insulin resistance, and uric acid is a potent marker for cellular energy depletion in general. High uric acid is also a powerful marker of hepatic insulin resistance and Non-Alcoholic Fatty Liver Disease (NAFLD), with an inverse relationship between these clinical problems and ATP. In other words, the lower the ATP levels in the liver, the higher the probability of fatty liver (NAFLD) or hepatic insulin resistance (Petrie, Patman et al. 2013).

Consider uric acid (UA) from a fresh perspective. Look at UA in a clinical context and track its changes over time. Don't be swayed by brief interactions with doctors or nutritionists; challenge their views. Corrupt behaviour in medicine and dietetics often originates from the top, where vested interests hold sway.

Lyon Diet Heart Study versus the Scandinavian Simvastatin Survival Study (4S). Diet versus Drug

It is amazing how we bury vital nutrition-based research that points the way out of this pandemic of deadly chronic metabolic diseases. The Lyon Diet Heart Study is a case in point. This dietary research was a pivotal study on the cardiovascular benefits of a Mediterranean-style diet and was supposed to be a 5-year study. However, amazingly, this study was cut short at 27 months because the results were so strikingly positive. Mortality was so greatly reduced that it became unethical to keep the control group on the pathetic staple food-heavy Standard American Diet (SAD) (Leaf 1999) that has been killing 100s of millions over decades.

Two landmark studies were published in The Lancet in the same year, where we can see the mortality benefits of a drug (a lipid-lowering statin) in contrast to dietary benefits. The two studies involved were the Scandinavian Simvastatin Survival Study (4S) and the Lyon Diet Heart Study. These studies were pivotal in shedding light on the benefits of drugs versus dietary management:

> *"Nearly twenty years ago, two landmark randomized clinical trials appeared in The Lancet, which forever changed the course of medicine for patients with coronary heart disease (CHD). The 4S study employed a cholesterol-lowering statin drug and reported a 30% mortality reduction. The Lyon Diet Heart Study utilized the Mediterranean diet and reported a 70% mortality reduction." (DuBroff and de Lorgeril 2015)*

With staggering diet versus drug benefits, why have doctors ignored these studies in favour of drug-only management? That mortality reduction of 70% versus a pathetic contrived 30% by a drug says it all. This dietary victory was over double (2.3x) the benefit of a statin drug. The diet also decreases the risk of cancer, diabetes, and Alzheimer's disease (DuBroff and de Lorgeril 2015). No drug can claim such benefits, so why are we throwing money down the drain with pointless drug management? Imagine the marketing blitz by Pharma if a drug had the power to do what diet did in the Lyon Diet Heart Study.

The Lyon Diet Heart Study is a triumph of a nutritional-based approach in preventing the biggest killer on the planet, and that is cardiovascular disease. The biggest cause of cardiovascular disease is insulin resistance, leading to all the fake labels like MetS or Type-2 Diabetes Mellitus (T2DM). In other words, the Lyon Diet Heart Study is triumphant proof that this underlying metabolic process can be stopped in its tracks and reversed. But remember that all these revered diets can be improved greatly by getting rid of staple foods.

The United States Food and Drug Administration (USFDA) warned after numerous statin studies that these drugs may increase the risk of diabetes and decrease cognition. Wow, we ignore a landmark study on a diet showing striking positive benefits in favour of drugs that have great potential to cause harm by actually speeding up the appearance of diabetes or triggering a decline in metabolic and brain health. It is not very clever to increase metabolic disease. Statins can reduce CoQ10, a vital component of the Electron Transport Chain (ETC), thus decreasing ATP production—yet another example of a class of drugs hammering cell energy production and tipping individuals into a diabetic state.

With the Cell Starvation Model (CSM), it is easy enough to see why statins could trigger diabetes or dementia as these drugs lower lipids, which are an energy resource or structural component for cells. Statins can decrease CoQ10, a critical point in the Electron Transport Chain (ETC) of mitochondria that will impair cell energy production, worsening bioenergetic decline.

Many mavericks in medicine look through the deceit of statins and call it out. Most doctors are not bad players and are longing for leadership and honest, ethical, conscientious and trustworthy medical guidance for their patients. How can this ever happen if we do not set up a department full of polymaths, such as a ***Future Generations Healthcare Commissioner (FGHC)*** whose sole purpose is a focus on population health, as discussed in the chapter ***Revolution Time***?

CHAPTER 3

Creating a starving cell is very easy in the 21st-century!

"Natural life is chemical." (Kovác 2008)

The Cell Starvation Model (CSM): Our metabolic "Rosetta Stone" or code breaker. Let's examine how easy it is to starve cells of energy

> *"Though at first glance the concept of the Starving Cell may seem counterintuitive, once the evidence is fully assembled, it may transition from far-fetched to self-evident."* (Golomb 2011)

There is no doubt that cellular bioenergetic, structural, and functional decline occurs as we age. Ageing is increased entropy in all its "glory" that has accumulated in cells, tissues and organ systems over time, creating cellular chaos in our skin, bones, brains and other organs. Cellular "hits" to energy and structural decay don't happen at the time of ageing or when overt organ damage presents to us, but this "biological rot" has to start somewhere, making all of us mere shadows of our former selves. Complex cellular systems need energy and nutrients to help generate that energy. Is this even arguable?

This process of cellular energy starvation develops for years to decades prior to any appearance of ageing or organ failure, where the process of cell bioenergetic decline leads to cell structural decline, with these two processes feeding on and reinforcing the other in a continuous ever-worsening vicious loop unless interrupted. Imagine a world of unbelievable health and longevity if we only focused on nutritional support from pre-pregnancy, childhood and throughout life.

Feast signalling doesn't help with both ageing and worsening cell and organ damage. Feast signalling occurs when we eat as if there is no tomorrow. High food energy intake, as I have mentioned previously, "paradoxically" shuts off energy production. I will discuss how this happens in this chapter under the NAD+/NADH redox couple. Most of the food consumed is packed with food calories (energy) but devoid of fibre diversity and micronutrients. Feast signalling is a surefire way to hasten ageing and organ failure. We are constantly causing glucose, triglycerides, inflammation, insulin, and IgF-1 to zoom upwards, and time and again, research has shown that such ad hoc food consumption and surges in the compounds mentioned above are associated with a decreased lifespan and increased risk of metabolic disease and cancer.

Feast signalling is a cell multiplication signal. This effect is shown in Appendix-33 - ***Lessons from the Laron Syndrome.*** When you keep on "poking the bear" by getting cells to multiply by constant food consumption, you can then trigger a range of metabolic, cellular and physiological changes. We are always producing abnormal cells that our immune systems have to deal with in our bodies. These are mutated cells primed to multiply abnormally. Cancerous cells need fuel like glucose to keep multiplying, and insulin and IgF-1 are the most powerful anabolic hormones in the body, supporting malignant cells in building components and new cells. So why poke this potentially cancerous and dangerous bear with the wrong food inputs?

These insulin/IgF-1 hormones can powerfully stimulate cell multiplication in various tissues, including skin, bone and organ systems. Dairy consumption does you no favours as it is a powerful stimulus in itself for the generation of high Insulin/IgF-1 levels. Both insulin and IgF-1 hormones work together either as "buddies" for good in our bodies or as "evil twins", damaging our bodies slowly, incrementally and cumulatively meal-by-meal and snack-by-snack.

It is no wonder then that research has shown conclusively in numerous cell and animal studies that ***famine-signalling,*** where we limit food energy intake as we do in ***intermittent or timed fasting,*** helps prolong life. Fasting allows all that cellular chaos and entropy to reverse and helps mitochondria repair themselves and ramp up energy-producing enzymes, receptors, signalling molecules, etc., all the things that are necessary for a functional cell to stay full of energy and low entropy.

Cellular energy decline drives insulin resistance and metabolic dysfunction. Poorly designed diets, promoting high Insulin-IGF-1 levels, accelerate ageing and chronic illness. Multiple factors gradually sap cellular energy and structural integrity. Prioritize essential nutrition to maintain cellular energy, thus keeping our cell "batteries" fully charged and keeping the cell 'lights' on.

This chapter will delve into the complexities of cellular energy production and highlight the fragility of these pathways. Our neglect of cellular energy requirements during the ongoing metabolic disease crisis is pushing humanity to a breaking point. The staggering number of metabolically affected individuals is rapidly escalating, placing us all at risk of premature suffering and mortality.

Our cells are a mass of complex chemical reactions requiring energy to break things down in cells or build them up

Life relies on optimal cellular bioenergetic pathways. Cellular life depends on the delicate dance of energy flows within cells and organs. Any disruption of the energy supply threatens our existence. Energy is thus vital and indispensable for optimal cell function and structural integrity; its scarcity can be lethal.

Cellular energy is fiercely guarded. Cells receive glucose, lipids, and amino acids for energy, repair, and steroid synthesis. Cellular energy flow is determined by evolutionary design. We cannot view anything in biological systems without seeing it through the lens of an evolutionary master plan and evolutionary survival intent for cellular actions and reactions.

Our cellular biochemistry and molecular mechanisms have been shaped by millions of years of threats from food scarcity, famine, climate change, infections and other factors.

> "***The organizing power of energy flow is hypothesized to be the origin of biological complexity and its decline the basis of "complex" diseases and ageing***" *(Wallace 2011)*

Interestingly, it was shown in ***normal-weight*** individuals with "Type-2 Diabetes Mellitus (T2DM)" that whole-body glucose uptake was reduced by up to a whopping 50% (Solis-Herrera, Triplitt et al. 2021). Imagine cells having their fuel (glucose) intake slashed by half. So, as you can see, once insulin resistance kicks in, the cell is in deep trouble regarding glucose availability, thus reducing ATP production and triggering accelerated structural decline in the cell. Insulin resistance hinders amino acid, fatty acid, and glucose uptake, so how can anything be built amid this energy crisis and building supply shortage?

Children born prematurely and those small for gestational age or who put on weight in the first year of life were at high risk of insulin resistance and future T2DM (Hofman, Regan et al. 2004). The cells of these children are already struggling with an energy deficit, so what do we do for these individuals born with such a high risk of insulin resistance and mitochondrial energy-producing handicaps? We put already struggling insulin-producing beta cells of the pancreas under even more stress by feeding babies insulin-demanding formulas with high carb loads, and high dairy intakes with the ***Glycemic Index (GI) – Insulin Dissociation*** problem. Foods that demand insulin but do nothing to support the nutrient needs for energy production are very damaging.

Modifying the five food groups: The "Golden Window"

The 5 food groups guide food intake: 1) Cereals and grains, 2) Meat and alternatives, 3) Dairy or alternatives, 4) Fruit, and 5) Vegetables and Legumes. We need to change our minds with regard to food inputs for babies and children as we set them up for a healthcare disaster in future. That our chronic metabolic diseases are set into motion in the womb and from childhood on is not arguable. It is a fact that doesn't need gaslighting and reductionism to tell us this, as populations are being shattered by the huge prevalence of chronic diseases that could have been halted from the baby stage onward.

Thank goodness we have companies now producing plant-based formulas that are gluten-free and dairy-free with all the necessary nutrients and not the damaging effects of staple foods that set children up to become disease-riddled adults. We have allowed staple food madness to determine the agenda. Imagine insulin-IgF-1 levels shooting skywards in a baby fed dairy milk of one kind or another or formulas almost invariably made from dairy, and then once weaned, they continue with insulin-IgF-1 spiking milk and then yoghurts, custards, and cheese. I hope we see far more plant-based formulas that do not spike all the damaging factors that occur after eating. Let's not set babies up for long-term failure in health.

Babies need a diversity of food fibre, phytochemicals, plant-based antioxidants, Omega-3s and Choline and a wealth of micronutrients at age-based higher RDAs and not foods packed with calories as this is totally unbelievable in a world where childhood obesity is soaring globally. Nutrients count, not the foods that house those nutrients.

In The Economist, 2024 in an article titled "***How to Raise the World's IQ***', it was stated that:

> *Many parents, even in middle-income countries, think it is enough to stuff an infant with stodgy carbohydrates but neglect protein and micronutrients. (Economist 2024)*

There are many other terms for "stodgy", such as stale, dull, unimaginative and uninspiring and yet these same terms can be used for the dietetic industry that makes parents believe they are depriving their children by not giving them "stodgy" glucose and insulin raising carbs when in fact this industry is sealing the fate of children with regard to both their physical and mental health.

So, how do you raise the world's IQ? You ensure adequate intakes of protein Omega-3, other essential fatty acids, Choline and micronutrient adequacy throughout a mother's pregnancy and ensure no nutrient at all is missing in the first 1000 days of a child's life. Nutrient adequacy ensures our cells are primed to be the energy-producing powerhouses they need to be, as just keeping them alive is an energy-intensive process.

This first 1000 days of a child's life is critical where nutrient adequacy is not negotiable. We sacrifice a child's life rather than subsidizing formulas or supplements that can help us stop this horrendous generation of chronic illness. We need to stop listening to conceited and arrogant professions that warn of potential side effects of food-based, nutrient-based approaches, driving us to drug-based approaches that produce the most horrific prevalence of dangerous or life-threatening side effects, putting enormous added strain on our healthcare systems. We have millions of years of natural evolutionary research on foods and nutrients, not the limited trial period of a drug alien to our cells that is dumped on healthcare systems without a whimper about potential side effect possibilities, which, as we know, surface after the release of those drugs.

As an individual, it is up to you to choose who is right. We have a drug-centric medical profession that has lost this war on chronic metabolic diseases, and we have a dietary industry that adds fuel to the fire by the promotion of damaging staple foods. Pushing people away from nutrient-based approaches is a deplorable strategy to bolster drug-based approaches.

The first 1000 days of a child's life is a period that spans the third trimester (from week 28) to the end of the second year of life, and this first 1000 days is regarded as the "***golden window***". It is in this critical period that IQ, learning, behaviour, mental health and future chronic disease are set. Without optimising nutrient support for both mother and baby, we condemn both to a life of poor metabolic health and cardiovascular risk as energy pathways will be incapacitated and without energy, as you are now aware, nothing gets built, repaired or restored, and this can lead to permanent structural damage in cells and organs from this very early stage in human development throughout life.

We allow entropy (decay, chaos, degeneration) to dominate organ development from this very early foetal stage, and this is reprehensible when all of this can be prevented. We must shift funds from useless drug management, as this is a waste of money, and move funds to avoid chronic illness by changing the face of dietary recommendations. The biggest bang for our buck will be a huge investment in prepregnancy and pregnancy to put the brakes on epigenetic programming and then on early childhood development. This investment in prevention will be unbelievably cheap in comparison to the expensive interventionist approach being used, which has undeniably failed.

Any nutritionally acquired damage that occurs in this golden window of opportunity after conception is likely to be permanent (Economist 2024). Once cells are permanently damaged, their ability to create energy will be limited, and their risk for chronic disease will jump skyward. These children will be born with a mitochondrial and cell structural handicap, and this will be discussed below.

Permanent cellular and structural damage in organ systems during development in the womb will mean a huge burden on healthcare systems in future when dealing with mental health or physical health problems, all because the system was too slow to act on prevention. Medical interventions are crude and clumsy, using drug tools that can never reverse this entrenched ongoing damage (biological rot) that was totally avoidable. How pathetic then that for a paltry $12 billion a year, we can fight malnutrition "***at scale***" (Economist 2024).

It is beyond doubt now that glucose-spiking foods can lead to diabetes, but do we consider this in childhood? We discussed this glucose-spiking risk for diabetes in the prediabetes chapter under "***Low-starchy carb diets***" and the huge benefits of a low-carb diet.

We "***carb-load***" with cereals that boost glucose and insulin, and then we boost insulin levels even further through dairy in formulas and ready-made food inputs that are grain and dairy-rich from this early childhood period onwards as adults. What hope, then, do we have in preventing metabolic disease? Keeping people ignorant of food-based impacts helps vested interests thrive at the expense of health.

1 in 3 children will develop diabetes in their lifetime

It is predicted that 1 in 3 children in the USA will develop diabetes in their lifetime (Moore, Zgibor et al. 2003). It is terrible that we condemn children to obesity, Metabolic Syndrome (MetS), fatty liver and diabetes all because we want to protect turf wars in the agricultural and food industry and support grain production and sales. In the next chapter, we discuss the fat-making, metabolic disease-driving impacts of fructose. Why are people so ignorant about the effects of fructose? All that gaslighting by "experts" in the pocket of the food industry? More on fructose in the next chapter.

We give babies high fructose fruit purees on weaning that can rapidly deplete cells of ATP, and do we even consider the long-term health effects of doing this? We also love giving children high fructose juices and dried fruit and then feeding them insulin demanding high carb loads like mashed rice, mashed potato, cereals, sugar, jam, honey, agave, and other grain-based foods that can drive glucose levels high where glucose can be shunted to fructose through a particular pathway. What is this high glucose to fructose shunt doing to fragile and developing brains long-term? None of these foods are essential for babies or in childhood, and yet we think we are damaging them if we avoid these foods.

We are, in fact, inflicting great damage by following dietetic advice or the lack of it. We don't need energy-packed foods or glucose-spiking or high fructose foods. But what we need is nutrient density, phytochemicals, antioxidants, amino acids, essential fatty acids and fibre-packed foods with enough energy from low sugar-spiking carbs that don't shoot glucose through the roof.

Professor Beatrice Golomb's seminal paper on cell starvation was a flash of amazing clarity for me and an "aha moment" as so many contradictions in managing chronic metabolic diseases made enormous sense finally (Golomb 2011). Cell starvation can be energy or nutrient starvation, and yet even high food energy inputs can choke off energy (ATP) production, as we will discuss.

The factors that work to cause insulin resistance in a wealthy country may be entirely different in a developing country. There is no uniformity. However, high-carb intakes from grains or sugar and fructose impacts are common in both populations.

All our cell energy-crushing factors work simultaneously. There is no polite queue of factors waiting to hammer cell energy production. Cells face a barrage of challenges—from nutrient overload depleting NAD+ and impairing energy production to micronutrient deficiencies affecting ATP enzymes and mitochondrial enzyme complexes. Specific food factors, like fructose, hinder essential energy-generating enzymes and can rapidly deplete cells of ATP. Additionally, severe anemias and environmental toxins cause intracellular ATP depletion, and many mediations are "energy bandits."

Medications often disrupt ATP production, especially antipsychotics that directly affect mitochondrial components, potentially triggering diabetes. In summary, when cellular bioenergetic systems decline, leading to reduced ATP, we risk triggering insulin resistance and Type-2 Diabetes Mellitus, as predicted by the Cell Starvation Model (CSM). This energy decline underpins metabolic dysfunction, driving chronic diseases, increasing mental health risks and affecting individuals, populations, and nations alike. Mitochondrial handicaps can happen from birth – a sad, very early state of compromised cellular energy production.

100s of millions are born with a mitochondrial handicap created by epigenetic programming in a mother's womb

In her excellent book, "***Every Patient Tells a Story***" Lisa Sanders, a professor of internal medicine at the Yale School of Medicine, states:

> *"Doctors are not known for their rapid embrace of the new ...... Physicians are so reluctant to change the way they practice medicine that it takes on average seventeen years for techniques well established by research ---such as giving aspirin to a patient having a heart attack --- to be adopted by even half of those in practice." (Sanders 2010)*

So, according to Professor Lisa Sanders, it took 17 years and a generation of doctors to die before aspirin was accepted at the grassroots level of medical practice, resulting in an untold number of deaths from strokes and heart attacks. So, how long will it take for the Cell Starvation Model to be accepted? Max Planck, the famous physicist, stated something very true that is encapsulated in *Planck's Principle*:

> *"A new scientific truth does not triumph by convincing its opponents and making them see the light, but rather because its opponents eventually die, and a new generation grows up that is familiar with it."*

We need to start educating this new generation of doctors and dietitians now. I have attended many conferences where the medical gurus on stage spruiking drugs looked overweight and unwell. I suppose they were following their propaganda.

In a study of children born to mothers with gestational diabetes mellitus (GDM), 21% of those followed up until 18-27 years of age had metabolic features of "prediabetes" and "diabetes" (Damm, Houshmand-Oeregaard et al. 2016). However, as we have discussed, these labels of "prediabetes" and "diabetes" are fake. Thus, this 21% figure would jump sky-high to perhaps 100% over this long-term follow-up if very early markers for insulin resistance and metabolic dysfunction were used rather than advanced glucose cut-off points like Impaired Glucose Tolerance (IGT) or Impaired Fasting Glucose (IFG) used to define "prediabetes" and even higher glucose cut-offs

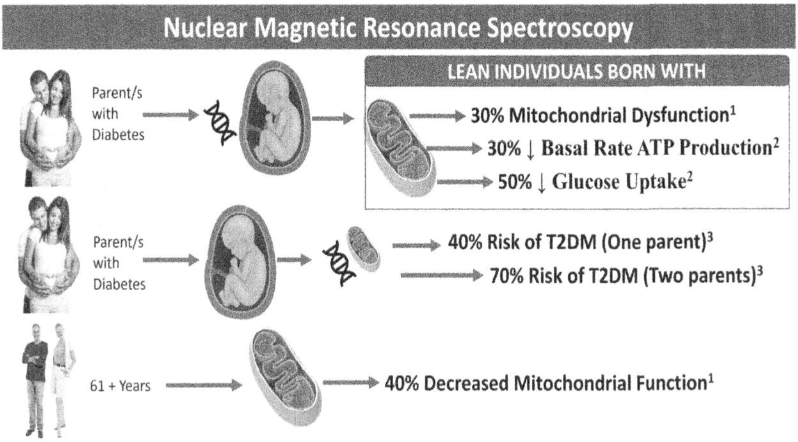

1. Lee, H.K., Cho, Y.M., Kwak, S.H., Lim, S., Park, K.S. and Shim, E.B., 2010. Mitochondrial dysfunction and metabolic syndrome—looking for environmental factors. *Biochimica et Biophysica Acta (BBA)-General Subjects*, *1800*(3), pp.282-289.
2. Petersen, K.F., Dufour, S. and Shulman, G.I., 2005. Decreased insulin-stimulated ATP synthesis and phosphate transport in muscle of insulin-resistant offspring of type 2 diabetic parents. PLoS medicine, 2(9), p.e233.
3. Ali, O., 2013. Genetics of type 2 diabetes. World journal of diabetes, 4(4), p.114.

to define "diabetes"—such a blunder in metabolic understanding.

Using ***Magnetic Resonance Spectroscopy*** to study mitochondrial function, it was found that insulin-resistant individuals born to parents with diabetes, even if lean, had a 30% reduction in mitochondrial function, a 50% - 60% decreased glucose uptake, and a 30% reduced baseline rate of ATP production (Petersen, Dufour et al. 2005). With rates of gestational diabetes tripling in just two decades, do we ignore the huge jump in populations of those born with an epigenetically programmed mitochondrial handicap? These affected individuals are at great risk of developing diabetes early in their lives? Why do we ignore their risk? We condemn these 100s of millions of individuals to a life of chronic illness and misery. We ignore this vital pregnancy period and the first 1000 days of life and thus pay the price for populations riddled with metabolic diseases.

As mentioned, gestational diabetes mellitus (GDM) has tripled in the past decades, and GDM is the fastest-growing type of diabetes in Australia. The highest increase of GDM was in women of normal weight (BMI less than 25) (Mnatzaganian, Woodward et al. 2022).

The fact these mothers were normal weight shows that the propaganda of obesity as the driver of metabolic disease is entirely wrong. I have mentioned that GDM is important because four (x4) generations are affected, including the mother.

GDM is like a mega-engine driving the explosive growth of metabolic disease in future generations. This intergenerational growth will be dramatic in the near future. How can it not be when one mum affects 3 future generations, and each child born can then affect the next three generations and so forth? It is easy enough to see that this will result in exponential growth of chronic diseases unless we wake up to this huge multiplier effect of GDM.

Our lack of an intense focus on prospective mothers baffles me. I propose dedicated prenatal clinics that assess early risks and offer comprehensive nutritional support, including subsidized prenatal nutrients. This approach can prevent intergenerational diseases and reduce the risk of mental health disorders, including Schizophrenia.

This intergenerational legacy means an explosion of metabolic diseases in the next two decades – our tsunamis of disease happening under our noses! Our legacy to future generations will be the ***Metabolic Singularity***, where there will be hardly a healthy human left, as Aldous Huxles presciently stated.

Insulin resistance (IR) at birth is the best predictor for developing diabetes in life (Petersen, Dufour et al. 2005). For example, 60% of these individuals with insulin resistance born to diabetic parents will have abnormal glucose tolerance by 60 years, and 36.5% will develop Type-2 Diabetes Mellitus (T2DM) by 60 years of age (Tattersall and Fajans 1975). Remember, as I have stated regularly throughout this book, that these statistics would skyrocket if we used early metabolic markers rather than redundant high glucose cut-off points that miss vast numbers with metabolic disease in the early stages of development. The numbers with a mitochondrial handicap would extend to 100s of millions of people and yet we don't even consider this risk in people.

Look at the graphic of mitochondrial handicaps, which shows a 40% decreased mitochondrial function in people 61 years and older.

Is it any wonder, then, that over 95% of our older adults have Type-2 Diabetes Mellitus, as shown in the Oxford Community Diabetes Study (Neil, Thompson et al. 1989)? Imagine all the factors that worsen this cellular energy problem for our seniors. Think of poor food intake in aged care facilities with limited funds for food, leading to micronutrient deficiencies due to malnutrition.

Five ultra-common factors exist to pull the rug from under cellular energy (ATP) production

We can look at five ultra-common factors to see how easy it is to create an energy-starved cell, but remember that all the other BIG-10 Womb-to-Tomb factors that rob cells of energy are also in play simultaneously. The four big factors are:

1. Massive insulin resistance prevalence in populations
2. High intakes of sugar (50% fructose), consumption of fructose-rich foods, or both consumed daily.
3. High food energy intake shuts off cell energy production through the $NAD^+/NADH$ redox couple.
4. Micronutrient deficiencies (hidden hunger).
5. Iatrogenic (medically induced). Many drugs decrease cell energy in many ways.

The graphic below shows you these factors colliding in cells to rob cells of energy. If there is insulin resistance, then our primary fuel source (glucose) used to produce ATP energy in cells is being blocked from entering cells by insulin resistance. So, we have this critical hit to energy production from less glucose entering cells.

But now, let's add fructose to this cellular energy hit. Fructose has its specific doorway into cells, which does not require insulin for this fruit sugar to gain entry. In that case, we have powerful synergistic factors working in cells that can rapidly deplete cell energy supplies. All of this is basic 101 understanding, and yet gurus of medicine and dietetics seem confused about such profound energy-depleting effects caused by the ultra-common factors mentioned above. Vested interests do you think driving this confusion to keep the business of disease prevalence running sky high?

Fructose is a highly effective ATP-depleting "machine." We have a double-whammy of insulin resistance along with fructose, which comes mainly from sugar (sucrose) saturating our foods and causing cell energy starvation. Sugar (50%) fructose is present in almost all foods, sauces, condiments, etc., and fructose consumption from high-fructose fruits, honey, agave, etc, is also extremely common. Now imagine the other BIG-10 Womb-to-Tomb factors also at play to pull the rug from cellular energy production. Gurus, you don't need to be confused. You just need to be educated, open your eyes to what is happening around you, and step outside the box.

If glucose is blocked from getting into cells by insulin resistance (IR), we will have a crash in ATP production. At the same time, fructose is richly present in many foods through not only sugar but other fruit sources. As you know, fructose rapidly depletes cells of ATP, making this one-two punch shown in the graphic a knockout blow for cell energy (ATP) production. Why aren't we seeing this one-two punch as clearly as the light of day? This one-two punch is a major cause of tiredness in people.

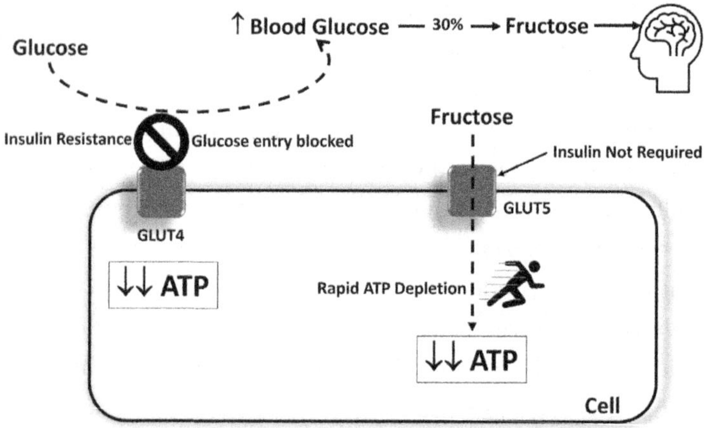

For people living on a knife's edge for life-threatening metabolic disease complications, small amounts of anything that decreases glucose levels within cells or worsens cell energy deficits will be all that it will take to tip them over the edge.

Type-2 Diabetes Mellitus (T2DM) is associated with a 60% increased risk of all-cause dementia from Alzheimer's to vascular dementia (Cholerton, Baker et al. 2016). Researchers have been scratching their heads trying to work out why there is such a high risk of dementia in those with high glucose levels. This huge glucose-to-fructose shunt in the brain is discussed in Chapter-1 and expanded upon in the ***Fiendish Fructose*** chapter.

High brain fructose levels will rapidly and persistently deplete brain cells of energy. Is it any wonder we have such a tremendously high risk of dementia and mental health disorders in those with insulin resistance or diabetes with either persistently elevated blood glucose levels or high blood glucose levels postprandially (after eating)? Insulin resistance of brain cells is strongly associated with all brain disorders. It doesn't matter if glucose is high due to a prediabetic or diabetic state or is high after eating high-carb foods. As Yale researchers found, high glucose blood levels from any cause can be shunted to fructose in the brain.

> *Energetics of the Brain: An Engine that Is Running Continuously at Full Speed. (Kovác 2008)*

The quote above says it all about the enormous and continuous energy requirements of the brain. Sugar taxes are now happening in many countries, and some cities in the USA have a soda (sugar-sweetened soft drink) tax. This sugar tax is a step in the right direction. Sugar (50% fructose) is how individuals commonly increase their fructose loads. Appendix-8 lists high fructose foods.

Tiredness is a very common presentation to doctors. "*Hey doc, why am I tired all the time?*" Doctors will check for the usual suspects, such as iron or B12 deficiency or organ failure, but often will come up empty-handed. Will a doctor ever think of this one-two punch described above or the conversion of glucose to fructose in the brain, depriving this organ of a huge amount of energy to stay functional? The worst thing a doctor can do is conclude that these individuals are depressed and then reach for that script pad in a 6-minute consultation and prescribe an antidepressant with so much potential for harm, including worsening mitochondrial function and cell energy starvation due to a quick fix solution.

Common cellular "shocks" driving cell starvation and structural decline. PEM and Hidden Hunger are major cell "shocks"

Common micronutrient insufficiencies and deficiencies are called "Hidden Hunger". We have greatly neglected hidden hunger, which is a global challenge affecting at least 2 billion people (Lowe 2021). To me, this is yet another gross underestimate. These common deficiencies include Iron, Iodine, Zinc and Vitamin-A (Lowe 2021). No one in a wealthy Western country is immune from a range of significant micronutrient deficiencies. These acute (short-term) and chronic (long-term) micronutrient deficiencies will drive biological rot throughout 100s of millions of lives.

Cellular energy pathways will simply NOT function without micronutrient adequacy as they are critical cofactors (minerals) and coenzymes (vitamins) for cellular energy production. These deficiencies are far from rare. They are highly common and often made far worse by many medications. Iron deficiency incredibly affects a staggering 1 in 3 people globally (Kumar, Sharma et al. 2022). An iron deficiency can truly hammer cell ATP production as it is vital for multiple enzymes needed for energy production. Iron deficiency is a true disaster in pregnancy for both the mother and the developing baby, causing long-term medical and behavioural problems.

We have injectable appetite-suppressing antiobesity drugs producing medically induced malnutrition, plain and simple. Without dietary inputs to offset this malnutrition, we will have weight loss but adverse outcomes. We will worsen already existing ***hidden hunger*** (nutrient deficiencies) in people undertaking drastic medical weight reduction. What could possibly go wrong? We already have up to a massive 99% of individuals in populations getting nowhere near their vegetable and fruit intakes, and these fresh foods provide the majority of vitamins and minerals needed by individuals. On top of this, we worsen vegetable and fruit intakes by medically decreasing appetite. Wow, how clever.

We can trigger fully blown diabetes with aggressive obesity management, and I will discuss an eye-opening research project that showed exactly this happening in the chapter "***That's no way to treat a metabolic marker.***" We treat obesity as a separate entity to this insulin resistance continuum when obesity is just another adaptation (branch) caused by energy-starved cells.

Protein and micronutrient-malnourished individuals can easily result from anti-obesity medications. But money matters.

These common micronutrient deficiencies can have serious consequences on cellular energy production. For example, zinc is vital for pyruvate transport to kick-start energy production in the mitochondria (Yang, Wang et al. 2017). Without enough Vitamin-A, a protein kinase enzyme cannot be activated in the mitochondria, thus impairing ATP synthesis (Acin-Perez, Hoyos et al. 2010). Suppose we add a very common problem of iodine deficiency, a vital mineral for thyroid function and energy regulation, to this mix. In that case, we have a huge synergistic effect of all these common deficiencies noted in populations worldwide, impairing cell energy production to produce an energy-starved cell that batters cell function and impairs cell structural integrity.

Now, let's add another common problem. Protein-Energy Malnutrition (PEM). Over 33% worldwide suffer from PEM, and many have stunted growth (De Onis, Monteiro et al. 1993). Without adequate protein intake that provides a wealth of amino acids, we risk overeating to meet our amino acid needs (Protein Leverage) and thus becoming overfat, overweight or obese. However, with PEM and a lack of critical amino acids, particularly Essential Amino Acids (EAAs), we risk cellular, tissue, biochemical and molecular deterioration, organ and vascular damage and organ failure.

Amino acids are needed to build proteins such as our energy-extracting enzymes or mitochondria and the Electron Transport Chain (ETC) - the protein/enzyme complexes in mitochondria. For this reason, I recommend using EAAs along with meals to ensure individuals have all the essential amino acids needed for cellular function and repair. EAAs should be incorporated into early childhood nutrition. They can also help repair and recover our microbiomes. We have dietary intakes riddled with holes in nutrition, which is not conducive to long-term health or a long life. I discuss EAAs in Chapter-7.

Adenosine Triphosphate (ATP)

ATP has three phosphate bonds attached to the adenosine backbone. When broken, each phosphate bond will release the energy trapped in that bond to power the work done by cells.

ATP needs three high-energy phosphate bonds to be an active energy supplier to cells, tissues, organs and our musculoskeletal system to drive cellular biological processes, movement and balance.

The first two bonds (gamma and beta) have equally high energy levels (LibreTexts 2023)

> *The phosphate loss from ATP to ADP to AMP and finally to adenosine signals energy depletion. ATP depleted of high energy phosphate then triggers cell energy crisis signalling by our cells through adenosine (and other signalling molecules), indicating that "we are starving."*

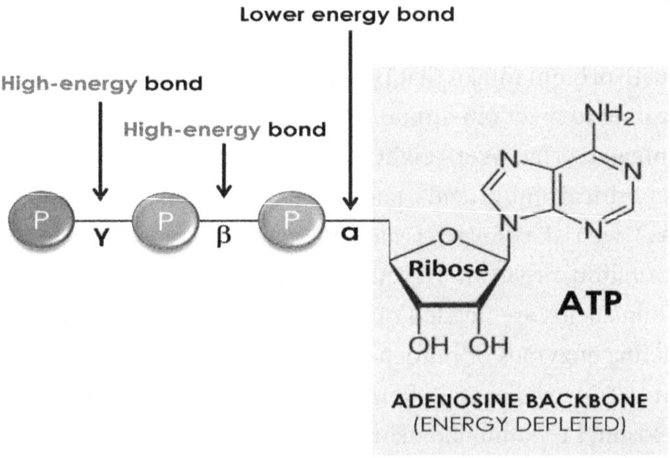

Amazingly, we can produce 40 kg of ATP in an average-weight person on a normal day

As I have discussed previously, this amount of ATP being produced is stunning (Acuña-Castroviejo, Martín et al. 2001). This huge amount of ATP is an affirmation of the amount of energy required by our cells to build, repair, and maintain all our cell "machinery" to stay functional and to keep entropy in check continually.

There are many moving parts in play with regard to energy production in cells. We have the glycolytic pathway and Krebs cycle, which involve many enzyme steps, with each enzyme needing a vast amount of micronutrients to function. So, as the author San-Millán stated, *"...disruptions of cellular bioenergetics..."* not just the mitochondria can lead to metabolic disease, and there are many steps involved long before our mitochondria join in on the action for ATP production. The term 'disruptions' refers to all the factors and steps involved in ATP energy production by cells prior to and including mitochondrial action. Energy production goes way beyond just the fuel needed for ATP production. No fuel gets burnt off as energy unless we have functional cells to do so. For cells to function, we need a myriad of micronutrients to ensure all our energy-extracting enzymes can work optimally.

Beyond micronutrients, many medications and toxic environmental chemicals can hammer these same enzymes in the glycolytic and Krebs pathways and our complex enzyme complexes in the Electron Transport Chains (ETCs) of our mitochondria to decrease ATP production. It is incredibly easy in the 21st century to create an energy-starved and structurally damaged cell.

Cellular energy and structural integrity are greatly intertwined. When cell energy falters, it sets off a metabolic dysfunction cascade, impacting biomarkers and leading to chronic diseases. Energy deficits worsen structural decline, creating a vicious cycle. All roads lead to microcirculation damage, the ultimate killer of organ systems.

ATP is actually magnesium-ATP (Mg-ATP)

When created, magnesium activates ATP. Magnesium is also critical for the formation of ATP in the first place, as ATP-synthase is the final point along the electron transport chain (ETC) along the inner mitochondrial membrane that produces the vast amounts of ATP needed for function and survival.

ATP-Synthase won't function without magnesium. Subclinical (unnoticeable) magnesium deficiency is of the most concern and is described as a "***public health crisis***" (DiNicolantonio, O'Keefe et al. 2018). The medical complications from deadly heart rhythms to mitral valve prolapse can stem from magnesium deficiency, even if that deficiency is subtle. There is much disrespect for the critical nature of nutrients in medical management, even when those deficiencies are not clinically obvious.

Since the 1940s, there has been a steady decrease in micronutrients in food, with a 21% reduction in whole milk, 24% reduction in vegetables, 82% reduction in polished rice, and 82% reduction in white flour, to name a few (DiNicolantonio, O'Keefe et al. 2018). Adding to this inherent micronutrient depletion in food is the stunning statistic that 95-99% of people are not getting anywhere near their vegetable and fruit intake, as I mentioned throughout this book, which is a major cause of vitamin and mineral insufficiency in populations including Australia (AIHW 2018). Such poor intakes of fresh foods make even the idea of an optimal diet being consumed by up to 99% of the population an absurd idea.

Magnesium levels are high in dark green leafy vegetables and, in fact, in many veggies and fruits. Fresh food indeed provides a wealth of many micronutrients. Do children eat their veggies? What about older or disadvantaged people who cannot afford fresh food? What happens in aged care facilities providing substandard food? In pregnancy – are pregnant women consuming "optimal" diets full of fresh vegetables and low-carb fruit? Governments are so short-sighted. Why are healthy fresh foods not subsidised? Why don't dietitians shout from the rooftops for far better food standards, not based on what their corporate masters of agriculture, governments and the food industry want them to promote?

Magnesium is a separate substrate in the ***ATP Synthase*** rotating ***nanomachine*** (Igamberdiev and Kleczkowski 2015). The role of magnesium is so critical to energy production, yet I have never heard magnesium routinely mentioned in clinical practice, at any medical meeting, even to people suffering from lethargy, heart rhythm disturbances or early insulin resistance. Usually, drugs come first in these medical meetings, and as for dietitians, all that matters is plates piled high with staple foods devoid of micronutrients such as magnesium.

Individuals with mental health problems are notorious for having poor diets for various reasons and, thus, will also have significant nutrient deficiencies that impair ATP production. Imagine then we add mental health drugs on top of micronutrient deficiencies that hammer cell ATP production. It is not clever in the least. Drugs are primitive interventions in mental health and can trigger diabetes from energy insults through impaired vulnerable enzyme systems and mitochondria.

When do we stop abusing those poor souls with mental health disorders with horrific drug interventions and begin restoring brain function through improving cell bioenergetics and reducing structural decline? We have rather adopted an uncivilized approach to managing mental health problems. I do concede that drugs may be needed but should never be used exclusively but only with a comprehensive nutritional plan.

Chronic and episodic cell energy starvation drives this metabolic disease disaster.

Cell bioenergetics is essentially about cell energy flows, i.e. how energy is formed and used, with the main form of power in the body being Adenosine Triphosphate (Mg-ATP), which I have described above. ATP powers cell-building functions (anabolic processes), protein synthesis, repair processes and waste removal.

90% of cellular ATP energy comes from mitochondria through oxidative phosphorylation (OXPHOS) (Sorriento, Pascale et al. 2014).

To get a better idea of OXPHOS, see Appendix-16 and 29. Without ATP, you can't blink an eye, move a finger a limb, or even breathe. ATP drives all our musculoskeletal and cellular activities in the body and brain, as well as anabolic (cell-building) processes in our trillions of cells.

Suppose cells lack the ATP power and building block supplies to create enzymes for the glycolytic Pathway, Krebs cycle or the protein complexes in the Electron Transport Chain (ETC). In that case, significant cellular energy and structural decline will follow soon after. Insulin resistance ("prediabetes") is tightly linked to this cellular energy and structural decay process.

> *"This bioenergetic perspective on disease provides a unifying pathophysiological and genetic mechanism for neuropsychiatric diseases such as Alzheimer's and Parkinson's Disease, metabolic diseases such as diabetes and obesity, autoimmune diseases, ageing, and cancer." (Wallace 2011)*

The Universality of Cellular Bioenergetic Decline Over Our Lifetimes: A Brief Overview

> *"The organising power of energy flow is hypothesised to be the origin of biological complexity and its decline the basis of "complex" diseases and ageing." (Wallace 2011)*

The term "Bioenergetics" was a book title published in 1956 by Albert Szent-Györgyi, the Nobel Prize winner who discovered Vitamin-C and Rutin (Vitamin-P, Bioflavonoids) and described oxidative stress (related to inflammation).

Australian researcher Professor Anthony Linnane, who studied at Sydney University and then went on to research cell bioenergetics at Monash University in Australia, published a paper titled: "***The Universality of Bioenergetic Disease.***" (Linnane, Kovalenko et al. 1998). This research studied muscle biopsies from the deltoid muscle of older people and found that 95% of skeletal mitochondrial DNA (mtDNA) was not intact. In other words, only 5% of the mitochondrial DNA appeared normal in older age groups.

It is mitochondrial DNA that is directly responsible for energy creation in the form of ATP. Is it any wonder that the Oxford Community Diabetes Study, as I have discussed in previous chapters, showed more than 95% of our older people suffer from diabetes? If we damage cell energy production, we set ourselves up for insulin resistance, diabetes and chronic diseases. These processes are continuums. This mitochondrial DNA damage didn't suddenly appear when we grew older.

There is irreversible cellular functional and structural decline following common (not inherited) damage to mitochondrial DNA caused by diet, environmental chemicals, and medications, leading to diminishing Oxidative Phosphorylation (OXPHOS) and diminishing ATP production (Li, Slone et al. 2020). See Appendix-16.

Thus, we can view mitochondrial DNA (mtDNA) damage as a continuum over our lifetimes, and these constant mtDNA hits come from many allostatic loads, as we have discussed. For example, many DNA toxic compounds (genotoxins) can preferentially accumulate in mitochondria, impairing their ability to create ATP and also damage mitochondrial DNA. In addition, many anti-psychotic medications can powerfully impair mitochondrial function. (Nadalutti, Ayala-Peña et al. 2022).

There are 1500 nuclear DNA mitochondrial genes required for mitochondrial structure and function (Li, Slone et al. 2020). We also have 37 mitochondrial DNA genes, all of which are solely involved in oxidative phosphorylation (OXPHOS) occurring in the Electron Transport Chain (ETC) (Nadalutti, Ayala-Peña et al. 2022). See Appendix-16 and 17.

So, all 37 mitochondrial DNA (mtDNA) genes are involved in cell energy production. Food factors can greatly damage mitochondrial DNA as well. Nutrient overload from energy-rich, nutrient-poor foods is so common in world populations that we neglect this as an important consideration in the creation of massive amounts of free radicals, Reactive Oxygen Species (ROS) and Reactive Nitrogen Species (RNS). The RNS forms when nitric oxide reacts with ROS to create these damaging RNS molecules. Thus, free radicals, ROS/RNS, are a by-product of the conversion of food to energy (ATP) and are yet another way food harms all of us meal-by-meal and snack-by-snack with food generating these free radicals that damage mtDNA.

In this process of creating free radicals, high-energy electrons escape the Electron Transport Chain (ETC) and react with oxygen to produce Reactive Oxygen Species (ROS) and RNS. Free radicals are any molecule that has an unpaired electron. These damaging molecules impair ATP production and can also damage mitochondrial DNA. This damage occurs every time we eat a meal or a snack, which is why intermittent fasting protects cells, tissues, organs and vascular beds. See Appendix-18. So much for food being benign.

There is a close proximity of the ETC components to our mitochondrial DNA (mtDNA), putting this mitochondrial DNA at risk of free radical damage (Nadalutti, Ayala-Peña et al. 2022). Mitochondrial DNA is solely involved in ATP production, as indicated in the quote above, so we damage the mtDNA just by the composition of the food we consume. Once again, our energy-dense, micronutrient-poor staple foods can be seen as mtDNA killers.

Thus, this exposed mitochondrial DNA is highly susceptible to free radicals generated by the food energy extraction process in mitochondria. It is easy enough to see how all food can take us out meal by meal. We must get rid of this notion that food cannot cause harm because it satisfies our primal needs, fills our bellies and gives us warm and fuzzy nostalgic taste sensations. It is this thinking that distorts our ideas of food and disease causation and prevention. Health depends on what we put in our mouths – every meal, every snack, every day.

For decades, it has been known that mitochondrial DNA is far more susceptible than nuclear DNA to inflammatory damage (Nadalutti, Ayala-Peña et al. 2022). This inflammatory ROS and RNS damage to mtDNA can then become persistent, and as a result, it has been suggested that ROS-induced mtDNA damage can be used as a biomarker for ROS-associated diseases, of which there are many (Yakes and Van Houten 1997).

Poor food choices contribute to food energy and micronutrient deficiency impacts, which damage both mitochondrial (mtDNA) and nuclear DNA. Poor food choice gradually reduces energy production and raises cancer risk over our lifetimes. Micronutrient deficiencies are a huge problem in a complex biological system such as a cell (Ames 2001).

The NAD+/NADH Redox Pair (Redox Couple). Too much or too little food damages us. Paradoxically, too much food incapacitates cell energy production (nutri-stress)

Our cells can be energy- and micronutrient-starved at the same time, even in the face of high food intake, where these foods are energy-rich but nutrient-poor and fibre-poor. This statement may seem paradoxical, but true. In terms of high food energy intake and turning off ATP production, it helps to think of constantly pouring fuel into a car tank, then permanently depressing the accelerator while in neutral, and then watching the engine heat up and burn out over time. The fuel in humans is food, and our engines are the trillions of mitochondria that won't survive being revved to the max constantly due to all those free radicals generated by the conversion of food to energy – our ATP. This is "***mitochondrial overheating***".

This NAD^+/NADH redox couple is a powerful regulator of cellular energy metabolism (Xiao, Wang et al. 2018). The cells then have a throttle mechanism in the NAD^+/NADH redox couple to limit mitochondrial "engine" burnout from food energy (fuel) overload. Without this redox mechanism existing to "choke" energy production, all of us will literally burn out all our mitochondrial "engines", which in turn would switch off all the lights in our cells. Food overload also permanently damages our mitochondria and protein-producing, 3D-activating organelle, the Endoplasmic Reticulum (ER). This damage is irreversible (Qiu and Schlegel 2018). When do people stop eating during the day? Just think of massive food energy intake in a mountain of pasta, rice, fatty food on a plate, or a family-sized pizza that many can devour by themselves.

In our rush to accuse obesity for all our metabolic sins, we often falsely quote that even a small amount of weight loss will result in highly significant metabolic dysfunction improvements. The often-quoted magical weight loss threshold to achieve this metabolic improvement is 5% to 10% of body weight. Individuals are often put on a dietary plan to lose weight. This plan means changing dietary inputs to decrease portion size or perhaps have healthy, nutrient-rich options. The very fact that food energy intake decreases (thus decreasing nutri-stress) will, in turn, improve the NAD+/NADH ratio, which then allows more ATP to be generated in mitochondria. So, more power will be available to a cell, which can now concentrate on anabolic (building) and repair processes and power reversal of entropy (cell decay), and this will decrease the famine signalling we have discussed to store body fat.

So, losing weight was just a side-effect of better dietary inputs and an improved cellular bioenergetic state. Increased cell energy will mean less metabolic dysfunction and improved insulin resistance, but we don't see these metabolic changes through the lens of improved cell energy and cell function. We simplistically attribute these metabolic improvements to weight loss.

By reducing food energy intake and improving nutrition for weight loss, we observe decreased blood biomarkers and improved microcirculation flow. These small blood vessels significantly influence vascular resistance, and so we see lower blood pressure as microcirculation stiffness and resistance decrease. As a bonus, weight loss through an enhanced diet ensures more valuable nutrient resources are consumed. Consequently, our power-generating energy pathways operate smoothly by providing essential vitamins and minerals for ATP production by our enzyme systems.

So, following what was stated above, this weight loss had nothing to do with the improvements in metabolic biomarkers, decreasing high blood pressure, etc. Weight loss as a metabolic biomarker itself occurred all because we shifted sick and distressed cells back to a normal state of energy levels, improved NAD+/NADH ratios, increased ATP levels, improved fat-burning and decreased structural damage all through cells being powered up and well-nourished. Focusing on weight loss through drugs can be deadly because medically-induced malnutrition works counter to cellular bioenergetic needs.

Interestingly, a ketosis diet generating Ketone Bodies from our body fat can help increase the NAD+/NADH ratio towards normal, improving mitochondrial function and cellular energy levels (Kolb, Kempf et al. 2021). I discuss such a diet in the final chapter, but the ketosis I am talking about is not the high-fat, high-animal flesh kind at all. It is far more gentle, timed, structured and far safer.

Insulin is the most potent anabolic hormone in our bodies

Many see insulin resistance (IR) as a public threat to humanity due to the increasing prevalence of this problem (Al-Qawasmeh and Tayyem 2018). Effective insulin action is vital to provide cells with fuel (glucose) and cell building blocks such as amino acids and fatty acids. As insulin resistance increases and fuel (glucose) diminishes in cells, we will have declining cellular energy, which will, in turn, increase cellular decay and disorder (higher entropy).

That insulin is our bodies' most powerful anabolic hormone is not arguable (Saltiel and Kahn 2001). Most practitioners equate insulin with glucose control, but insulin's action is far, far greater than that. The term “anabolic” describes the synthesis of compounds in cells, from proteins and hormones to signalling molecules, neurotransmitters, synapses, membranes and enzymes, along with myriad other biological compounds needed for cellular function.

This anabolic action of insulin extends to creating the protein-enzyme complexes like the ones found in the Electron Transport Chain (ETC), critical for ATP production and also for receptors, cell organelles, cell structural components and ultrastructural cellular components. Insulin action is also necessary for the building of cell and cell organelle membranes. Our trillions of mitochondria depend on the building blocks provided by the normal action of insulin. So, there are many critical, non-negotiable anabolic processes powered by insulin's action. We have to build these components from scratch, so even a mild building supply or micronutrient shortage in cells is disastrous as structural decay and deterioration are set into motion for obvious reasons, and entropy increases to the point of organs losing function and ultimately failing.

As our metabolic dysfunction progresses, our insulin hormone becomes less and less functional as insulin is a protein molecule that requires building itself and storing in our beta cells. Thus, insulin, by not working as it should (insulin resistance), shoots itself "in the foot," and therefore, as you can see, this will be a vicious cycle of diminishing creation, storage and weakening insulin action. What hope will cells have? Our cell-building (anabolic) processes become more and more impaired. Yet when does medicine consider nutrient needs and rescue? When does it ever consider providing nutrient building blocks such as amino acids or micronutrients to support and boost the reversal of structural decay and to support protein synthesis, as insulin itself, as mentioned, is a protein? Ignoring nutrient needs for cells is gross negligence to me.

Insulin was discovered in 1921, so we have over 100 years of knowledge about this critical and powerful anabolic hormone. Even with a century of knowledge about insulin action and inaction, medicine has mangled this insulin-resistant metabolic disease process. So, for anabolic (cell protein and cell structure building) processes to occur in our cells, we need:

1. **Energy Supplies:** in the form of ATP from glucose or from lipids and even amino acids. Without energy, cells grind to a halt and may become irreversibly damaged. In insulin resistance, we lose our primary fuel (glucose) as insulin resistance blocks glucose from entering cells. Shouldn't we get around this by providing a fuel like ketone bodies that can be a significant source of ATP for cells that don't require insulin in the least to get into cells?

It seems obvious to me that we should.

2. **Building supplies:** Glucose is used to create glycogen, glycolipids, ribose, deoxyribose, neurotransmitters, neuromodulators, and proteoglycans. Amino acids are needed to produce proteins, enzymes, organelles, membranes, neurotransmitters, and hormones. Lipids like cholesterol are used in membranes and are used to make steroids, hormones, and Vitamin D. Lipids also act as cell messengers. So you can see how disastrous it is that poorly functioning insulin action creates havoc in cells by blocking both energy and all our cell-building supplies.

Our energy and building supplies are the result of normal insulin action. If insulin action falls apart, our cells fall apart as they become metabolically dysfunctional, and this starts our slow and inexorable journey towards biological damage and a high entropy state.

Carbohydrates, lipids and proteins ultimately break down into glucose, the primary metabolic fuel for mammals and the universal fuel for the fetus (Nakrani, Wineland et al. 2020).

Impaired insulin action impairs glucose utilisation in the brain, impairing and leading to bioenergetic failure and hypometabolism (low metabolism) in brain cells (Sharma and Singh 2020). If insulin works well, the cells have all the glucose (fuel) they need to create ATP and power cell functions. However, when insulin resistance occurs, we have a decreasing amount of glucose entering cells, thus impairing ATP production and, therefore, diminishing the power required for anabolic functions.

No ATP energy = No power to drive anabolic processes to build cellular components = high entropy

Insulin works through various cell membrane transporters to allow the entry of nutrient components (Saltiel and Kahn 2001).

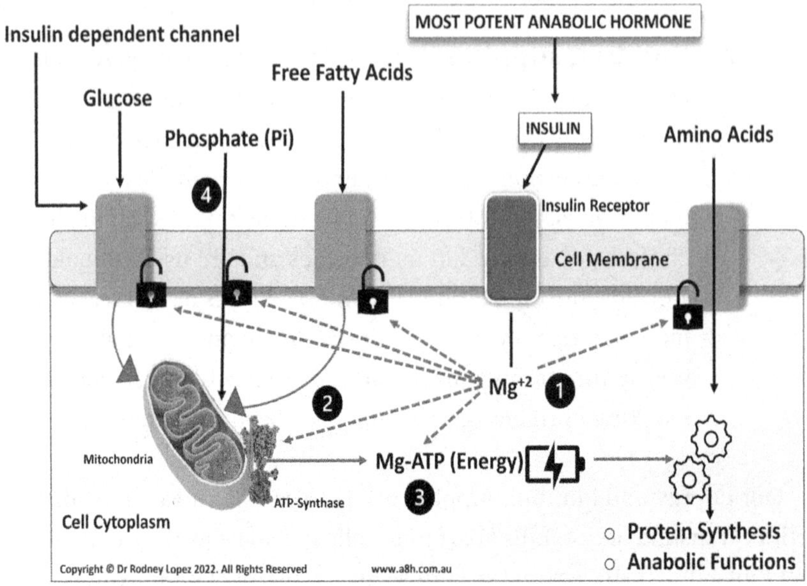

Follow the points in the graphic above.	
1.	Magnesium is critical for insulin signalling. Up to 72% of Australians may lack magnesium (ABS 2015). Similar or worse figures exist in other countries. In the graphic on insulin's action, you can see it unlocks insulin action at the insulin receptor, affecting transporters across the membrane (Saltiel and Kahn 2001). Magnesium deficiency is thus one of the many common nutrient factors causing insulin resistance, which works in synergy to affect insulin signalling. Magnesium deficiency is strongly associated with Type-2 Diabetes Mellitus and is a direct factor in insulin resistance (IR). There is an inverse relationship between Magnesium and diabetes. The lower the magnesium, the higher the risk of T2DM (Gommers, Hoenderop et al. 2016). This vicious cycle occurs as insulin resistance (IR) will increase kidney excretion of magnesium, thus further lowering magnesium. Thus ↑ IR > ↑ Kidney Magnesium Excretion > ↓ Magnesium > ↑↑ IR > ↑↑ Magnesium excretion > ↓↓ Magnesium and so on – it is a vicious

	cycle (Gommers, Hoenderop et al. 2016). The two up arrows mean progressively worsening problems. So why isn't it standard practice to recommend magnesium in insulin-resistant disease states? Safety? Well, that is laughable when you compare the safety of an ESSENTIAL mineral to the huge and life-threatening risks of Adverse Drug Reactions (ADRs). See Appendix-35 for this foolish notion of nutrient safety. We are putting people at great risk by not supplementing with magnesium and placing them at cardiovascular risk, high blood pressure and arrhythmias (abnormal heart rhythms). It is as if only drugs count. Such naïve thinking only drives the failed drug-centric model. One huge flaw with medical research using vitamins or minerals such as magnesium is the researchers' lack of knowledge. Their mindset is looking for a quick drug-like response, but nutrients are not drugs and don't work in a drug-like fashion. With magnesium found mainly in intracellular compartments (inside cells), it takes a very long time to reach a steady state (balance), and in fact, it can take 40 weeks or more for this steady state to occur (Ismail, Ismail et al. 2018). Using poorly bioavailable forms of magnesium in the wrong doses and for the wrong time interval will create major errors in research findings, thus reinforcing the ignorance and bias of doctors and dietitians regarding supplementation, which could be life-saving.
2.	ATP Synthase is a biological machine (a nano-motor) described as one of the most beautiful molecules in biochemistry and is the final step in the Electron Transport Chain (ETC) in mitochondria. Our mitochondria are the Mg-ATP powerhouses in cells, producing around 90% of our ATP. Therefore, ATP-Synthase enzymes are an amazing **biological rotatory nanomachine**. Without magnesium, ATPase will not work. Look for a diagram of this amazing complex in this chapter. Without magnesium, ATP-synthase will dramatically decrease the production of ATP, showing the critical nature of minerals like magnesium in keeping us alive and our cells' supply of ATP sufficient. What hope do cells have of not becoming starved of energy when essential minerals like

	magnesium are lacking? This mineral is just one of many minerals needed for energy extraction of food and ATP production and should reinforce how easy it is for cells to become energy deficient, either chronically or episodically. Hopefully, doubters of the Cell Starvation Model (CSM) are seeing how impactful just one mineral can have on the action of insulin and energy production. Insulin resistance results in a decreasing fuel supply (glucose), and on top of this cell fuel supply problem, we then have a hamstringing of mitochondria's ATP-Synthase by a lack of magnesium. This combination is a recipe for disaster regarding cell ATP (energy) production. See Appendix-29.
3.	Magnesium-ATP (Mg-ATP) is the molecule produced, not just ATP, as we often abbreviate this molecule (Igamberdiev and Kleczkowski 2015). For ATP to work, it must be activated by magnesium (Mg^{2+}) to form Mg-ATP (Mildvan 1987). What is not appreciated is the gigantic amount of Mg-ATP produced by the body daily. *It has been estimated that forty kilograms (40 kg) of Mg-ATP are formed and broken down in the average body every day (yes, 40 kg)* (Acuña-Castroviejo, Martín et al. 2001). Normal insulin action regulates intracellular magnesium levels (Paolisso, Scheen et al. 1990). Even phosphate (Pi), critical for Mg-ATP production, has limited entry into cells when we have insulin resistance. So the "nothing green will touch my plate" mentality for 95-99% of those in society with extremely poor vegetable and fruit intakes simply diminishes magnesium and phosphate levels. Where is that "optimal diet" when you need it? Our cells thus suffer, and cellular energy decline puts us at great risk for insulin resistance. So much negative cellular impact is caused by only one mineral deficiency, such as magnesium. Yet many people have multiple mineral and vitamin deficiencies simultaneously. Because of the tremendous need for magnesium to produce Mg-ATP, it is recycled by absorbing it from the kidneys, but if we have increasing excretion of magnesium due to worsening insulin resistance, we are then in trouble in terms of cellular energy production and structural

	decay. Is the 101 principle of magnesium loss due to insulin resistance ever in the minds of GPs, Dietitians, Endocrinologists, and other specialists? No, they tell you to eat an "optimal diet" or give you guidelines that are lacking and highly superficial.
4.	Phosphate (Pi) transport into skeletal muscle cells is thought to occur similarly to glucose transport. This phosphate transport is "severely blunted" in insulin-resistant patients (Petersen, Dufour et al. 2005). With 40 kilograms of ATP needing to be produced in our bodies every day, you can see how critical ongoing phosphate supply is to ATP generation. ATP contains three (x3) phosphate bonds that must be broken to release the energy trapped in those bonds required to power cell activity. Insulin resistance thus impairs many aspects of cell energy production. Besides highly intelligent pioneers who understand bioenergetic systems, the practice of medicine seems blind to cell energy deficits at the grassroots level of medical practice. This cell starvation process is driving the insulin resistance continuum and the chronic disease pandemic, killing 100s of millions over decades. We have no choice now but to look at this whole diabetes and chronic disease mess from this bioenergetic angle. Our focus should be to restore cell balance (allostasis) by stopping dangerous food impacts and preventing nutrient deficiencies. We can only achieve optimal cell power and balance by providing optimal supplies of vital nutrients, enabling cells to become functional again. We need an alternative fuel source if glucose cannot get into cells. I describe this alternative fuel in the final chapter, where we side-step this fuel supply issue. The established failure of drugs to halt or reverse this ever-increasing disease process now demands that we view insulin resistance as a result of gradual and progressive cell bioenergetic failure over years and decades in humans that drives the insulin resistance continuum. Nutrient supply is key to halting this destructive process of cell energy deficits, not drugs that do nothing to nourish a cell and never will. Drugs are not nutrients and never will be! See Nutrient Rescue in the final chapter.

The Electron Transport Chain (ETC)

You don't have to understand the nitty-gritty of cell energy production but to get a general idea of ATP production.
The Electron Transport Chain (ETC) is where most ATP is produced in our trillions of mitochondria. One glucose molecule produces 32 to 34 ATPs from Pyruvate through Glycolysis in the cell cytoplasm (Cooper 2000). However, it is stated that 36-38 ATP can be produced based on some variables from one (x1) glucose molecule.

Once formed, pyruvate produced in aerobic conditions (oxygen available) would usually be shunted through the Krebs Cycle, also known as the Citric Acid Cycle, to make two critical compounds, NADH and $FADH_2$, each containing high-energy electrons that zip through the ETC to power ATP production. See Appendix-17, 29. Just keep in mind that 90% of ATP is produced through the mitochondrial Electron Transport Chain via oxidative phosphorylation (OXPHOS). (Sorriento, Pascale et al. 2014).

The Electron Transport Chain (ETC) needs a wealth of nutrients to function and produce ATP in mitochondria

All enzymes involved in energy production, of which there are many, and the vital multi-protein enzyme complexes in the ETC along the inner membrane of mitochondria demand a never-ending wealth of nutrients to function. To think, as medicine and dietetics do, we can slap food on a plate due to our taste preferences, and then those food preferences will meet all our requirements for an abundance of vitamins, minerals, and trace elements needed to support these energy-producing pathways is fantasy thinking.

Taste preferences can drive large amounts of food energy intake but not necessarily a high nutrient intake. Often, the foods consumed are made up of nutrient-poor ultra-processed foods (UPFs) that can taste savoury and protein-rich, but such foods act as "***protein decoys***", causing protein energy malnutrition (PEM). No protein means no amino acids to build cellular components. In other words, leaving nutrient intake to chance, as most do by using taste preferences and consuming a very limited number of food choices, can be a disaster for cellular energy production.

There is such a conceit and disregard for supplementation in the medical and dietetic worlds, putting lives at risk. Such scorn is not deserved as multiple research outcomes have shown significant health benefits from the use of nutrient supplementation. Supplementation in a world full of horror food inputs that are micronutrient insufficient can fill in any nutrient gaps. If safety is used as an argument against supplements, then nothing comes near the deadly nature of medical drug treatments. This drug risk is highlighted in Appendix-25, 26, and 35. I do agree, though, that taking a supplement and thinking this will fix all our chronic illness problems is also laughable.

Supplements should always be taken on the advice of a practitioner who knows what they are talking about and always in conjunction with a meaningful and well-structured whole-food diet, and this doesn't mean all the damaging staple foods out there. In an ideal world, this would be a doctor or dietitian, but in this real world, both these groups are untrained and unfit for this purpose, driven by vested interests that distort their perspectives. These professions have been trained to push drug treatments or staple foods. Supplementation should be used to ensure we are never deficient of even one critical nutrient and should never be taken without a well-designed and meaningful diet, as we need to avoid all the damaging after-eating (postprandial) food impacts I discuss in this book, and we also need a wealth of phytochemicals and fibre from whole food.

To think about our pregnant and lactating mothers, children, our senior population, those with acute or chronic diseases, acute trauma and recovery, or those who exercise a great deal, or work in physically demanding jobs will meet all their nutrient requirements by chance or from limited food intake is definitely comical. For those taking multiple medications, it is well-documented that many of these drugs can interfere with vitamin or mineral absorption (think powerful PPI antacids). If we then consider appetite suppressants such as GLP-1 anti-obesity injections, creating medical malnutrition or anyone with eating disorders or mental health illnesses preventing them from eating well can all benefit from a well-designed diet that includes supplementation. To think that this wide-ranging group of vulnerable people don't need nutritional support in the form of supplementation is truly distorted thinking and puts all these groups in their 100s of millions at huge risk for cellular energy and structural deterioration. When do we wake up to the fact that nutrients are not negotiable for good health?

At many points in this book, we discuss the critical nature of the mitochondria in energy production. In reality, it is the Electron Transport Chain (ETC) components found along the inner membranes of mitochondria that are the crucial points for ATP generation. We have a vast pool of mitochondria in our 37.2 trillion body cells, where we may have thousands of mitochondria in each cell, except Red Blood Cells (RBCs), which lack them. Mitochondrial numbers are thus astronomical.

All cells with mitochondria can produce ketone bodies, which can bypass the restriction of glucose entering cells due to insulin resistance. If we can't fix insulin resistance, we can then work around it. However, we can fix insulin resistance by supporting our cells to make them functional again by ensuring that they have ketones as a fuel source to "spark" that recovery through the energy needed to repair cells.

Apart from Vitamin-B12 and folate (B9), which can be stored in the liver, the other B-group vitamins cannot; thus, we all need adequate B-group vitamin resources daily, including those vitamins stored in the liver. As you can see from the table below and Appendix-7, our ability to produce energy is critically dependent on a steady supply of B-group vitamins.

ATP Synthase is the most beautiful enzyme and an ancient rotatory nanomachine

Appendix-17 provides information about this amazing rotating enzyme "motor" that creates a wealth of ATP and sits at the very end of the Electron Transport Chain (ETC) that powers most of our 37.2 trillion cells and produces huge amounts of Magnesium-ATP. This amazing rotating nanomotor won't work without magnesium.

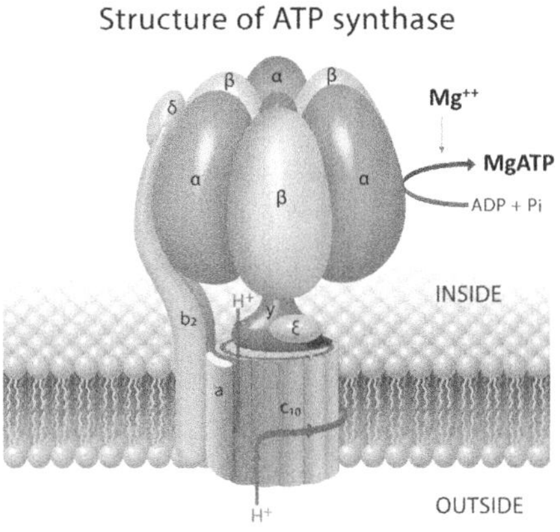

> *"All enzymes are beautiful, but the ATP synthase is one of the most beautiful as well as one of the most unusual and important"* (Boyer 1997)

The mighty multivitamin

A 2024 article in the peer-reviewed medical website Medscape discussed the use of multivitamins and colorectal cancer (CRC) mortality. Even a moderate intake of multivitamins 3 – 5 times a week showed a 45% lower risk for cancer-related mortality. This moderate intake of a multivitamin also showed a lower risk for all-cause mortality, as did a dose of a multivitamin of 6 – 9 a week.

To complicate matters like most research does, this study showed that 10 or more multivitamins a week showed a 60% higher mortality. However, this association is very complicated. Is it the supplement, or is it the fact that many seriously ill people start to take multivitamins all of a sudden and maybe high doses? Also, supplementation in the presence of a bad diet will never work, and bad diets can cause a lot of harm and death. Multivitamins can only outrun a bad diet for so long and can't overcome the sins of bad lifestyle and dietary inputs forever, which distorts these adverse statistics on the use of multivitamins. For some in the medical profession and certain medical and dietary gurus who run victory laps at the failure of nutrient support, all because of brain-dead interpretations of such conflicting micronutrient research findings. It helps no one and can do a great deal of harm. What is the alternative? Failed drugs?

The caveat is whether the supplements used covered all the necessary critical micronutrients. Did these multivitamins have active forms of the B-group vitamins, and were they highly bioavailable forms of vitamins or minerals, or were the research multivitamins cheap and not well absorbed? Did the supplements used only have beta-carotene or mixed carotenoids? Did the Vitamin-E component have only one or all of the Vitamin-E isomers? We will discuss flawed beta-carotene studies later and cancer risk. No multivitamin on the planet will offset a cancer-causing diet, keeping in mind virtually all our staple foods have cancer-causing properties, as we have discussed in "***Lessons learnt from the Laron Syndrome***" (Melnik, John et al. 2011).

When gurus of medicine and dietetics dismiss or denigrate supplementation, they push people into hazardous drug management with huge risks involved. Do these gurus dismiss the need for nutrient resources altogether? Can cells ever survive or function without nutrients? As a medical practitioner, I never see mentioned in anyone's medical files a detailed plan for dietary management along with a script for diabetes, hypertension or weight loss. So what do these supplement-dismissing gurus have in mind for populations that have the worst nutritional inputs in the history of humankind? We have diseases largely caused by dreadful dietary inputs, so shouldn't we concentrate on nutritional factors as our primary focus? Diseases do not happen because of a "drug deficiency".

Red meat, processed meats, cheese, refined carbohydrates and eggs increase the risk of bowel cancer (Ryan-Harshman and Aldoori 2007). These foods are backed by the most powerful and highly influential food boards, such as Egg, Meat & Livestock, Poultry, Dairy and Big-Food and Beverage. Imagine a drug achieving this equivalent of slashing bowel cancer rates with multivitamins, as stated above. This drug would be promoted far and wide, with an army of reps seeing doctors and seeing it as the best thing since the lightbulb was invented. So why aren't we hearing about this amazing multivitamin effect in preventing bowel cancer, one of the most rapidly increasing cancers in younger individuals under 50 years of age?

The previous section discussed horrific Adverse Drug Reactions (ADRs), and Appendix-33 discusses the horrors of staple foods.

Nutrients and cellular ATP production

As mentioned, it is absurd to think we get a full complement of micronutrients from that fabled "optimal diet". Just throw food (any food) onto a plate, and voila, we will have all the nutrients we need to drive our cellular machinery. It is a flight of fancy!

Without adequate nutrient intake, we put our 37.2 trillion cells in great jeopardy. The trillions of organisms in our gut microbiome also depend on our food and nutrient intake. When you view the table below, also look at Appendix-7 and Appendix-17 to see where micronutrients work in the Krebs cycle and Electron Transport Chain (ETC) in mitochondria. It is easy to see how very common micronutrient insufficiencies and deficiencies can incapacitate cellular ATP production, thus significantly weakening cells and driving an increase in entropy. It is an absolute injustice to hoodwink people that they can get all the nutrients they need from staple foods. This thinking sets the scene for chronic metabolic diseases. All the micronutrients mentioned in this table are not negotiable and are critical for cell energy production.

Nutrient - Respiratory Chain Impacts		
Nutrient	Component Affected	Comment
CoQ10	CoQ10	CoQ10 is a vital component of the Electron Transport Chains (ETCs) in mitochondria. It can be synthesized in the body or acquired in the diet. Statins can interrupt production. CoQ10 decreases with ageing. The electron transport chain

		produces significant free radicals at this CoQ10 point (Scientific American 2006).
Iron-Sulphur	Aconitase Krebs Cycle	Aconitase works at two locations in the Krebs (Citric Acid Cycle). Iron and sulphur deficiencies affect the critical first steps of ATP formation (Haddad and Mohiuddin 2021).
Iron Electron Transport Chain	Complex-I (NADH CoQ reductase) Complex II (succinate-CoQ reductase) Cytochrome-B (Complex III); Complex-IV Cytochrome-C (Cyt-B; Cyt-C) (Oexle, Gnaiger et al. 1999).	Iron is at the heart of cytochrome redox-active proteins in the Electron Transport Chain (ETC). Iron is also a part of a heme molecule. Complex I (NADH-CoQ reductase) requires Iron-Sulphur. Complex II (succinate-CoQ reductase) contains both heme and iron sulphur. Complex-IV –has two heme groups and copper ions. Aconitase and three other Krebs Cycle enzymes become impaired with iron deficiency – citrate synthase, isocitric dehydrogenase, and succinate dehydrogenase.
Magnesium (Mg)	ATP Synthase Mg-ATP (each ATP molecule needs Mg. We produce Mg-ATP, not just ATP)	ATP-Synthase is located at the end of the respiratory chain, generating ATP in large quantities. However, ATP Synthase does not work without Magnesium as a cofactor. According to the Australian Bureau of Statistics, 1 in 3 Australians over 2 years do not meet the requirements for magnesium intake. In addition, 72% of females and 61% of males aged 14 to 18 did not meet the estimated average requirement (EAR) for magnesium intake (ABS 2015).
Omega-3's (DHA, EPA), Choline	Mitochondrial membranes	Mitochondrial membranes are bilipid layers made up of phospholipids such as phosphatidylcholine. Omega-3s are vital for membrane fluidity and receptor function. Cell signalling is highly dependent on fully functional membranes. Cell membrane fluidity is a "pacemaker" for cell metabolism (Hulbert 2007).
Vitamin-A *Avoid in pregnancy*	Protein Kinase Activation	Vitamin-A has recently been shown to be critical for not only mucosal immunity but also for energy homeostasis. In addition, low Vitamin-A will impact Pyruvate Dehydrogenase (PDHC) and

		pyruvate utilization in the Krebs Cycle (Acin-Perez, Hoyos et al. 2010). Vitamin-A is a common worldwide vitamin deficiency, putting everyone at risk, especially when intakes of beta carotene are low due to such incredibly low vegetable intakes. Beta carotene can be converted to Vitamin-A in the body.
Vitamin-D	Gene transcription Multiple sites of action	Vital for mitochondrial integrity and protection of mitochondria from Reactive Oxygen Species (ROS) (Ricca, Aillon et al. 2018). Vitamin-D supports Oxidative Phosphorylation (OXPHOS) and optimal ATP production. Remember winter months and low Vitamin-D levels. Do children have adequate Vitamin-D levels?
Vitamin-B1 (Thiamine)	Pyruvate Dehydrogenase Complex (PDHC)* *Also affected by Vitamin-A (see above)	Vit-B1 is the 'spark' for oxidative phosphorylation in the mitochondria where pyruvate forms Acetyl CoA through PDHC action. Acetyl CoA enters the Krebs Cycle to kick-start ATP generation.
Vitamin-B2 Riboflavin	FADH2/FAD	FADH2/FAD and NADH/NAD^+ have major impacts on ATP production (Haddad and Mohiuddin 2021). $FADH_2$ passes on electrons to Complex-II (Feher 2017)
Vitamin-B3 (Niacin; Nicotaminde)	NADH	Passes on highly charged electrons to Complex-I (Feher 2017)
Vitamins B1, B2, B3, B5, B6, B8 and B12 + Iron and Magnesium	Eight oxidations in the Krebs Cycle from Acetyl-CoA to energy in the form of NADH & FADH2	NADH and $FADH_2$ kick-start the creation of ATP from their high-energy electrons that enter the mitochondrial respiratory chain for ATP extraction at the abovementioned locations. (DiMauro, Quinzii et al. 2007).
Zinc	A critical mineral affects around 300 enzyme systems, but	For example, zinc is vital for pyruvate transport to kick-start energy production in the mitochondria (Yang, Wang et al. 2017), Pyruvate transport is crucial for ATP production and is impaired if Zinc is deficient.

Iron deficiency is a profound energetic insult to cells. Iron deficiency in pregnancy and children is immensely common and dangerous

Iron deficiency is the most common nutritional deficiency globally, affecting a massive 30% of the world's population (Kumar, Sharma et al. 2022). In research studies, iron deficiency depleted ATP in heart cells by a whopping 74% (Hoes, Grote Beverborg et al. 2018).

Missing iron deficiency in children and prospective mums should be seen as gross medical malpractice due to the massive physical and mental impacts that iron deficiency can inflict long-term. Iron deficiency is very common in heart failure and is not a mineral deficiency to miss. Imagine a failing heart with less and less energy due to a mineral deficiency that is so easily corrected.

Mental health disorders are also skyrocketing in populations. An article in the Medical Journal of Australia (MJA) states the mental health of young Australians is "rapidly declining", but this is a worldwide trend (McGorry, Coghill et al. 2023). Sure, there are many stressors, from climate change to wars or COVID-19, robbing people of life, opportunity and mental health stability. These stressors, however, are not the only problem. With metabolic disease also skyrocketing, we have brains that are damaged and unprepared for such stressors. A brain that lacks micronutrient support and energy becomes less and less resilient to handle any stress in life.

A huge correlation exists between mental health disorders and metabolic disease. Appendix-34 summarises brain impacts caused by metabolic disease. Imagine then these poor souls suffering mental health disorders with undoubtedly poor nutritional intakes and, in all probability, a wealth of nutrient deficiencies.

A study was published showing an incredibly high prevalence of iron deficiency in a wealthy country like Australia. This study showed that an astonishing 75% of infants between 6 and 12 months and 1 in 3 toddlers suffered from iron deficiency (Moumin, Netting et al. 2022). Where is that "optimal diet" when you need it? Considering how long an iron deficiency may exist before it is diagnosed, this is staggering as there would be a very long period of biological damage caused by unrecognised iron deficiency. Early childhood impacts can leave a lasting health legacy.

Iron deficiency is a huge micronutrient crisis if we consider potential ***permanent cellular damage*** due to our cellular energy being hammered. Such damage will not be recognised at the time, even after years or decades of iron deficiency neglect, but will manifest as behavioural problems, mental health disorders, dementia or organ failure later in life. Iron deficiency progresses slowly in children, but waiting for anaemia, pale skin, and lethargy to manifest is a sheer disaster. Any child with a behavioural problem should be assessed for a nutrient deficiency such as iron. Our "biological rot" is worsened by deficiencies like iron deficiency.

The dangers of iron deficiency range from anaemia that cannot deliver enough oxygen to the brain or heart, as iron is vital for the oxygen-carrying capacity of haemoglobin, to shortness of breath, irregular heart rhythms, worsening of heart failure and even death if the iron deficiency is severe enough. Researchers have established that iron deficiency can have a long-lasting effect on the brain and cognitive outcomes that persist long after iron deficiency is treated (Lozoff, Beard et al. 2006).

I have discussed that 60% - 70% of oxygen supply to tissues and organ systems is delivered by our vital microcirculation networks (Munoz, Lucas et al. 2020). If we then add microvascular disease, which is a continuum leading to progressive blockage of blood supply to tissues and organs, we now have a multiplier effect where the oxygen supply for energy production is made worse by the decreased oxygen-carrying capacity of red blood cells due to iron deficiency. All micronutrient deficiencies will be magnified greatly by a failing microcirculation network that shatters the delivery of these critical nutrients to cells, tissues and organ systems.

It is important to remember that just because someone has a significant deficiency, such as iron, this does not mean that the other ATP-depleting factors are not in play as well to make the effects of that iron deficiency far worse simultaneously. When is this multiplier effect ever considered? We seem to think that these factors wait in queue for a green signal to act.

In children, we have fussy eating, creating a nutrient intake nightmare. Where are they getting their iron from? Iron deficiency is common in children, and where do they ever eat an "optimal diet"? From the stodgy cereal (carb-rich) gruel dietitians want them to eat to the iron-deficient and insulin-elevating dairy "coming out of their nostrils"? The fact that cow's milk may be deficient in iron doesn't seem to stop this practice in babies. The dairy "police" will always use fear tactics to ensure the dairy industry survives. There are many negatives to using dairy, and sadly, a well-designed plant-based diet is not even considered in babies. Dietitians will use baby growth concerns against plant-based formulas, which is ridiculous when that formula provides alternative fuel sources in the form of good fats and amino acids that can be converted to glucose to drive growth needs. It is downright deception to think animal-based food is required in order to survive. Food is not essential. Only the nutrients and energy within those foods are crucial. Are we setting babies and children up for cancer in future, feeding them animal flesh to prop up the Meat & Livestock industry? Such nutrition recommendations for children belong to the Dark Ages, in my opinion. Women are at high risk for iron deficiency due to menstrual blood loss that spills over into pregnancy, where iron deficiency accelerates in pregnancy due to the demand of the fetus.

From a common iron insufficiency problem to a deficiency in omega-3 intake to reduced intake of all the other nutrients needed in appropriate quantities - we risk these little lives by not supplementing them, leaving it to chance, believing that parents have a brilliant knowledge about foods and the specific nutrients they contain. Interestingly, dietitians failed to ensure that 43 meals met even the Recommended Daily Allowances for the *Arkansas Diet Manual (Dollahite, Franklin MS et al. 1995).* Ouch!

We discussed the 3-fold increase of gestational diabetes with higher consumption of animal flesh heme iron in the BIG-10 Womb-to-Tomb list. Insulin resistance plus iron deficiency is a tragedy for pregnant women and their developing babies, who need huge amounts of energy for growth and development.

Bioenergetic failure is well established in insulin resistance syndromes like Metabolic Syndrome (MetS), where bioenergetic failure will trigger insulin resistance (Carré and Affourtit 2019).

No lingering mineral deficiency will end well for cells. Iron is critical for various components along the energy-extracting pathways in cells that produce ATP. The Electron Transport Chain (ETC) has twelve (x12) iron-sulphur (Fe-S) complexes and several iron-containing heme molecules to function (Jeong, Crooks et al. 2011). Also, a critical enzyme, Aconitase, in the Krebs Cycle, the pathway before the Electron Transport Chain (ETC), requires four iron-sulphur complexes (x4 Fe-S) (Meyron-Holtz, Ghosh et al. 2004). Not only is Aconitase affected by iron deficiency, but we also have three other Krebs Cycle enzymes that become impaired with iron deficiency – citrate synthase, isocitric dehydrogenase, and succinate dehydrogenase (Oexle, Gnaiger et al. 1999).

Now imagine the Aconitase enzyme being further inhibited from higher uric acid levels as well as iron deficiency due to fructose impacts. Do people with iron deficiency watch their sugar intake (50% fructose) and high fructose (fruit, fruit juice, dried fruit, honey, agave, soda) consumption? So, we have two extremely common factors in sugar/fructose consumption producing higher uric acid levels and iron deficiency that profoundly affect cell energy production and work simultaneously to undermine ATP production. Appendix-1 shows the sequence of events with fructose leading to high cellular uric acid levels.

An Austrian study showed that 12% of pregnant women suffer from an iron deficiency at the beginning of pregnancy, but iron deficiency accelerates to 65% as the pregnancy progresses due to the additional iron needs of the mother and developing fetus (Zeisler, Dietrich et al. 2021). It is truly sad when this one factor can be so easily prevented. Other findings have shown that 40%-50% of pregnant women and children after birth suffer from iron deficiency (Bastian, von Hohenberg et al. 2019).

So, why is iron deficiency (ID) so important? "***From a human health perspective, early-life ID affects ~ 40%-50% of fetuses and***

children, resulting in long-term neurobehavioral dysfunction." *(Bastian, von Hohenberg et al. 2019).* The same authors state that gestational iron deficiency: "***increases the risk of significant psychopathologies, including schizophrenia, autism spectrum disorders, attention deficit hyperactivity disorder, bipolar disorder, and depression in the offspring later in life.***" *(Bastian, von Hohenberg et al. 2019)* We need to keep in mind the impacts on the mother as well.

It has been found that iron deficiency can have a striking 74% reduction in intracellular ATP levels (Hoes, Grote Beverborg et al. 2018).

Research has shown that chelating iron (removing iron) from cultured nerve cells resulted in an immense 84% lowered Glycolytic Pathway capacity and that ATP production in those cells was lower by 21% (Bastian, von Hohenberg et al. 2019). See Appendix-29, which shows where glycolysis fits in with the Krebs Cycle and then the mitochondria's electron transport chain (ETC) to produce ATP.

Optimal nutrient intake in the pregnant woman and the first 1000 days of a child's life are critical (Scott 2020). Nutrient deficiencies at this early stage could massively impact the high prevalence of chronic diseases and mental health disorders in the long term—such a wasted opportunity for prevention. The greatest gift you can give yourself, a newborn and a growing child, is to ensure no one lacks even one micronutrient. Please have your iron levels checked.

So, what tests should you have done to see if your iron levels are OK?

According to new findings published in the Lancet Haematology, figures for iron deficiency in both women and young children may be greatly underestimated (Mei, Addo et al. 2021). This underestimation is because we are using an outdated means of testing for iron deficiency. The *Lancet Haematology* researchers mentioned above stated that the WHO guidelines for using ferritin to detect iron deficiency are greatly misleading as Ferritin is a marker of more advanced iron deficiency.

Ferritin levels can rise due to inflammatory conditions (a so-called acute phase reactant). As the *Lancet Haematology* paper discussed, haemoglobin **and *soluble transferrin receptor (sTfR)*** are far better indicators. If sTfR and haemoglobin are used as indicators of iron deficiency rather than ferritin, it would mean that 30% of women and children in the USA could be considered iron deficient, thus identifying and enabling iron supplementation to begin at a crucial time (Mei, Addo et al. 2021).

Heartburn anyone? Let's use a Proton Pump Inhibitors (PPI) and pull the rug from iron and other micronutrients

Using powerful antacid PPIs for heartburn can block mineral and vitamin absorption. We thus magnify the effects of already present poor diets and already existing micronutrient deficiencies (hidden hunger) by the thoughtless use of drugs that can rob cells of critical nutrients. Micronutrient deficiencies can significantly impact cell energy pathways and cell signalling mechanisms, as you now know. Thus, iatrogenic (medically caused) cell starvation is yet another huge detrimental issue caused by drugs that often should never be used long-term and yet precisely, this is what is done in real life. Never use these PPIs around pregnancy. Medicine is adding to this pandemic of chronic diseases.

Shockingly, you can get these PPIs over the counter. PPIs can cause mineral and vitamin deficiencies that range from barely noticeable to obvious. Pharma-influenced research will always downplay this problem. The term "mild" deficiency should never be used. A cell either gets the nutrient resources it needs for optimal function or doesn't. The Cell Starvation Model predicts these PPIs will cause Type-2 Diabetes Mellitus, heart and vascular disease, renal failure and dementia. And so, research shows exactly this. The long-term use of PPIs does indeed increase the risk of "diabetes" by a huge 24% (Yuan, He et al. 2021), and there is a significantly higher risk of developing dementia in individuals who use PPIs over 4 years (Northuis, Bell et al. 2023). Remember, if we used early biomarkers for metabolically related illness instead of sledgehammer glucose cut-off points, this 24% risk would soar skyward.

Because medical researchers and professionals seem unaware of the underlying bioenergetic impacts of micronutrient deficiencies, they never determine how and why these complications occur. Biased PPI research is understandable as PPIs are a multibillion-dollar industry. Paid research by Pharma through their guns-for-hire medical gurus will always paint a rosy picture of these and other drugs.

PPIs are incredibly potent antacids and can decrease intragastric hydrogen by several hundred to thousand-fold and decrease intragastric pH by several units (Heidelbaugh 2013).

It is easy enough to see how PPIs can pull the rug from energy-producing pathways by depleting vital cofactors and coenzymes needed for the enzymes of energy-producing pathways to function. Getting dementia or heart disease in exchange for treating GORD/GERD (reflux) seems like a very steep price to pay.

We must have an acidic pH in the stomach to absorb B12, which must be cleaved from the surrounding dietary protein by stomach acid. For example, Pepsin, the stomach enzyme needed to free Vitamin-B12, can only be created if powerful stomach acid acts on pepsinogen to produce the active protein-digesting enzyme pepsin. This stomach acid also changes the redox state of minerals like magnesium, calcium, and iron, enabling them to be absorbed. Imagine the huge risk of 1 in 3 people worldwide having iron deficiency and, on top of this, taking a PPI that impairs the absorption of iron, magnesium and other minerals plus worsening Vitamin-C and B12 adequacy, all needed for energy production.

Stomach acid is powerful and can sterilise food, eliminating pathogens or organisms that can disrupt the gut microbiome. That gut bowel overgrowth can occur (dysbiosis) with PPI use should come as no surprise. It is a warning sign of how damaging PPIs can be to someone. Is the gut microbiome important? Yes indeed!

The medical profession often ignores the concept of subclinical (unnoticeable disease) caused by barely measurable reductions of vitamins or minerals. It has been found that 80% of those in the USA purchase a PPI without a script or any medical evaluation (Heidelbaugh 2013). You can buy a PPI over the counter in Australia and many other countries, and this is a horrendous practice that hugely benefits pharmaceutical corporations, but at what price to society?

PPIs can cause a deficiency of iron, magnesium, Vitamin-B12, and Vitamin-C. (Heidelbaugh 2013)

So, the three micronutrients affected by PPIs – iron, magnesium and Vitamin-B12 -can all profoundly impair cell ATP production. Iron deficiency can markedly impair Complex-IV of the Electron Transport Chain (ETC) by 95%, and Vitamin-B12 can significantly impact the Krebs Cycle that feeds into the ETC of mitochondria (See Appendix-7). We have discussed how critical magnesium is to insulin action, ATP-Synthase and ATP production – See Appendix-29. So, one powerful PPI drug can have multiple and terrible effects on cell energy networks. Yet all of this will be downplayed in medical research, and foolish doctors hand PPIs out like lollies.

PPIs are just one example of several medications that can cause profound disease in individuals through micronutrient impacts. It has been stated that anywhere from 1 billion to 10 billion biochemical reactions occur in a human cell every second (Hunyady 2022). Even if we take the lower figure of 1 billion reactions per second, and if we use the often quoted 37.2 trillion number for cells in the human body (Bianconi, Piovesan et al. 2013), we have 1 billion reactions occurring in our 37.2 trillion cells every second. This figure is an astronomical number of reactions every second of our lives, and without adequate nutrient support, it is easy to see how the human body can significantly deteriorate over time.

Many of our elderly take PPIs even though 20% to 29% may already have a Vitamin-B12 deficiency (Heidelbaugh 2013). Sad. Drug sales have become more important than nutrient adequacy in individuals at a vulnerable time of their lives. Atrophic gastritis in older adults, caused by various factors such as Helicobacter Pylori or autoimmunity, damages the lining of the stomach and is present in the general population, but there is a much higher prevalence in older individuals. Atrophic gastritis impacts Vitamin-B12 and iron absorption, and the low gastric acid levels in this disease process affect the absorption of many other minerals (Cavalcoli, Zilli et al. 2017).

How absurd is it then that doctors rarely consider this common decreased gastric acid output problem of atrophic gastritis in older people that often results in achlorhydria (a total lack of acid) and decreased intrinsic factor (IF) production leading to decreased Vitamin-B12 absorption? This gastritis can frequently present as indigestion, so the knee-jerk reaction by doctors or pharmacists is to recommend a powerful PPI acid suppressant to individuals with already suppressed acid production. Go figure. So clever (not)!

We foolishly use PPIs in babies and children

How dreadful then that despite all of the risks of a medication that in the vast majority of cases cannot be justified when other far less damaging options are present, we regrettably give these incredibly potent PPIs to babies under three months of age to "calm" them down from presumed reflux - GORD or GERD. Yet, gastroesophageal reflux has never been proven to cause excessive crying and irritability in babies. We use PPIs in babies based on another hypothesis (guess), like our failed glucose and lipid hypotheses for diabetes, heart and vascular disease.

Lacking evidence doesn't get in the way of using drugs in a clinical circumstance when money can be made. Only when it comes to nutrients will the medical and dietetic professions cry out loudly that we need a few centuries of research on nutrient safety, and yet no cries whatsoever when we release drugs rapidly into populations with little testing after paying the ferryman (a drug regulator) their dues to get this drug across the "river" and into populations. On the flip side, those who cry out about nutrient safety forget nutrient trials began when human beings started walking the earth and consuming food. Our early human ancestors have been involved in nutrient safety trials from the moment food was placed in their mouths over millions of years. Can any drug trial match that?

A lack of evidence hasn't stopped these powerful PPI drugs from being used in highly vulnerable and nutrient-dependent children based on a presumption of GORD/GERD (Smith, Israel et al. 2013).

A paper published in JAMA has shown a 34% increased risk of serious infections in children given PPIs (Lassalle, Zureik et al. 2023). How will immunity (as a super-system) with a voracious appetite for nutrient and energy resources function if it doesn't have all the nutrient resources it needs in vast quantities when activated? Is it any wonder, then, that depleted nutrient levels and a competing immune system in children will result in serious infections? It is deplorable that PPIs are given to babies and children at a stage when they depend on a complete and adequate supply of micronutrients every second of every day!

Only drug-dazzled researchers and medical gurus under Pharma's thumb would argue that PPIs in children have no potential adverse effects when we know PPIs trigger iron. calcium, magnesium, Vitamin-C and Vitamin-B12 deficiencies. Yet, all these deficiencies, even if mild to undetectable, can have profound consequences on DNA and cancer risk (Ames 1999, Ames 2006) (Ames 2001). Iron deficiency, for example, can have a marked impact on pregnancy and childhood outcomes without manifesting as anaemia (Liu, Barks et al. 2021).

PPIs can seriously impact nutrient levels, such as life-threatening low magnesium levels (hypomagnesaemia) (Regolisti, Cabassi et al. 2010). Please remember the critical role of magnesium in not only ATP creation but also ATP activation. PPIs are commonly handed out in medical practice, and individuals are kept on this long-term mindlessly. This practice shows the medical profession's disregard for critical nutrients in disease causation and the irresponsible set-and-forget mentality with regard to medications.

The North American Society for Pediatric Gastroenterology, Hepatology and Nutrition and the European Society for Paediatric Gastroenterology, Hepatology, and Nutrition (ESPGHAN) have called for an end to giving PPIs to babies unless there is a compelling medical reason to do so (Smith, Israel et al. 2013). Hopefully, this dreadful practice will end soon, but doctors often don't follow medical advice or evidence-based research. It is as if the doctors know better, so why bother with recommendations that may interfere with their way of practising medicine or their bottom line?

How dreadful that a PPI would ever be considered in babies when safe age-appropriate thickeners can be used for formulas such as alginate, mucilage, or gums that can be used instead to prevent presumed but unproven acid reflux. These natural compounds could also act as valuable prebiotics for the gut microbiome. This approach as well may not help a cranky baby, but it certainly won't harm them and, in fact, will help their critical immune-enhancing gut microbiomes and not destroy the vitally important gut microbiome.

PPIs may even make babies crankier through a detrimental effect on the gut-brain axis. It is well-established that PPIs can cause gut dysbiosis. Ahh, but wait, how will Pharma make billions of dollars from this healthy approach? How will corrupt researchers and medical gurus make a dollar to fund their lifestyles through paid research or strut stages in conferences? How do GPs get through their allotted 6-minute consultations without a script?

As we are constantly told, the first 1000 days of a child's life after birth are critical to developing tissues and organ systems, including the brain and IQ (Scott 2020). So, what are we doing with PPIs given to babies at a crucial time of brain and body organ development? We undermine vital micronutrient adequacy in childhood for no good reason. We instead put them at long-term risk for dreadful diseases.

It is not surprising that a paper written in The Journal of Clinical Endocrinology & Metabolism in 2022 stated that:

"Regular and prolonged use of PPIs is associated with a higher risk of diabetes. Physicians should therefore avoid unnecessary prescription of this class of drugs, particularly for long-term use." (Ciardullo, Rea et al. 2022)

Not proven, not proven, not proven: Well, prove it to me!

The tobacco industry needed a way to confuse populations and professions. So what they came up with was the following:

"Devised in the 1950s and '60s, the tobacco industry's strategy was embodied in a script written by the lawyers. Every tobacco company executive in the public eye was told to learn the script backwards and forwards, no deviation was allowed. The basic premise was simple—smoking had not been proven to cause cancer. Not proven, not proven, not proven—this would be stated insistently and repeatedly. Inject a thin wedge of doubt, create controversy, and never deviate from the prepared line. It was a simple plan, and it worked." (Brownell and Warner 2009)

What a corrupt industry, using unethical lawyers to devise this strategy, even as vast numbers of people died from tobacco-related diseases. We now have something very similar from the dietetic associations: "***There are no good or bad foods.***". Anything and everything is fine to eat "***in moderation***". This thinking mimics what the National Rifle Association (NRA) stated in the USA: "***The only thing that stops a bad guy with a gun is a good guy with a gun.***" The sentiment is clear enough for the food industry to borrow from and twist to suit their needs. Is it OK for anyone with insulin resistance who cannot tolerate glucose to consume sugar daily? Can they have a can of sugar-sweetened soda or have sugar-rich desserts? Is this "moderation"?

So, as populations are getting sicker and sicker, we borrow disingenuous and dangerous arguments and punchlines from other associations that have blood on their hands. For the 100s of millions with insulin resistance in populations, how dare we ever say that sugar or fructose or high-energy foods can ever be consumed in moderation? Can a person with diabetes on the brink of a catastrophic cardiovascular event have ½ a can or one can of sugar-sweetened soda a day? How absolutely dumb to even think this way, but I guess if you are embedded in the sugar industry, you will tell people it is OK to do so. I say it is up to dietetics to prove it to us, not empty rhetoric designed to sell grains, dairy, sugar, fructose, sugar-sweetened beverages, etc. Prove that "moderation" is safe – Prove it, prove it, prove it!

Three selfish super-systems that hog energy and nutrient resources

Energy balance is critical to our survival. In times of crisis, such as an infection or physical trauma, we have a hierarchy for energy utilization, and in this instance, the immune system has the highest rank (Straub 2017).

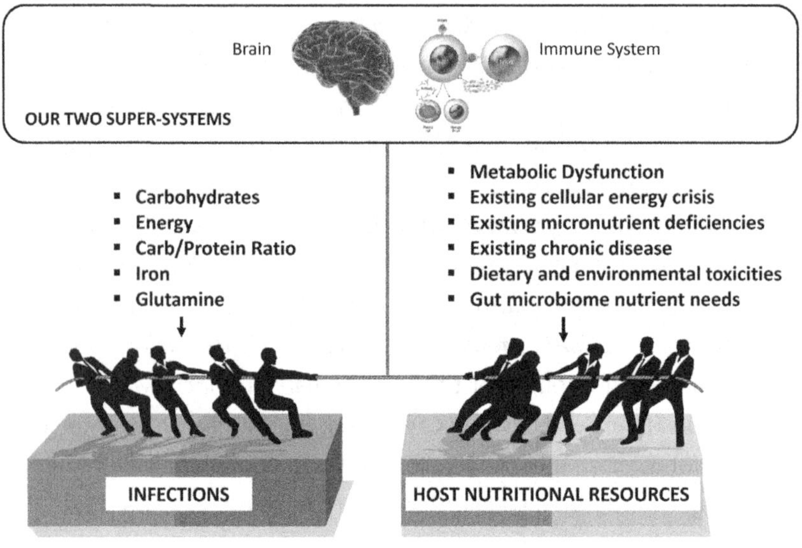

Two ever-present selfish super-systems compete for energy and nutrient resources. These ever-present energy and nutrient-hogging systems are the brain and immune systems. These energy hogs can draw energy and nutrient resources from already struggling insulin-resistant cells caused by all the factors driving disease in the 21st-century. Remember, we often have decades before we see the metabolic markers of insulin resistance rise. Metabolic function is fragile, with many common cellular "shocks" that will disrupt this metabolic function, tipping us over into metabolic dysfunction.

We must consider that background systemic inflammation from various sources in the body means our immune system will be constantly activated and thus voraciously consuming nutrient resources, drawing them away from already struggling cells starved of nutrient resources and energy. No doubt, a common presentation to a doctor is lethargy, and immune super-system activation should be considered a factor adding to this misery of ever-present tiredness. There is a third super-system, which is conditional on pregnancy.

So the three energy and nutrient-hogging systems are:

1. **The immune system:** Especially when activated.
2. **The brain:** Constant background glucose demand working at full-throttle.
3. **Pregnancy & Foetal Demand:** This foetal super-system is conditional on pregnancy to meet the baby's developmental needs and breastfeeding demands.

This foetal demand draws energy resources from already affected cells in the mother struggling to meet her energy and nutrient needs. This nutrient tug-of-war can trigger decompensation in pregnancy to provoke frank diabetes if nutrient resources are not provided in adequate amounts throughout pregnancy and breastfeeding for the mother and baby. Who thinks of this nutrient resource tug-of-war between the fetus and pregnant mother?

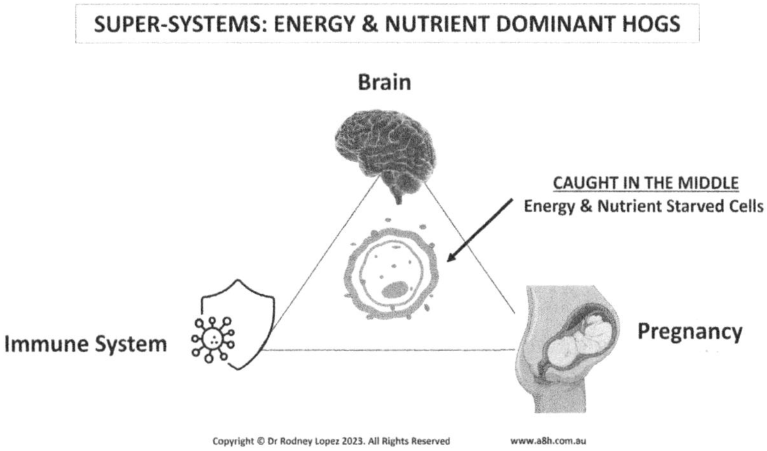

The activated immune system can consume 25%-30% of the Basal Metabolic Rate (BMR) (Straub 2017, Almajwal, Alam et al. 2018). This energy consumption is a huge drain on energy and nutrient resources by an activated immune system. When is the immune system never activated?

There are many sources of inflammation, from deep visceral fat pouring out inflammatory chemicals to PM2.5 particles embedded in our lungs from bushfires to other air pollution particulates and inflammation from postprandial (after-eating) impacts. We must remember that we have background insulin resistance (IR) in vast numbers in populations globally, where IR is a known driver of oxidative stress and inflammation. Monumental numbers already have metabolic markers for insulin resistance in populations globally, indicating IR, metabolic dysfunction, and inflammation are rampant problems in populations.

The brain makes up only 2% of body weight but consumes a whopping 20% of the body's total energy expenditure (Cunnane, Trushina et al. 2020). Imagine these energy hogs against the background of all the other energy-robbing factors discussed in the BIG-10 Womb-to-Tomb list. The brain's preferred energy source is glucose, but it can also use ketone bodies during fasting produced from fat utilisation. Inducing ketosis is a very clever way to overcome the barriers caused by insulin resistance for body and brain cells. We should all assume that insulin resistance will be our fate. The Oxford Community Diabetes Study showed that almost 100% of our older population suffers from overt diabetes, and we should proceed with this fate in mind (Neil, Thompson et al. 1989).

Immune cells are also at the mercy of insulin resistance (Makhijani, Basso et al. 2023). Immune cells suffering from insulin resistance, along with other mechanisms, explain why those with insulin resistance, MetS, and Diabetes are at high risk for several severe infections and cancer. It makes sense to use nutritional ketosis to supply immune cells with the energy they need to fight off disease and cancer. We will discuss this in more detail in the final chapter.

Gestational diabetes has tripled over the past two decades (AIHW 2019). So imagine mothers at huge risk for diabetes where the fetus becomes a super-system, drawing energy and nutrient resources away from the mother. Insulin resistance in these mothers is already limiting fuel (glucose) entry into cells and decreasing cellular access to the building resources they need. How easy is it for the mum to decompensate to overt diabetes in pregnancy, with the fetus now making matters worse by competing for nutrient resources, increasing that mum's cell starvation pressures? How negligent that medicine and dietetics don't have a laser-like focus on nutrient adequacy from preconception to breastfeeding. Nutrient adequacy is haphazard around pregnancy, and the risk of nutrient inadequacy is unnecessary and irresponsible.

The prevalence of prediabetes in women post-GDM can be just over 50%, a hugely unacceptable statistic. Yet, for a woman who develops gestational diabetes (GDM), the risk of T2DM after birth is twenty times (20x) the chance of a woman who does not have GDM (Shivashri, Hannah et al. 2022)—huge impacts caused by a super-system that is the fetus competing with the mother for resources.

Post delivery and breastfeeding in a mother at risk of diabetes, we should strongly consider a nutritional ketosis diet, ensuring that the mother gets every nutrient under the sun along with the necessary calories through a thorough, mindful diet. A high-carb diet has no place in this circumstance. Breastfeeding, it is stated, requires 400 calories to 500 calories above the mother's needs. Is it any wonder that a woman with gestational diabetes is at such massive risk for diabetes or heart attacks and strokes after birth when ridiculous high-carb recommendations are made to insulin-resistant mothers who can't use that glucose as fuel to power ATP production anyway?

There is a 70% risk of a woman with gestational diabetes mellitus (GDM) developing diabetes (T2DM) from 6 weeks after delivery, with a high risk of T2DM to 28 years. However, the highest risk for T2DM is a mere 3 to 6 years after delivery (Shivashri, Hannah et al. 2022). Nutrient adequacy and a ketosis diet should extend for years beyond child delivery and breastfeeding. Being proactive seems anathema to the medical profession, which appears very silent on nutritional adequacy due to the drug-centric model, failing all of us and failing women.

COVID-19: Immune Supersystem Activation Energy Demands & Triggering Diabetes.

Dietetic advice should not harm, but the opposite is true. Long Covid can potentially tip many early in the insulin resistance continuum to frank diabetes and chronic diseases prematurely. For example, those recovering from COVID-19 had a 40% increased risk of developing diabetes (Xie and Al-Aly 2022). Many who landed in an intensive care unit due to COVID-19 were found to have diabetes. Note the term "diabetes" as a late blood glucose cut-off point. Imagine the percentage jumping skyward from 40% if we used early markers of metabolic dysfunction rather than the fake diabetes glucose cut-off point. We have yet to see the legacy of COVID-19 in the decades to come.

The question often posed is, "Why are people developing diabetes after COVID-19?" but this question is redundant if we consider the Cell Starvation Model (CSM) and all the factors leading to insulin resistance from the womb to the tomb. It should be obvious that monumental numbers were already affected by insulin resistance long before COVID-19 struck. All COVID-19 did was activate the immune super-system even further, which then hogged nutrient resources to deprive already struggling insulin-resistant energy-deprived cells, thus triggering cell starvation and diabetes. COVID-19 only unmasked the already smouldering "prediabetes" problem in people's lives that medicine ignores.

The Cell Starvation Model predicts the effects of COVID-19.

An insufficient intake of Vitamin-D can impair mitochondrial OXPHOS

OXPHOS is the process that generates around 90% of all ATP needed for cells (Sorriento, Pascale et al. 2014).

We now know that Vitamin-D has a critical role in mitochondrial oxidative phosphorylation (OXPHOS) energy metabolism, and we also know how vital magnesium is to OXPHOS in the final stage of ATP production by ATP-Synthase. The ATP-Synthase enzyme is dependent on magnesium for it to work, as I have discussed. However, many are unaware of magnesium's vital role in Vitamin-D metabolism. Doctors and dietitians are not trained to see the amazing nutrient interrelationships and synergies involved in the human body.

Virtually all stages of Vitamin-D metabolism are magnesium-dependent (Dominguez, Veronese et al. 2021). This magnesium-Vitamin-D interrelationship is shown in Appendix-20. Both magnesium and Vitamin-D are common deficiencies and will affect cell energy metabolism in everyone, with a special impact in pregnancy because a mother competes with the developing baby for nutrient resources, as discussed above.

Up to 40%, according to one evaluation of those living in the UK during winter months, suffer from Vitamin-D deficiency (Calame, Street et al. 2020). The Australian government-sponsored Healthdirect, which provides health information to the nation, states that 1 in 3 (33%) Australians suffer from mild, moderate or severe Vitamin-D deficiency (HealthDirect 2022).

As I have stressed in this book, there is no such thing as a "mild" micronutrient deficiency. The term "mild" is a disgrace when used by medical or dietetic practitioners. When we consider a so-called "mild" increase in blood glucose, we fail to recognise that we are well along the insulin resistance continuum to even reach this "mild" glucose cut-off point. We either have optimal nutrient resources or not. Therefore, the assumption that a mild deficiency cannot produce profound cellular impacts with long-term complications is completely wrong and a mindless concept.

It is important to know that although negative bioenergetic impacts are in constant action due to all the BIG-10 factors, we have episodic (acute) hits like iron deficiency, magnesium deficiency or Vitamin-D deficiency that exacerbate cell energy production along the course of a lifetime. Each episodic hit will heighten cellular energy and structural damage and impact ATP production in the long term, thus triggering or exacerbating insulin resistance. These nutrient impacts set us on a path to insulin resistance from a very early age. Long-term damage can occur from any significant micronutrient deficiency.

Cells undergoing an energy crisis and structural decline will need warning signals (biosignals) and adaptations to survive

When cells undergo any crisis, from a virus invading our cells to trauma, the cells send out distress signals that can be seen as a cry for help. This crisis signalling allows the body to respond appropriately in various ways depending on the crisis involved. Cellular energy decline is a serious existential threat. It is no wonder that evolution is so concerned with energy expenditure, conservation, and storage that it has developed an exquisite signalling system to warn us of a threat to cells. This energy vigilance and alarm signalling has been honed in our ancient human ancestral cells and passed down to present-day humans over millions of years.

The central theme in this book is that cells start to lose the ability to create energy in the form of ATP programmed in the womb and then from birth onwards by all the factors I have mentioned. With ATP in decline, cells do not have the power to drive cell anabolic (synthesis) functions, repair themselves or create cellular balance through allostatic and homeostatic mechanisms. These cellular insults are not conducive to cells surviving unless the body notices these adverse impacts and then takes action to reverse these effects.

Cellular anabolic (building) functions require significant energy (ATP) inputs to drive biochemical and molecular processes and reverse entropy (decay). We will look at all our biomarkers, including glucose and others, as sources of energy or as cell building blocks. The body adapts to cells in crisis and calls upon these biomarkers to support these cells suffering an energy crisis. Declining energy levels will then lead to distress signalling. There are many signals for low cellular energy, but these are complex. I have shown four important signals in the graphic above – Adenosine, Uric Acid, Inflammation and Ketone Bodies.

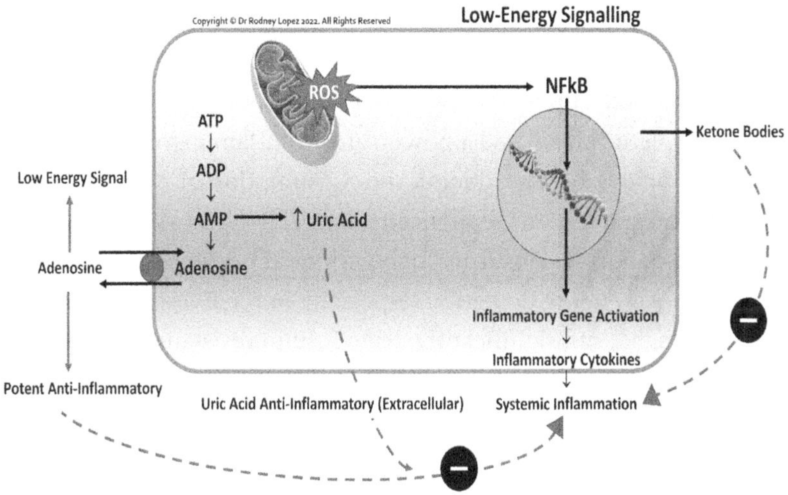

ATP is Adenosine Triphosphate, which means x3 phosphate bonds. Once all three phosphates are removed to provide cells with energy, we are left with the energy-depleted adenosine backbone. It thus makes sense that adenosine is a low-energy signal. Adenosine can also be seen as an adaptation to a cellular energy crisis, not just a signal, because adenosine is a potent anti-inflammatory molecule (Cronstein 1994). This anti-inflammatory effect of low-energy signalling compounds is important as inflammation drives most, if not all, diseases. Adenosine is also a neurotransmitter involved in neuromodulation, supporting brain health and energy balance (Chang, Wu et al. 2021).

ATP decline will also affect the synthesis and repair of our mitochondria. As a result, mitochondria can decrease in number (reduced mitochondrial biogenesis) and become structurally weak and defective, making the mitochondria susceptible to Reactive Oxygen Species (ROS). Damaged mitochondria can trigger inflammatory genes and lead to systemic inflammation. Inflammation thus becomes a marker for cellular distress and energy decline indicative of mitochondrial distress.

Vitamin-D, I would like to mention, has a powerful role in diminishing this ROS damage to mitochondria (Ricca, Aillon et al. 2018). As a potent anti-inflammatory, adenosine can offset increased inflammation caused by mitochondrial deterioration (Cronstein 1994). The same applies to uric acid as an adaptation, acting as an energy-depleted signal and a powerful anti-inflammatory outside cells. Uric acid is a by-product of the consumption of ATP to provide energy. You can see this sequence from ATP → ADP → AMP → Uric Acid in Appendix-1. Unsurprisingly, uric acid becomes a potent biomarker for energy depletion, especially in the liver, an organ that, when damaged, can significantly drive insulin resistance (Petrie, Patman et al. 2013).

Like adenosine, uric acid acts as both a biosignal of ATP depletion and as an adaptation to offset the increasing systemic inflammation that occurs with insulin resistance and metabolic dysfunction affected cells. Uric Acid is often raised in MetS or diabetes. Likewise, Ketone Bodies (KBs) are produced in cell starvation, and these also act as a signal of cell starvation, but KBs also have powerful effects on dampening inflammation by activating many anti-inflammatory gene sets (Kolb, Kempf et al. 2021).

Uric acid is a powerful antioxidant, but only outside cells. Inside a cell, uric acid is a prooxidant (causes damage) within cells (Sautin and Johnson 2008). This antioxidant adaptation of uric acid can be distributed widely in the body to dampen pervasive inflammation associated with the insulin resistance continuum and cellular damage. All of this is a delicate balance trying to restore cellular energy, function and balance.

CHAPTER 4

Fiendish Fructose: Swift ATP depletion, insulin resistance, fatty liver

A gene that doesn't even work allows fructose to decrease cell energy (ATP) rapidly. Fructose increases risk of insulin resistance, high uric acid, overfat, overweight, obesity and fatty liver

"Nothing in biology makes sense except in the light of evolution," Theodosius Dobzhansky

Right under our noses is one of the biggest "energy bandits" found hidden in many foods that we take for granted and see as benign. Fructose will make you overfat, overweight or obese. Fructose is designed by evolution to help us store fat in our bodies, making us chubbier all over, from our bellies and hips to even our faces. Fructose consumption has increased dramatically in the last 40 years and parallels the obesity and metabolic disease pandemics.

Sugar is our nemesis. Both components of sugar (sucrose), i.e. glucose (50%) and fructose (50%), can be toxic to us, but what are governments and public health bodies doing to protect all of us? We get most of our fructose from sugar, which drenches the vast majority of the foods we consume. We have powerful food corporation interests working against us, and one of the biggest problems is the fact that governments also depend on taxes and duties derived from foods that create sugar and sweet beverages, sauces, condiments, grain products, etc., that contain sugar, and governments always seem to be under pressure from food lobbyists.

The dietetic industry succumbs to the influence of government pressures and food corporations and then convinces us that all foods are just fine. Fructose, unlike other factors, causes rapid depletion of ATP in many cells, including the liver and skeletal muscle. Both tissues are strongly linked to insulin resistance and are impacted by fructose. Fructose metabolism can be seen in Appendix-1.

It is interesting that in liver cells, high fructose levels can slash ATP production by a whopping 50% to 80%, and ATP levels can remain low for 20 hours after a fructose load. So if ATP stays low for 20 hours, will people stop eating sugar-packed foods over these 20 hours to allow ATP to go back up to normal levels? Not likely. So, with low energy levels in our liver and skeletal muscle, how can we not inch our way towards fatty liver and insulin resistance meal by meal, snack by snack?

This same research paper reported that protein synthesis in those liver cells exposed to fructose was cut by over 90% (Latta, Künstle et al. 2000). Without protein synthesis, how do you repair cell components or make new cell components, create membranes, synthesise hormones or reverse cell entropy (decay, chaos, deterioration). These changes in cell metabolism are not random but occur due to evolutionary design that wants your body to store fat as an energy source by impairing a cell's ability to burn food and create ATP. Fat storage is an evolutionary survival mechanism.

Thus, any excess calories consumed will not be burned into energy (ATP) but diverted to fat formation and storage for a "rainy day". It is important to know that we don't have to be outwardly overweight or obese, but we can be ***overfat***, which is far more common, and thus, we can see ourselves as being of normal weight and think that all is fine with regard to our health. Looks can be deceiving, right? Deep, hidden abdominal (visceral) fat is dangerous.

Now imagine the impact of this decreased level of protein synthesis caused by fructose on cell structure and ultrastructure. Fructose is behaving as an ***entropy driver*** towards more cellular decay and deterioration. We may be living in the 21st century, but we have to live with the legacy of a genetic mutation 15 million years ago designed to make us store fat due to the impending loss of fruit and fructose-rich forests at the time this uricase mutation occurred. As you will learn, those lush forests have now been replaced by 21st-century "lush forests" consisting of supermarkets and convenience stores full of foods rich in sugar and fructose-containing foods.

That fructose loading can lead to insulin resistance even in young, healthy, normal-weight men should be a huge alarm signal for all of us (Aeberli, Hochuli et al. 2013). The evidence against sugar and fructose is compelling and crushing, and yet we allow dietetic gurus to continue deceptive practices and gaslight the negative impacts of sugar, which is our main exposure to fructose, all to keep the current health-destroying food industry churning along as if there is no concern in the world as populations get sicker and sicker.

All governments who lack courage seem to care about are the duties and taxes generated by sugar extraction from foods like beets, sugarcane, sweet sorghum, or corn, as well as taxes from sugar-rich foods and beverages sold. They fear the wrath of food boards or food corporations that want to maintain the status quo irrespective of the damage to population health.

Fructose has been called "***a weapon of mass destruction***". Fructose is the "mother" of ATP-depleting factors – a super "energy bandit". ***In fact, up to 80% of ATP depletion in cells can occur within 5 minutes*** (Latta, Künstle et al. 2000). This reinforces the rapidity of cell energy loss by fructose. If fructose from sugar isn't part of a particular food you are about to eat, then it will be in the sauce or condiment or the accompanying foods, such as buns, bread, fruit juice, sugar-rich sodas, desserts, etc., that you have with that meal.

We have to remember frequent hits of fructose from that morning coffee or tea with sugar to that fruit juice at lunchtime or fruit snacks during the day. All these foods are a fructose hit to cell energy production. If we accept that our diseases later in life are programmed in childhood, then we need to look at all the sugar and fructose impacts we inflict on babies and children through fruits, fruit juices, fruit purees, dried fruit, honey, jam, fruit bars, fruit salads or the fruit we put in lunch boxes. We are priming our children for chronic illnesses. We think weaning babies by feeding them fructose-packed purees or juices is a good thing. It is not!

Let's look at how this fruit sugar became a menace to humankind.

Pure, White and Deadly: The story of sugar. We are advancing one funeral at a time

Nutritional advice by doctors and dietitians has been one big, messy situation. Both groups jumped onto the "***glucose hypothesis***" or "***glucotoxicity***" bandwagon as the fall guy for diabetes complications. This glucose hypothesis has been a miscalculated guess that ignored many other adverse impacts, such as fructose hits leading to poor prediabetes and diabetes outcomes, let alone all the after-eating impacts created by all food after-eating.

We now know that our "*glucose hypothesis*" and "***lipid hypothesis***" have failed us. How foolish have we been to see the biological damage caused by insulin resistance as due simply to glucose or abnormal blood lipids like LDL (the "bad" cholesterol)? We want simple solutions, I guess. We will discuss LDL later.

Suppose glucose or lipids are the "monsters" that we have made them out to be driving diseases. In that case, if these guesses (hypotheses) were correct, and by targeting them with pharmaceuticals, we should have seen diabetes and chronic diseases plummeting by treating them over the decades with drugs. Why, then, in fact, are these diseases exploding worldwide despite glucose or LDL-lowering drugs?

We have our professions to blame for wanting a simple answer where they don't consider multiple factors working in synergy as cell "energy bandits" leading to structural damage. We continue to fail to take into consideration ultra-common factors like fructose or after-eating impacts. However, suppose we view these simplistic notions about glucose or lipids like LDL as enemies. In that case, we can then start a pharmaceutical war on these biomarkers, and this drug war has made pharmaceutical companies unbelievably rich and enabled the medical profession to see more and more patients crammed into appointment schedulers to make a dollar as it is easy to end a 6-minute consultation with a script of one kind or another.

Professor John Yudkin, a professor of nutrition at Queen Elizabeth College, London, wrote a book in 1972 titled "***Pure, White and Deadly. How sugar is killing us and what we can do to stop it.***" After a short honeymoon period of acceptance after the book's release, it was subsequently discredited. Professor Yudkin's reputation was tarnished after the food industry and prominent nutritionists conspired against his findings and conclusions. Typical of vested interests and "experts" on the take from corporations and professionals wanting to protect their turf at any cost, including destroying the reputation of a professional. He died in 1995, a forgotten and forlorn man discredited by the corrupt, selfish and ugly behaviour of vested interests and those professionals paid by these vested interests who couldn't care less about the brilliance of mavericks who see beyond the petty (Leslie 2016).

There should be no doubt that sugar and fructose can lead to childhood and adult obesity, diabetes, hypertension, high uric acid levels and fatty liver, along with many chronic diseases. Gaslighting and keeping people ignorant is the mantra of food corporations and corrupt dietary "experts". All for profits. People are getting wiser and reading widely about all things nutrition. We also have social media that can make mincemeat of companies or professionals seen as bullies when the public's mindset has changed dramatically against certain foods, the food industry, vested interests, corrupt professionals and the drug industry.

People are now witnessing the failure of medicine, Pharma and dietetics every day as their health fails, or they see family members suffering from chronic diseases or dying suddenly and the fact they are seeing healthcare systems crumble around them. Professor Robert Lustig, a US paediatric Endocrinologist, sugar and fructose researcher interested in childhood obesity, read Prof Yudkin's book and stated:

"Holy crap, this guy got there 35 years before me." (Leslie 2016)

This character assassination shows what happens when you threaten food corporations and drug-centric approaches and where the ugly nature of humanity's self-interest kicks in. It is now getting harder to discredit someone when a massive amount of information is available to lay people in the palms of their hands. It's a pity the mavericks of yesterday did not have this social media power to crush the ugly hearts of "experts' driven by greed.

The aisles of supermarkets have greatly changed by nutrition-savvy people. The world is moving away from disease-producing staple foods and wants replacement foods for managing chronic diseases as they are witnessing the gigantic failure of drugs in preventing horrific chronic metabolic diseases. Companies and the dietetic profession should be aware that as the world changes, you either adapt or perish. A showdown looms in the near future as novel foods surge ahead and will replace destructive staple foods.

Just think about the tobacco industry, where even as late as the 1960s and after millions of deaths, heart attacks, strokes and limb amputations, only 1/3 (33%) of doctors believed the case against tobacco was established (Proctor 2012). Sound familiar?

Fructose: An ancient genetic change 15 million years ago in our ape ancestors is now a "killing machine" in the 21st-century

A genetic change 15 million years ago occurred as an adaptation for Great Apes to survive a cooling climate change that threatened their environment and food supply. Still, this mutation that offered an advantage to these Great Apes (our ancestors) has created a colossal maladaptive nightmare in the era we now live in. We are now in a warming period, but we have other dietary, epigenetic, and environmental threats that made matters worse in the 20th century and now in the current 21st century. Fructose worsens the effects of all these cellular insults.

The fructose supply in that cooling period 15 million years ago endangered the survival of Europe's lush forests that had an abundance of fructose-rich fruits. Evolution intervened and silenced the uricase gene, and this was a means of survival, selecting those with this gene silencing to survive and thrive. The mechanism involved was an incredibly clever way of hijacking cellular biochemistry to store body fat as a means of ***energy storage***, all for a "rainy day" in the presence of a looming threat to the food supply.

This uricase gene silencing made fructose a "***weapon of mass destruction***" in the modern era, producing monumental adverse healthcare outcomes for humankind (Basaranoglu, Basaranoglu et al. 2015). We are all paying the price in terms of our personal health and population health. This negative health outcome won't stop until governments dare to mandate changes regarding sugar and fructose intakes. As I have mentioned, sugar is 50% fructose and 50% glucose, and sugar is the main way we consume fructose (Tappy 2017). Hidden sugar contaminates virtually all foods.

That we have not acted on sugar and high fructose foods is simply alarming. The biochemical and molecular impacts of fructose are well-known and striking. In the previous chapter, we looked at the one-two punch provided by insulin resistance, where we not only had glucose being blocked from entering cells by insulin resistance, thus limiting fuel supply to produce ATP, but we also had fructose entering cells freely as it didn't require insulin action thus rapidly depleting cellular ATP as well.

Are those with insulin resistance, MetS or diabetes ever told in no uncertain terms that this one-two punch to ATP production in struggling insulin-resistant cells is a very bad idea? Are doctors or dietitians aware of this one-two punch? Instead, they are told that sugar can be consumed in moderation and that small amounts won't harm you. All such statements are designed to keep the wheels turning in the sugar industry. Where are the long-term, not short-term, studies to show there is no harm over a long period caused by consuming harmful foods in moderation? Beware of corrupted research that pushes an agenda.

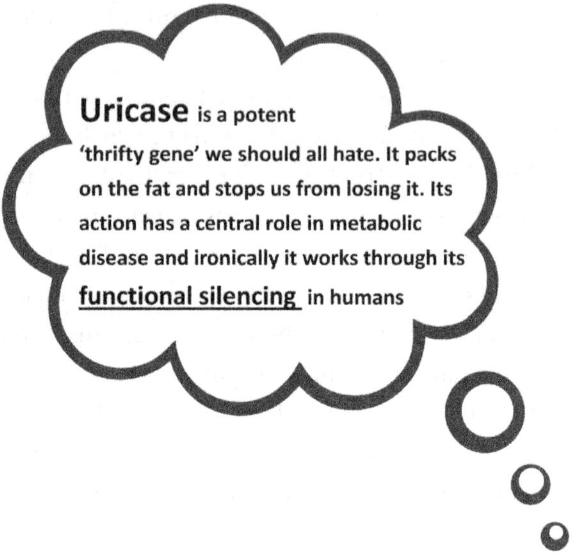

To make matters worse, the dreadful alliance of dietetics with grain producers push carbs of all kinds to populations that are exploding with insulin resistance and cannot tolerate glucose spikes. These grain-based carbs and other starchy carbs like potatoes and legumes are just glucose in disguise, and glucose can be converted to fructose. No starchy carb is something essential in our diet. They are all glucose in disguise, plain and simple, and our bodies can readily create glucose in many ways.

Just think of all the things you see in these shops, from sugar-sweetened sodas, sweets, chocolates, pastries, desserts, dried fruits, packaged fruit in syrup and fruit juice wrapped in shiny, colourful packaging to attract modern apes (humans).

That fructose can generate a significant and highly damaging Reactive Oxygen Species (ROS) load, leading to mitochondrial and cell dysfunction, is not disputed. This increased generation of ROS damages the very mitochondrial DNA (mtDNA) that codes the organelle for energy production. Uric acid increases rapidly after fructose consumption and can increase intracellular ROS by a staggering 200% (Madlala, Maarman et al. 2016).

Fructose contributes not only to substantial cell bioenergetic decline but also to this expanded list of fructose-related problems: overfat, overweight, obesity, insulin resistance, cancer, non-alcoholic fatty liver disease (NAFLD), hypertension, metabolic syndrome (MetS), gout, and Type-2 Diabetes Mellitus (T2DM). As a result, fructose contributes to a wide range of preventable chronic metabolic diseases, crushing our healthcare systems currently.

Uricase silencing 15 million years ago has been a "gift" that keeps on giving

We have an evolutionary genetic misfortune in that uricase gene silencing affects all of us. Humanity's altered and non-functional gene is called a pseudogene (Kratzer, Lanaspa et al. 2014). This gene silencing is also called a "***loss of function***" mutation. The human gene we have inherited through evolution has been deactivated, preventing uricase from lowering uric acid levels in humans. As a result, blood uric acid levels in humans are much higher than those of mammals that express this uricase gene.

Uricase gene silencing causes immense trouble in modern times and millions of deaths through the effects of being overfat, overweight, obesity and the induction of insulin resistance. Anyone suffering from gout should know the uric acid-spiking impact of sugar and fructose-rich foods. Do doctors understand this fructose-gout connection? Yet just two (x2) glasses of high fructose fruit juice increases the risk of gout by a massive 81% (Underwood 2008).

Is it acceptable that doctors are so ignorant about nutrition? Should we radically change undergraduate teaching?

Uricase - Our legendary 'Thrifty Gene'?

We have long sought a fall guy for fatness. We are all seeking a single 'fall guy' to point the finger at for our expanded waistlines. Does Uricase have all the hallmarks of being that 'fall guy?

Indeed, this uricase mutation has features that a 'Thrifty Gene' should have. We have all theorised about fat accumulation caused by a gene that programs us to store fat energy (Johnson, Nakagawa et al. 2013). Interestingly, an inactive (silenced) gene, not an active one, fits the bill for a thrifty gene.

However, fructose works in conjunction with other dietary factors such as high starchy carbs (glucose), high sugar (glucose + fructose), and high fat and protein intakes. Fructose does NOT work in isolation from other factors that create cell starvation. Other dietary factors magnify cell energy depletion. Even a "moderate" fructose intake can cause havoc in cells. The BIG-10 Womb-to-Tomb factors act simultaneously and synergistically with fructose to deplete our cell's "battery" of energy.

Toxic environmental and medication exposures, along with micronutrient deficiencies, epigenetic programming and mitochondrial dysfunction, all add to our cell energy woes. So, multiple factors converge simultaneously to create the havoc we see in healthcare today. Is it that hard to see how cell energy systems can be extremely compromised day to day? As we have discussed, energy conservation in cells should be our absolute focus through supplying cells with an abundance of nutrient resources.

Targeting sugar and fructose should be a priority at the government and public health levels. We live sedentary lifestyles like sloths in our artificial fructose-rich "Garden of Eden". Also, unlike whole fruits, our sugar and fructose consumption from Frankenstein foods lack micronutrients and fibre. But this does not mean whole fruits are not potentially damaging to energy-stricken cells that are subject to insulin resistance. Consume low-fructose fruits, as shown in Appendix-8, but never overdo them.

You can see how, in a world of food surplus, we can paradoxically create energy-starved cells.

In her outstanding paper on cell starvation, Professor Beatrice Golomb made the following statement that is worth repeating multiple times:

"Though at first glance the concept of the Starving Cell may seem counterintuitive, once the evidence is fully assembled, it may transition from far-fetched to self-evident" (B. Golomb, 2011

Fructose-induced fat accumulation deep in the abdomen (visceral fat) and in the liver (fatty liver or NAFLD/MASLD) can trigger and worsen insulin resistance and, as a result, cause the many hallmarks of metabolic dysfunction, the Metabolic Syndrome (MetS) and Type-2 Diabetes Mellitus (T2DM) affecting populations worldwide. Remember, as insulin resistance worsens, we choke off our supply of fuel (glucose) to cells, with fructose acting on top of this fuel blockade, aggravating cell bioenergetic decline. Fructose adds significantly to our relentless biological rot.

A sobering thought is that 1 in 3 young Australians 25 years and older have Metabolic Syndrome (MetS) (Cameron, Magliano et al. 2007). MetS is a prediabetes syndrome that puts colossal numbers of individuals in populations at high cardiovascular risk. Why have we dreadfully allowed young individuals to be at such a high risk medically? If the diets of these young people are not changed, we then condemn them to a life of disease and a high risk of early death.

Why we haven't taken action on sugar restrictions is a disgrace. All we do is protect farming practices and industries and never the health of populations. Are these reasons enough to allow the deaths of millions of people to occur yearly to save farming traditions, industries and taxes? How downright absurd is this way of thinking? We must change the very nature of foods to be less damaging.

The uricase story may also explain why we are at such a high cancer risk through the Warburg effect enhanced by this silenced gene and fructose effect. Fructose enhances the Warburg effect, which can drive many cancers (Fini, Lanaspa et al. 2021).

Think twice about eating that box of mangoes in the summertime or pouring colourful cereals out of a box. Dessert anyone?

So, let's look closer at uricase, our non-functional gene in humans

Uricase is an enzyme found in all three life domains but not in humans. If we had the uricase gene, we could convert highly insoluble uric acid into a soluble molecule (allantoin) for excretion. Uric acid, you now know, causes the common problem called gout, an extremely painful acute inflammatory condition of a joint, often in the big toe, but can affect any joint and cause kidney stones.

Because the gene is silenced (non-functional), this uricase gene makes us susceptible to higher uric acid levels enhanced by dietary factors such as fructose or high purine foods. For example, higher uric acid levels predict not only our risk for gout but also uric acid kidney stones, fatty liver (NAFLD), MetS, hypertension, high triglycerides, cardiovascular disease and diabetes (Johnson, Lanaspa et al. 2011).

All the disease risks mentioned above can occur due to high sugar (50% fructose) and high fructose intake. Fructose has a knack for increasing uric acid levels within cells (intracellular uric acid), leading to rapid depletion of the cell's ATP supply. In this intracellular compartment, uric acid (UA) acts as a prooxidant (increases oxidation and damage), but interestingly, uric acid is an antioxidant outside the cell (Sautin and Johnson 2008). Remember the 200% increase in intracellular reactive oxygen species (ROS) I mentioned above, which is caused by uric acid within cells. This increase in ROS can lead to mitochondrial DNA (mtDNA) and mitochondrial damage. Such ROS damage worsens ATP production levels. The body needs to neutralize these damaging ROS compounds through various mechanisms, including an optimal antioxidant system.

A high uric acid level is an independent marker for cardiovascular disease. Some experts think the loss of uricase enzyme action may be tied to our inability to create Vitamin-C, which was lost 40 million years ago. Vitamin-C is an antioxidant that helps decrease oxidative stress caused by energy extraction from food to ATP, mainly from mitochondrial Electron Transport Chain (ETC) activity. Vitamin-C neutralises Reactive Oxygen Species (ROS) and free radicals. High uric acid levels outside cells seem to take the place of Vitamin-C to a certain extent. The loss of uricase activity in humans 15 million years ago may thus have been an adaptation to offset this loss of Vitamin-C synthesis in our bodies because of uric acid's effective antioxidant capacity in the extracellular compartment (outside cells) (Johnson, Lanaspa et al. 2011).

So, in a nutshell, because a cooling climate threatened to diminish a major food supply (fruit and fructose), fat (energy) storage became the dominant evolutionary advantage to store energy as fat at a time of threatened food scarcity – a looming famine. This clever biochemistry hijacking mechanism by uricase silencing condemned humanity to body fat-storing, and fat-storing should be seen as an adaptation to cell starvation pressures.

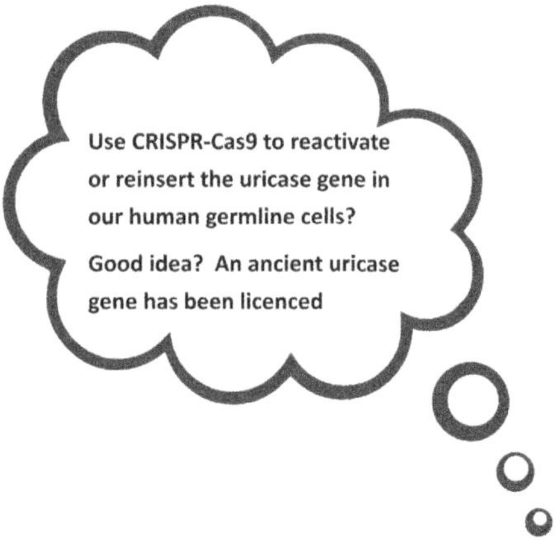

Fructose is a weapon of mass destruction, rapidly depleting cellular ATP and making us fat

A research paper was published in 2015 with the title "***Carbohydrate Intake and NAFLD: Fructose as a Weapon of Mass Destruction.***" (Basaranoglu, Basaranoglu et al. 2015)

Along with other harmful inputs, fructose helps drive a medical catastrophe of unparalleled historic proportions that will define healthcare this century and into the next unless public health agencies take action. Fructose is also driving another related pandemic of Non-Alcoholic Fatty Liver Disease (NAFLD), or simply "fatty liver", that can lead to deadly cirrhosis or cancer of the liver. NAFLD is the liver manifestation of metabolic syndrome or MetS

(Flisiak-Jackiewicz, Bobrus-Chociej et al. 2021)—the damaging effects of fructose and fatty liver, as mentioned, parallel that of the obesity, insulin resistance and diabetes pandemic.

NAFLD and metabolic dysfunction are so intertwined that the name changed in 2023 to ***Metabolic Dysfunction-Associated Steatotic Liver Disease (MASLD)*** to move away from the "alcoholic" part of the name and hence the stigma of being diagnosed with NAFLD. So, we change the name but not the nature of the disease. Fatty liver adds to the burden of chronic systemic inflammation. This fatty liver-driven inflammation affects the whole body, worsens insulin resistance and is another vicious cycle (Luo and Lin 2021).

Such inflammation adds to other sources of systemic inflammation. An activated immune system, as discussed previously, voraciously consumes energy and nutrient resources, drawing energy and nutrient resources away from already struggling cells that are trying to survive. These struggling cells become even more deprived as they have been struggling in the womb and from birth, trying to work out how to prevail in a toxic world and end up competing with an activated immune system due to so many factors.

Fatty liver is an independent risk factor for insulin resistance and cardiovascular disease (Basaranoglu, Basaranoglu et al. 2015). Fatty liver is also a condition that can lead to deadly liver cancer. The rise of NAFLD (MASLD) is expected to have a prevalence of 33.5% in the adult US population by 2030. Just think of this: 1 in 3 people in the USA, in half a decade, will have a fatty liver process that is silent and potentially deadly, all due to what is being consumed as "healthy" staple food options, many soaked with sugar and fructose.

20% of NAFLD cases are classified as the more advanced form of liver-scarring problem termed ***nonalcoholic steatohepatitis (NASH)*** (Estes, Razavi et al. 2018). I wish someone could tell me how the medical and dietetic professions can move forward, oblivious to the unequivocal failure around them, unaware and blindfolded to the blatantly obvious factors driving this pandemic of chronic diseases, including fatty liver.

NAFLD follows the progressively skyrocketing insulin resistance and obesity pandemic worldwide. High sugar and fructose consumption add to this chronic fatty liver pandemic (Dietrich, Geier et al. 2023). NAFLD/MASLD is yet another continuum that we can prevent, halt, and reverse, yet we take no action (Stahl, Dhindsa et al. 2019). We ignore all these continuums and wait till it's too late to act, but when we do, our action is pathetically inadequate as we have only weak and ineffective drugs to use in the insulin resistance process that leads to obesity, MetS and fatty liver. Drugs will never reverse fatty liver if we don't stop the damaging inputs.

A pooled prevalence rate of 25.24% for NAFLD was found worldwide, and 30% was reported in Middle Eastern and South American countries. However, Mexican Americans see a staggering 70% (7 in 10) prevalence rate of NAFLD due to a high consumption rate of beverages with high fructose corn syrup (HFCS).

Fructose consumption supports visceral fat accumulation, and this deep intraabdominal fat acts like an endocrine organ pouring out a large array of chemicals that affect the rest of the body and is associated with low-grade systemic inflammation (Kershaw and Flier 2004). This body fat inflammation helps to drive damage to our microvascular (small blood vessel) beds and, in turn, our macrovascular (large blood vessel) systems. Remember, we add to this cell, tissue, vascular, and organ damage day by day due to factors we can all avoid.

The moral of this story about fructose is the absurdity of our inaction in taking a stand on sugar consumption, which we know is 50% fructose, and not warning populations about the dangers of sugar and high fructose intakes. When do we start to warn people about all the hazards of staple foods? When do we stop killing millions of people for a handful of industries and jobs?

Brain glucose to fructose conversion: A dementia warning. Fructose created from glucose is a bioenergetic threat to our brains

It is a known fact that those with diabetes and high blood glucose levels are at high risk for many forms of dementia, including Alzheimer's and vascular dementia. We were unaware of a large hidden risk until now. This discovery was made by Yale researchers who published a paper in 2017 and thus wiped away a lot of the mystery of why those with metabolic diseases like diabetes are at such a super high risk for dementia, although other significant factors are involved as well.

This Yale University paper established that fructose can be created in our brains from high blood glucose levels (hyperglycaemia) and that the concentration of fructose is twenty times (20x) higher in the brain fluid (cerebrospinal fluid) than in the blood as a result of elevated blood glucose being converted to fructose in the brain (Hwang, Jiang et al. 2017).

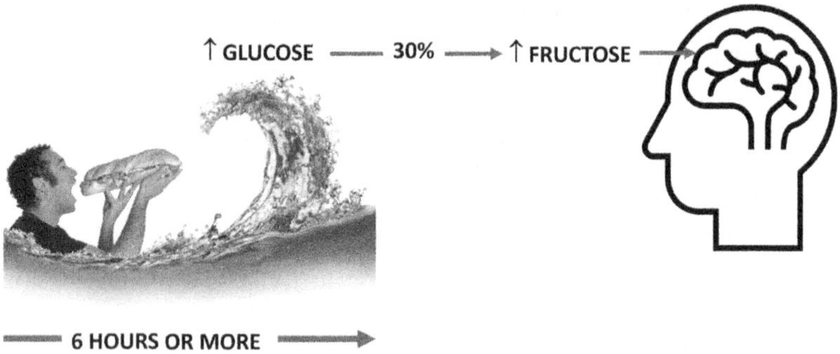

Each high-carb meal, as mentioned, creates a ***"mini diabetic event",*** as shown in point (1) in the graphic, as insulin resistance (IR) blocks glucose entry into cells. So, glucose builds up in the bloodstream as a result. Low glucose entry into cells decreases the fuel needed for ATP production, so insulin resistance (IR) is a major "energy bandit". What we never hear about is how the powerful ATP-depleting effect of fructose (point 2) magnifies the energy-depleting effects of insulin resistance (IR) and glucose restriction as a fuel for ATP production.

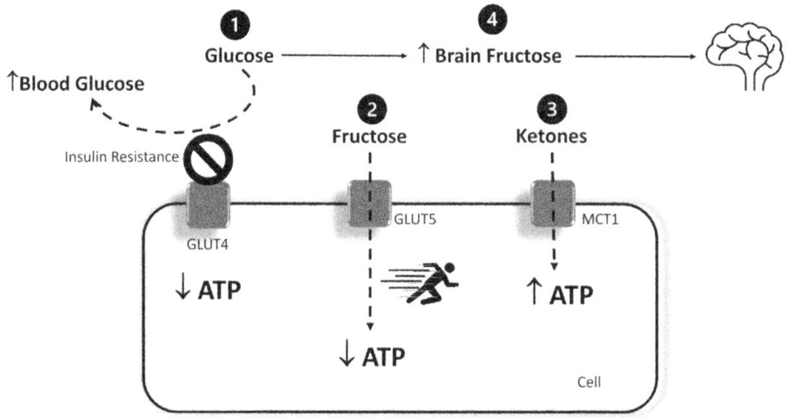

We thus have a synergistic impact, robbing cells of energy. Both IR and fructose will deplete brain cells of energy, and now we know that after eating, glucose spikes can be significantly converted to fructose (point 4), further robbing brain cells of energy. Our only hope to restore energy in these cells is ketones (point 3).

Postprandial (after-eating) surges in glucose are no different to a glucose infusion through a vein used by researchers to establish this high blood glucose-to-fructose shunt in the brain. These after-eating glucose surges happen three or more times a day, especially when high starchy carb loads are consumed. People with diabetes have a constantly elevated glucose level to drive this glucose to fructose conversion in their brains, made worse by after-eating glucose surges. Compared to non-diabetics. Someone with diabetes has a massive

25% to 91% higher risk of developing dementia (Huang, Zhu et al. 2022). Both glucose and fructose are damaging to our brains.

Importantly, these Yale researchers showed that this jump in brain fructose level occurred from a mere 20 minutes of a glucose infusion. This glucose infusion used by Yale researchers mimics what happens after eating, especially when consuming starchy or simple carbs. High carb loads will mean high blood glucose levels soon after eating – the postprandial or after-eating effect studied over decades. These same researchers stated that ***ANY*** sugar or carb consumption that raises glucose would trigger fructose formation in the brain through the ***polyol pathway***.

Elevated blood glucose after eating a mound of starchy carbs can linger for hours or even 24/7 in those with insulin resistance and trigger high brain fructose levels (Johnson, Gomez-Pinilla et al. 2020). So, I wonder why we are expecting a tsunami of dementia in the coming two decades. It should be obvious, shouldn't it?

When someone has high blood glucose levels (hyperglycaemia), up to 30% of this glucose can be shunted to fructose through the polyol pathway throughout the body and brain (Hwang, Jiang et al. 2017). This high level of glucose → fructose conversion is a grim fact that puts not only people with diabetes but all of us at great risk for dementia, neurodegeneration and mental health disorders. It is now well established that mental health disorders and abnormal metabolic health like insulin resistance are strongly linked and have bi-directional properties. Why aren't we using this knowledge in managing those with mental health problems and only using primitive psychiatric drugs that make matters worse?

The "grains-are-good" mantra still exists in the minds of dietitians. It is an unwanted remnant of the Green and Farming Revolutions from the 1960s onward that produced volumes of cheap grains. We have used "bliss points" to hook people to keep on consuming highly damaging foods that raise blood glucose levels.

Grains are NOT essential. No starchy carb is vital. Dietetics puts a spin on grains and has shifted to a "***whole grains are good***" mantra. Sure, whole grains added to a pathetic Western diet will have a positive impact. Anything with extra fibre or micronutrients will have a positive effect when given to individuals consuming horror staple foods depleted of fibre or nutrients – this is no-brainer logic but doesn't mean those foods are great and won't ultimately cause biological damage. This perverted logic about whole grains taken out of context of default and ugly diets skews nutritional research towards a positive result to push the "grains are good" agenda.

However, it doesn't mean whole grains can't have negative impacts from carb loading. Glucose elevation after grains consumption, whether whole grains or not, in a "normal" or insulin-resistant individual can stay elevated for 6 hours or more or never come down but stay elevated 24/7 (Ceriello 2003). How deceptive. Grains are cheap, can be stored for long periods, feed impoverished populations and are a way to boost food energy. But at the same time, these grains are a double-edged sword that damages the health of populations that consume them. It is time to rethink grains.

Neurodegeneration and mental health disorders are seen as bioenergetic decline now (Palmer 2022). Just imagine how we can slash chronic diseases, neurogenerative diseases like Alzheimer's and mental health disorders with a professionally guided diet untainted by vested interests that ensures nutrient adequacy through supplementation and consuming foods without the glucose-spiking effect in blood after eating.

Fructose is more glycating than glucose

Not only does fructose damage our cells by depleting them rapidly of ATP energy, but fructose also causes great cellular damage through glycation (glucose or fructose damage) to proteins. ***Fructose, in fact, is 7 – 10 times more glycating than glucose*** (McPherson, Shilton et al. 1988) (Guilbaud, Niquet-Leridon et al. 2016).

So think of highly damaged proteins like beta-amyloid in Alzheimer's or synuclein in Parkinson's disease, not to mention many other brain proteins damaged by this glycation process through the effect of glucose or fructose. Fructose causes neuroinflammation and oxidative stress, both destructive processes in the human brain that can damage brain proteins (Spagnuolo, Iossa et al. 2020). Imagine those with mental health disorders consuming sugar-sweetened sodas or high-energy drinks riddled with sugar and, hence, fructose to try and overcome their lethargy and clouded minds. By doing this, they, in fact, make lethargy and brain function many times worse. How sad we treat those with mental health disorders so primitively.

Sugar soaked foods

So, we now have sugar and fructose-rich foods coming from supermarkets or convenience stores instead of luscious fructose-rich fruits hanging from a tree 15 million years ago. The problem is that we now can't metabolize fructose the way the Great Apes did before the uricase mutation. Fructose now simply pulls the rug from under cell energy production and ensures we become fatter.

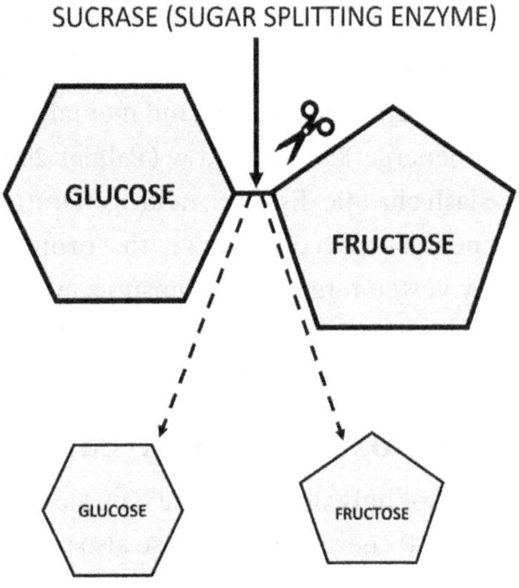

Sugar or sucrose comprises two sugars joined together - 50% glucose and 50% fructose. We find sugar to some extent in virtually all our foods, whereas in non-diet soft drinks or sodas, we find an abundance of sugar and, hence, fructose. Is it any wonder that sugar-rich beverages are such a huge risk for diabetes? Consuming 1 – 2 or more sugar-rich beverages can increase Metabolic Syndrome (MetS) and diabetes risk by at least 26% (Malik, Popkin et al. 2010). Even though this 26% is not a small risk, always take these statistics with a grain of salt. Early biomarkers would make this risk percentage skyrocket.

Toxic breakfasts

In countries like the US, sodas are high in fructose due to damaging high fructose corn syrup (HFCS). Honey or Agave syrup can also provide a big hit of fructose, with Agave syrup being up to 90% fructose. Ouch! Imagine the huge glucose and fructose hit when we add honey or agave to a bowl of glucose-spiking cereal from a colourful cardboard box.

Cereals out of a box have been highly destructive to the health of individuals. Don't think oats, steel-cut or not, are benign, as they provide a huge carb hit to start your morning made worse by insulin-spiking milk and then adding further insult through sugar and fructose from honey or agave added to that bowl of cereal. Let's not forget the custom of having a glass of fructose-rich fruit juice like orange or pineapple juice. Muesli is also a huge risk because the components are made up of glucose-spiking cereals and fructose-rich dried fruits. And yet, these are regarded as "healthy" options. So, much for propaganda to keep selling grain-based or fruit products.

We have been conned into eating grains to the extent we do. As mentioned before, humankind has become "canaries" pecking at grain-based foods every day. Dementia occurs due to many impacts acting on the brain. A high glucose and fructose hit every morning will greatly add to this daily brain cell damage, let alone all the damage done to our vascular systems, one breakfast at a time.

We are adding milk that spikes insulin levels even further to the insulin-IgF-1 spiking effects of all cereals in oats or cereal-based muesli. I have discussed how simply keeping insulin levels high can trigger insulin resistance (Del Prato, Leonetti et al. 1994). Fructose, on the other hand, doesn't spike insulin but causes far more damage than glucose through glycation, which, as mentioned, is a whopping 7 – 10 times worse than that produced by glucose discussed above.

Any disbelieving gurus of medicine or dietetics who think foods cannot damage us in the way is living in an alternate universe. We have been conned into believing staple foods can be consumed till they come out of our ears and there will be no damage.

Vegetable-rich foods for breakfast are far healthier and have nutrient, fibre, and antioxidant densities far greater than any grain product. Avoid eggs, bacon, sausages, mounds of baked beans, hash browns, or any other sugar-soaked breakfast, such as pancakes drowned in maple syrup for breakfast. A breakfast disaster!

Choline's impact on the starving cell and NAFLD

Micronutrient deficiencies like Choline, an essential nutrient deficient in many populations, don't aid this fatty liver - NAFLD/MASLD pandemic. In fact, choline insufficiency in many people is adding to this misery of fatty liver that can drive insulin resistance even deeper. Having enough choline, an essential micronutrient necessary for health and positive pregnancy outcomes, supports the transportation of triglyceride-rich VLDLs out of the liver, helping prevent fat accumulation within the liver.

Choline is incredibly cheap and also essential in our bodies, so it is pretty daft not to recommend choline intake when someone has fatty liver, along with advice on limiting sugar and fructose consumption. Choline supplementation in pregnancy may actually prevent mental health disorders such as Schizophrenia (Ross, Hunter et al. 2013).

NAFLD/MASLD is an extremely common feature on routine abdominal ultrasounds or abdominal CT findings. But if fatty liver is reported, when does a doctor ever recognise this as a manifestation of metabolic syndrome (MetS)? When do doctors who get these imaging reports mention Choline as an aide to help prevent fatty liver progression to liver scarring, cirrhosis and liver cancer (Corbin and Zeisel 2012)? When will a doctor warn about sugar and fructose consumption to help reverse fatty liver? Dreadful ignorance in the medical and dietetic professions.

I don't say negative things about doctors, just for the heck of it. I am one of them. These are "holes" in their training as drug pushers in interventionist medicine and medical management of chronic diseases. Doctors can be far more than what they have become. We need to address these holes in training as they are destroying lives.

An unbelievable 10-29% of individuals with fatty liver may progress to cirrhosis (Basaranoglu, Basaranoglu et al. 2015). Cirrhosis is advanced scarring of the liver, a life-threatening complication that requires drastic liver transplantation to save their lives, and fructose is a leading cause of fatty liver.

Without adequate choline, we are at high risk of developing NAFLD/MASLD because triglycerides bound to VLDL, the transport vehicle for triglycerides, cannot be exported out of the liver due to the lack of choline (phosphatidylcholine). These triglycerides then stay trapped in the liver, causing it to swell and also causing the liver to become inflamed and ultimately extremely scarred.

The fact is that a recent 2022 study has shown a whopping 81% reduction in visceral obesity-related fatty liver disease using a

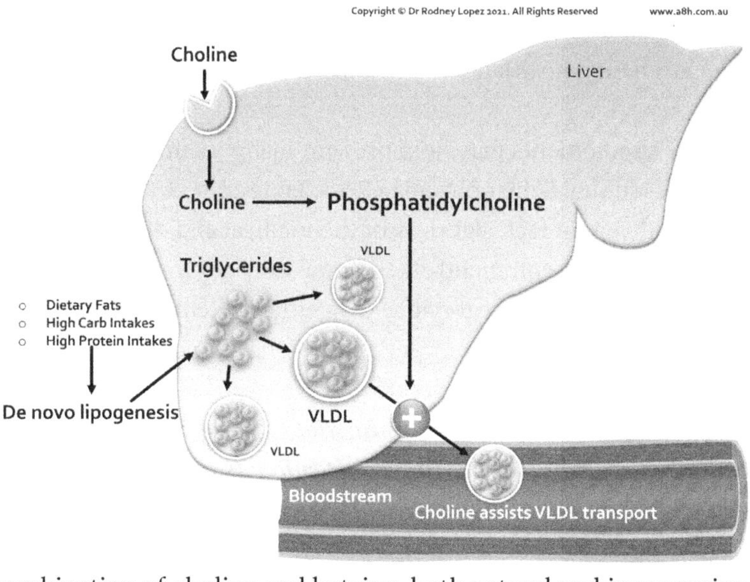

combination of choline and betaine, both natural and inexpensive substances (Chang, Wu et al. 2022). It could take decades before a bright spark in medicine with enough clout in public health can start a choline revolution for fatty liver and pregnancy outcomes.

Choline, as mentioned, is a cheap essential nutrient the medical profession ignores as a treatment option. How can Pharma make money if 1) something is cheap and 2) it is a natural compound that you can't put a registered trademark on - so how can a corporation say this compound is mine and then make a ton of money by holding people hostage who may need such a compound? For individuals, choline is in lecithin, and you can get cheap supplements. Therefore, choline should be regarded as a pharmaconutrient, as it can potentially change outcomes in NAFLD/MASLD.

We can't expect Choline to do all the heavy lifting without optimising dietary impacts affecting this fatty liver process. Why use any drug if we have a safe, essential nutrient that can do the trick?

Choline is a common deficiency in someone consuming a Western diet and a risk to public health (Zeisel and Da Costa 2009). The widespread risk of choline deficiency reinforces how silly that throwaway line is by nutritionists, dietitians and doctors who say to their clients, "***Just go and eat an optimal diet***", and all will be fine. In addition, Choline is a common deficiency in pregnancy and can be a disaster for mental health issues for a developing fetus in the long term.

Choline supplements may help prevent many mental health problems, including Schizophrenia (Ross, Hunter et al. 2013). It is short-sighted and, in fact, sightless of the medical and dietetic professions not to recommend an essential nutrient in pregnancy, as nutrient adequacy is not negotiable. You either take it or suffer the consequences. The thought of safety issues of a nutrient is arrogant and redundant and causes tremendous harm.

"The importance of choline in the diet extends into adulthood and old age. In a study of healthy adult subjects deprived of dietary choline, 77% of the men and 80% of the postmenopausal women developed signs of subclinical organ dysfunction (fatty liver or muscle damage)" *(Zeisel and Da Costa 2009)*

So, how does fructose rapidly deplete our cells of ATP?

If you want some detail on this amazing evolutionary impact on uricase and how it depletes cells of energy, please read on. Follow the steps in the graphic to see evolution in action.

This graphic looks complicated, but once you get the picture, it is incredibly satisfying to see evolution in action to overcome the threat of famine. At the same time, this uricase mutation has helped drive so many chronic diseases we are struggling with currently, including overfat, overweight and obesity, insulin resistance, MetS, diabetes, fatty liver and abdominal (visceral fat). So, let's see this fat-making machine and evolution in action.

Notice the glucose to fructose shuttle on the top of the graphic and how glucose from high starchy carb intakes increases our brain's fructose, as we have discussed. Just follow the numbers in the graphic and view the explanation below. Skip this section if you don't want the details.

Follow the steps outlined below using the graphic to get your bearings and see this fat-making "machine" in action, a gift from our Great Ape ancestors to us in the 21st-century.

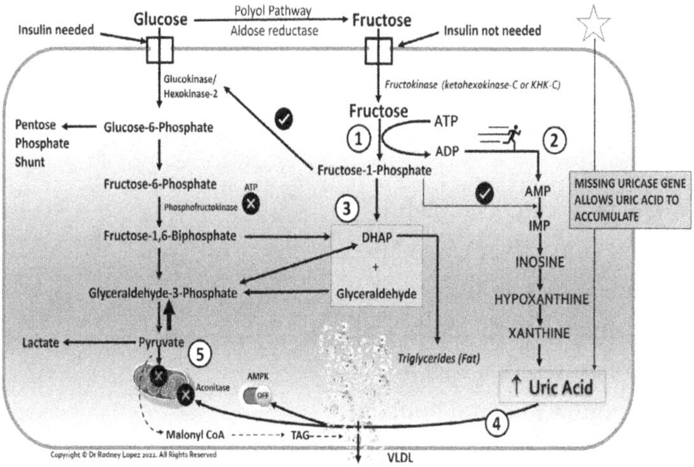

The ATP-depleting mechanism in action. It's easier than it looks.

(1) Fructose can enter a cell without help from insulin, unlike glucose, which needs insulin to open the door for it to gain entry. We can view insulin resistance as a defective lock and key mechanism so the glucose door doesn't open as well as it should if insulin action is faulty (insulin resistance). By preventing glucose from entering cells, glucose can build up in the blood to affect tissues and organs. Remember, if glucose builds up in the blood, 30% of that can be shunted to fructose through the polyol pathway in the brain within 20 minutes of becoming elevated (Hwang, Jiang et al. 2017).
Fructose doesn't need a similar key but enters the bloodstream through the intestinal GLUT2/GLUT5 receptors. Once in the blood, fructose makes its way to the liver (~ 70%) and other tissues to be metabolised. Once inside a cell, fructose is rapidly metabolized and converted to Fructose-1-Phosphate.

Unlike the glucose pathway, fructose has no 'brakes' to stop this reaction.

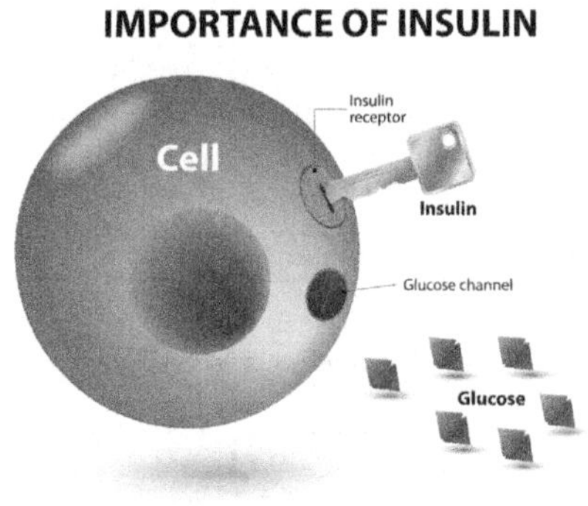

The liver can become full of fat (fatty liver), and fat-forming metabolites can be distributed to the body and increase visceral (deep abdominal) fat and body fat in general. All of this drives insulin resistance and metabolic dysfunction. The conversion proceeds rapidly and keeps going quickly, consuming all the ATP. So you can now see how that uricase gene mutation 15 million years ago can disable oxidative phosphorylation (OXPHOS) in our mitochondria so that energy can be diverted to triglyceride (TAG) or fat formation.

(2) The rapid conversion of fructose to Fructose-1-Phosphate (F1P) requires phosphate from ATP. So ATP is the phosphate donor. Because the process is so fast and where there is no negative feedback or braking mechanism to stop this fructose to F1P conversion, ATP is thus rapidly consumed. An energy-weak cell cannot consume ATP to build things, so the focus is on fat formation. ATP loses the terminal (energy-rich) phosphate to form Adenosine diphosphate (ADP). Once ADP has donated its phosphate to fructose for fructose-1-phosphate formation, we are left with Adenosine Monophosphate (AMP), which has one final phosphate bond that can be donated for this process. Once AMP donates its last phosphate, we are left with Adenosine's backbone molecule, an energy-depleted remnant. Adenosine then accumulates in an energy-starved cell and can diffuse outside of a cell to become a low-energy warning signal. AMP will also collect and proceed down a pathway to create uric acid. Uric acid increases inside cells because we don't have uricase to lower it due to gene silencing, as we discussed. Increasing uric acid inside cells creates havoc with cellular energy-extracting enzymes in the Krebs Cycle, disabling the Krebs Cycle and mitochondria.

(3) Fructose creates dihydroxyacetone phosphate (DHAP), the primary precursor to produce triglycerides (body fat), also known as triacylglycerol or TAG, which is how fat is stored in our bodies- See Appendix-9. Triglycerides are a high-energy food substrate that can accumulate inside cells and increase fat accumulation in the liver (Non-Alcoholic Fatty Liver Disease or NAFLD). Triglycerides can also be transported to other body parts as an energy source. This accumulation of intracellular fat switches off the Insulin/PI3K-AKT pathway, preventing the translocation of GLUT4, our main insulin glucose transport receptors, to the cell membranes (Petersen and Shulman 2006). Without GLUT4 in cell membranes,

insulin-dependent glucose entry into cells is limited, thus limiting our main fuel for ATP creation (insulin resistance). Decreasing cellular glucose entry will then worsen energy production, increasing cell starvation.

(4) Uric acid accumulates inside the cell and switches off the Krebs Cycle by inhibiting the critical Aconitase enzyme. This enzyme is involved in the first two steps of the Krebs Citric Acid Cycle, thus impairing energy extraction from food through the electron transport chain in the mitochondria, where typically 90% of ATP is formed.

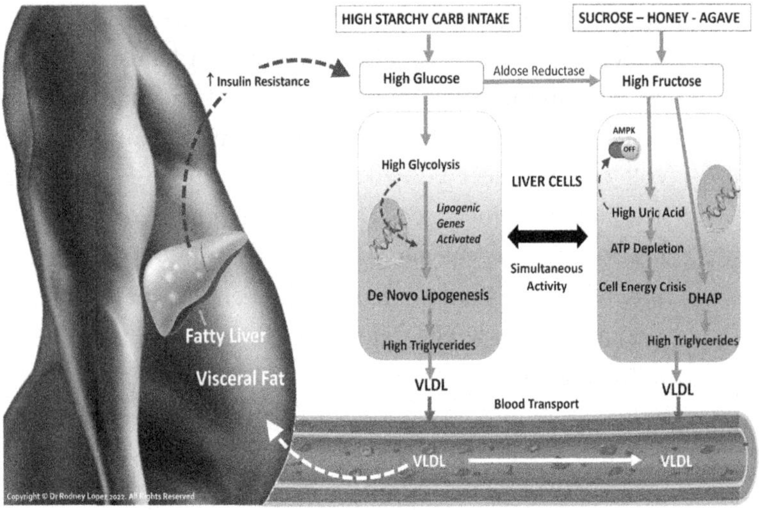

(5) Switching off Aconitase leaves pyruvate nowhere to go as the Krebs Citric Acid Cycle in the mitochondria has been disabled by uric acid (Aconitase inhibited) – See Appendix-7. Pyruvate can proceed to DHAP via Glyceraldehyde-3-Phosphate, as the thicker arrow shows in the graphic in point 5. You can see how clever evolution is by switching off the uricase gene, forcing metabolites to go down the fat-forming pathways. Metabolites from glucose metabolism in the pre-mitochondria glycolytic pathway build up as the mitochondria become impaired by uric acid.

We must remember that people are still eating high-energy foods that can't be metabolized as would normally occur because fructose has turned off the normal energy-ATP-producing pathways. So excessive food energy consumed when fructose has disabled OXPHOS is shuttled to fat. If you are one of the unlucky ones born to one or more parents with diabetes, your mitochondrial handicap will worsen the processes discussed above. These glycolytic metabolites trigger lipogenic (fat-forming) genes to create fat that will accumulate inside the cell and also be transported outside the cell for fat storage and build up in the liver to cause Non-Alcoholic Fatty Liver Disease (NAFLD), or abdominal adiposity visceral fat especially if choline is deficient. See Appendix-9.

Uric acid also switches off AMPK, a cellular low-energy sensor that would generally boost ATP production (See Appendix-2). Uric acid's effect is to push fructose and glucose towards fat formation and energy storage.

Glucose can also be converted to fructose through the Polyol Pathway, as mentioned above, thus enhancing this effect further, driving more fat formation - so much for high-carb consumption pushed by dietetics.

Insulin resistance further depletes phosphate and ATP production

It is well known that Non-Alcoholic Fatty Liver Disease (NAFLD/MASLD) can increase insulin resistance and elevate insulin levels in the blood (hyperinsulinaemia) even in lean individuals with normal glucose tolerance (Marchesini, Brizi et al. 1999).

High blood insulin levels can, by themselves, downregulate cell signalling, worsening insulin resistance (Del Prato, Leonetti et al. 1994). We know that insulin resistance can also severely restrict phosphate entering cells, and this was studied in skeletal muscle, where this mass of skeletal muscle has a major impact on systemic insulin resistance (Petersen, Dufour et al. 2005). With diminishing phosphate, how is ATP even formed, with each ATP requiring three (3) phosphate bonds?

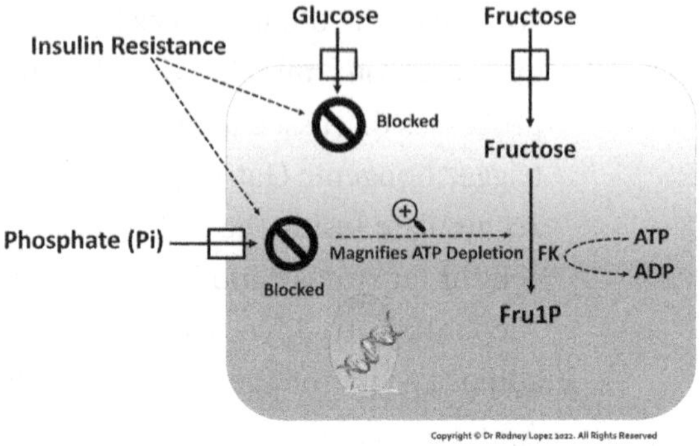

With no brakes to stop fructose-1-phosphate (F1P) forming, phosphate and ATP are rapidly depleted. A vicious cycle leads to more and more phosphate depletion inside cells. A perfect storm to create energy-starved cells.

CHAPTER 5

That's no way to treat a metabolic biomarker

Highly predictable blood biomarker changes occur in insulin resistance (IR). Why?

"Nothing in Biology Makes Sense Except in the Light of Evolution"
The quote above was from Theodosius Dobzhansky

A biomarker war has been fought for decades now. We have long fought drug-based battles trying to lower glucose or LDL cholesterol. We have also tried to lower triglycerides or stamp out the fires of inflammation. Still, despite staggering sums of money spent on pharmaceutical warfare against the blood biomarkers of diabetes and chronic metabolic diseases, all that has happened is that Big Pharma has become unbelievably wealthy. There is nothing new here.

The sad fact is that in this metabolic disease warfare, nations have become poorer and poorer, and populations have become sicker and sicker. So, the efforts to combat glucose and blood fats like LDL, decrease inflammation, or lower blood pressure have been a dismal failure overall, and why failure? Chronic metabolic diseases never tumble down to lower and lower levels but skyrocket up and up despite these pharmacological approaches. This failure can be gaslighted but not denied, as the prevalence statistics of metabolic diseases will unequivocally contradict anyone who dares to deny these bleak statistics. So, we must accept pharmaceutical failure as an undeniable certainty.

As I mentioned earlier, biomarkers do not change randomly. The changes in glucose, triglycerides, LDL, VLDL, and HDL, and we can also include high blood pressure (hypertension) in this basket of biomarker changes; all of these act "poster boys" for metabolic diseases and are highly predictable. The amazing predictability of biomarker changes should be our key to understanding that these changes are by evolutionary design and not random events that make no sense. Any biochemical or molecular changes that occur should be seen as survival mechanisms, plain and simple.

These biomarkers have been used historically to diagnose, monitor, and assess risk. Still, since metabolic diseases have exploded since 1960, we have used a divide-and-conquer mentality focusing on just one metabolic biomarker as if they are totally independent of other biomarker actions or external factors. Such thinking is absurd, and yet this has been the exact way medicine has progressed, using a divide-and-conquer approach, choosing one biomarker to point the finger at and then declaring war on that biomarker. Such simplicity is not how chaotic systems work in the real world and not how diseases progress as if they are driven by one biomarker hit at a time. There are no singular hits like glucose or lipids driving this trainwreck. ***What we do have are multiple hits, all working simultaneously to steer this runaway train.***

Metabolic markers are not a gift from the Gods to the pharmaceutical industry. They are adaptations or can be seen as a cry for help by cells struggling to maintain adequate energy levels or to reverse cell decay or entropy, which is a neverending battle.

This divide-and-conquer approach has been a complete failure. It is "Biochemical and Molecular Dualism" in action. With prevalence statistics continually rising higher and higher, it would be wildly optimistic to claim that our focus on blood biomarkers has had any meaningful impact on metabolic disease prevalence.

Thus, in the face of complete failure on a grand scale, i.e. at a population level globally, the fact we are allowing the use of drugs that do nothing to modify the biological rot discussed is insanity to me because at the end of this rot lies all the crushing chronic metabolic diseases we need to deal with but don't know how to.

The blood biomarker profiles are incredibly reliable in their predictability

Read what follows as a summary of blood biomarkers and what they mean through the lens of the Cell Starvation Model. This summary can then be a foundation for what you will learn in this chapter. This chapter will be an eye-opener for you as you begin to understand how medicine and pharma have gotten this all wrong.

Metabolic networks are highly connected, and thus, the predictability of biomarker changes is not surprising. Such predictability will have survival benefits as honed through millions of years of evolutionary biochemical and molecular challenges.

The high level of predictability of biomarker changes persists until metabolic decompensation occurs, where our beta cells burn out and die and where biomarker changes now become more and more unpredictable as chaos and decay (increasing entropy) overwhelm our systems all because of utter neglect in not supporting cells through nutritional means from a very early stage in metabolic disease development.

In insulin resistance and metabolic dysfunction, you can bet your bottom dollar that the following will happen in the continuum before decompensation and dysregulation occur:

1. **INSULIN** levels will rise (hyperinsulinaemia). This insulin increase is to try to overcome poor insulin receptor (INSR/GLUT4) sensitivity. High insulin levels become a "battering ram" to push glucose (fuel) into cells. The smart thing to do when insulin is not working is to bypass it and provide an alternative fuel source to glucose if glucose struggles to get into cells because insulin is behaving badly. Ketones fit the bill very nicely. They are discussed in the final chapter.

2. **BLOOD GLUCOSE.** Glucose is our major fuel source for cells and will rise with insulin resistance. Glucose entry into cells is blocked due to insulin resistance, and so glucose increases in the blood. A higher glucose (fuel) level outside cells can increase the chance of some fuel getting into cells (another battering ram). Is it any wonder that glucose will increase to help power cell energy (ATP) production? Let's forget about glucose and instead help cells power themselves with ketones. Don't forget that high blood glucose will turn "off" our brain cell energy due to the blood glucose to fructose shunting.
3. **TRIGLYCERIDES.** Will rise – triglycerides are a blood fat and an important energy source, and a metabolic shift to fat as an energy source if glucose availability is low. The backbone of triglycerides (glycerol) can be converted to glucose through gluconeogenesis, which is the reason why carbs for glucose are not essential. It is no wonder we see a high triglyceride level in insulin-resistant states to help power cells when our primary fuel for ATP production (glucose) is being denied entry into cells by insulin resistance. Carb foods can significantly increase triglycerides. So, carbs increase blood fat.
4. **VLDL.** Is triglyceride-rich. VLDL is a hallmark of insulin resistance, and it will also rise. VLDL is a source of high-energy triglycerides. A high VLDL is predictable in cell starvation states as the body adapts to cells needing energy as ATP starts to decline in cells.
5. **LDL** (a major cholesterol carrier). Will increase. Cholesterol is needed for cell and organelle membrane integrity and repair, bile acid production, Vitamin-D and steroid production. Cholesterol is an important structural component for cells and steroid synthesis. So, it is no wonder LDL increases in structurally damaged cells with increasing entropy as cell energy drops.

6. **HDL. Will *decrease***, preventing reverse cholesterol transport and thus keeping cholesterol near cells and not taking cholesterol back to the liver for processing. Lower HDL is an attempt to keep cholesterol in the vicinity of cells to be used for structural repair and membrane construction and restoration, along with all the other cholesterol tasks mentioned above to keep cells functional. Is it any wonder that HDL will decrease to help cells survive and stay functional? Why haven't we focused on the critical functionality of biomarkers and only seen them as enemies? Will increasing HDL then improve or worsen cell survival? Please read on.
7. **HYPERTENSION. Blood pressure will rise** to improve blood delivery of oxygen, micronutrients, and energy substrates to starving cells. Increasing blood pressure is the body's attempt to "push" blood, fuel, oxygen and micronutrient delivery through increasingly damaged and obstructed microcirculation networks. We described the critical nature of a damaged microcirculation in the chapter on prediabetes and how this factor itself is enough to explain why blood pressure rises in insulin-resistant states. It is truly astounding that we don't see hypertension in this practical sense for cell survival. In other words, hypertension, like all the different biomarkers, is part of an evolutionary adaptation process for survival. It is an established continuum.

   A lack of blood and nutrient supplies to create ATP energy and support cellular repair is of the highest order of threats to cells and organs. So, is it any wonder that blood pressure rises when our smallest blood vessels (our microcirculation networks) are being hammered and blocked? In my chapter on prediabetes, we saw how very small decreases in blood vessel diameter produced huge changes in blood vessel resistance, needing more pressure to get blood through. This adaptation is cell survival 101.

If blood can't get through, then delivery of oxygen, fuel and cellular building blocks, along with waste removal, are all impaired. This increase in vascular resistance that drives blood pressure higher is our punishment for not preventing blood biomarkers, inflammation, postprandial impacts and oxidative stress from damaging our small blood vessels over time.

Small blood vessel damage occurs long before any glucose cut-off point. Hypertension should be seen as a wake-up call that microcirculation damage exists. We need to see microcirculation damage driving hypertension and not the other way around, although one worsens the other in a bidirectional fashion. In my mind, most of what we call "***essential hypertension***" or high blood pressure of unknown cause is a foolish designation when we consider early microcirculation damage and where, over eons of time, in human history, we have used damaging staple foods that can trigger small vessel disease meal-by-meal. We have neglected our microcirculation networks as the simultaneous killer of cells, tissues and multiple organ systems.

8. **INFLAMMATORY MARKERS.** Why do inflammatory markers increase while anti-inflammatory markers decrease in our insulin resistance metabolic dysfunction continuum? Is this just a random finding that happens to occur in almost everyone with metabolic dysfunction? Is there no advantage to inflammation from a biological perspective? Can these ratios of inflammatory to anti-inflammatory markers change without evolution having a hand in this? Inflammation is associated with vasodilation, i.e. the opening up of blood vessels. The opening up of blood vessels means more blood flow to cells and organs. Is this an advantage to stiff and narrow microcirculation networks? Opening up these damaged small vessels is a huge advantage. Will inflammation then help to lower

> blood pressure by widening small blood vessels? The answer is a resounding yes. So inflammation has distinct advantages in metabolic dysfunction that threatens to block our small vessel pipelines to biological tissues. To think these markers occur as targets for Pharma shows the conceit of corporations who will only want to see any marker as a target to declare war on. This twist on perspective is a huge money-making ploy that will never see biomarkers as an advantage, only as a disadvantage that needs correction. I will take a look at this war on inflammation, and like all the other biomarker wars that have been fought, the results are not that great for individuals. Inflammation has a purpose that has gone over our heads in our rush to use drugs in biomarker wars.

Cells undergo energy and ultrastructural deterioration in an insulin-resistant state for years to decades before manifesting as any chronic illness (end-organ failure). Thus, weakened cells may be unable to use any nutrient resources presented to them initially. Therefore, we must use ***nutrient rescue*** with dedicated nutrient resources to rebuild weakened "limping" cells over time. All our cells have moved towards a high entropy (decay) state due to slowly starving cells, so without an alternative fuel source like ketones, our cells are destined for death or senescence. It is not as if we have found a brilliant way to overcome this insulin resistance blockade with a drug, thus allowing glucose to once again get into cells easily. No drug has overcome this insulin resistance blockade in a meaningful sense. Drug (and dietary) failure is why metabolic disease is skyrocketing in prevalence globally.

We must "nudge" cells slowly but surely back to health. Sledgehammer approaches won't do. We can't force a cell to become functional after years to decades of neglect as medicine expects. They will have to gradually utilise nutrient resources as the damaged cellular machinery is repaired or replaced, which will then enable more and more nutrient resources to be used. The take-home message is that through ***nutrient rescue*** and then ***nutrient maintenance***, we can put the brakes on these biomarkers "biting" us. We can stop them in their tracks, but not by drugs. Getting cells back to a functional state should be seen as a no-brainer nutritional support approach to prevent this chronic disease pandemic from inflicting so much misery and death.

That insulin resistance can predate and damage cells over decades is not in doubt (Petersen, Dufour et al. 2004). It will take many months to many years to get injured cells back to optimal function. We can then move on to a maintenance phase with nutrient support.

Biomarkers as energy or repair resources

Biomarkers must be seen as evolutionary designed adaptations for survival. Their huge predictability and the very nature of these biomarkers as either energy resources or cellular building supplies should be shouting at us that these biomarkers have functional and survival value.

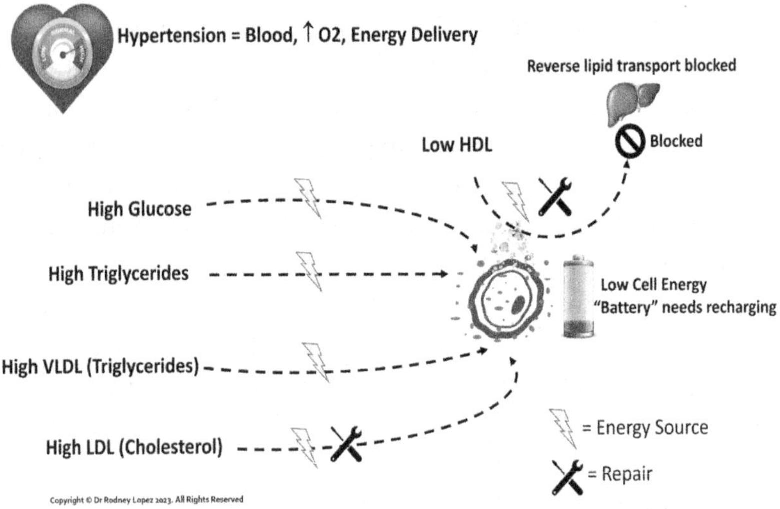

Most lipid transporters are a mix of lipids. VLDL is rich in triglycerides, an important source of energy for ATP production. In contrast, LDL is a rich source of cholesterol that is a structural component in cell membranes and is used to create steroids. LDL can also supply triglycerides (an energy resource). So, some carriers can be seen more as energy supplies and others as structural supplies for structural repair and anabolic functions.

We must have a far more enlightened view of metabolic biomarkers. This biomarker predictability remains until the metabolic house of cards topples over as the pancreas beta cells fail or tissues and organs start to fail, and biomarkers shoot through the roof and become chaotic. This decompensation is highly predictable and easily avoidable.

Our biomarkers are Janus-faced (two-faced) destroyers of biological tissue

We need to see biomarkers in three phases. All of these phases are a part of a continuum of change.

1. **The Early Phase:** Biological damage occurs at a scale we cannot measure with our limited technology currently.

2. **The Crossover Phase:** In the crossover from early to late phases, we do have telltale increases in blood biomarkers or very early microvascular changes. It is at this point we need to act and not wait for blood biomarkers to "bite" us.

3. **The Late Phase:** Biological damage occurs at a noticeable scale. Biomarkers produce noticeable biological rot and microvascular assassination of organ systems. Organ complications start to appear.

We must remember that shifts in metabolic markers as a result of cells undergoing energy and structural decline caused by the many womb-to-tomb factors discussed are magnified by the after-eating (postprandial) effects discussed. So if glucose is increasing due to cells becoming increasingly damaged and distressed by all the factors never addressed, then glucose will be pushed higher in the bloodstream with each starchy carb meal and snack. The same is true for other biomarkers, such as triglycerides or inflammatory markers.

As I have mentioned in previous chapters, biomarkers cannot be seen as an enemy as this is naïve. In this early phase, they should be seen as adaptations for struggling cells trying to overcome bioenergetic and structural decline. Biomarkers are a lifeline to distressed cells as an energy source, i.e. fuel (glucose, triglycerides) or structural components (cholesterol, phospholipids) or the building block for steroid synthesis (cholesterol). Biomarkers have a function, but for some reason, we have never seen them as such, only as playthings to be crushed by pharmaceutical means.

Thus, drugs can be seen as working counter to evolutionary adaptations occurring to support struggling cells in an energy or structural sense. So, suppose you ever see a drug that has created a medical disaster, i.e. increased medical complications like a heart attack or a stroke. In that case, it is easy enough to know why this happens if we view a drug as taking away precious nutrient resources that cells crave at a time of struggle.

So, in the early phases of metabolic disease, we need to see biomarkers as supportive, but they do have features that can damage us the longer we allow them to stay abnormal. The biggest risk of biomarkers that behave badly is that they constantly hammer our blood vessels, adding to plaque formation or making the lining of these blood vessels stiffer, limiting blood supply to organ systems. Vascular disease progresses as a continuum, and thank goodness that we are seeing all of this now as slow, incremental, and cumulative damage – our SIC continuum process.

But why do we continue to target biomarkers with drugs? In the crossover phase, these biomarkers start showing their "teeth" and thus begin the slow and relentless biological rot that will take all of us towards chronic metabolic disease. This "bite" of metabolic markers is an established continuum of risk. The longer we leave these biomarkers to "do their thing", the more likely we will suffer early chronic illness or suffer a catastrophic cardiovascular event that takes us out. Who among you reading this book is going to escape these diseases in your lifetime unless you know how to avoid the biomarker impacts that can prevent these medical disasters?

The moral of this story is to build the technology to find the extremely early changes in metabolic dysfunction and to take action at this point, but technology holds us back, and so practically, we need to take action in the early crossover phase. We negligently don't bother with early signs of disease and so "manage" advanced stages of metabolic biomarker changes and risk. I want to discuss how these biomarkers damage us all, but ultimately, all roads lead to damaged microvascular disease networks, the destroyers of organ systems.

Drugs vs drugs research and not drugs vs diets

With drug trials, what you will see is a battle for supremacy between one drug versus another or between drug classes in our divide-and-conquer biomarker approach. What you won't see is a battle between a drug and a comprehensive diet, so why would this be the case? As we saw in the prediabetes chapter, when we compare the action of a drug (an ant) such as a statin in the 4S study versus a diet like the Lyon Diet Heart Study (a steamroller), we see that this steamroller crushes the ant.

It was interesting then that both the 4S paper and the Lyon Diet Heart Study were published in the Lancet in the very same year. And so a drug company wouldn't dare undertake a trial between a drug and a great diet and then publish it with fanfare because that would be humiliating for any drug company that does so. It is far better to compare one pathetic drug against another pathetic drug and squeeze as much benefit out of that drug as possible and state: *This drug, in comparison to that drug, will decrease the risk of kidney disease by X or heart attacks by Y*, and so on.

Presenting research findings in this way as a drug-to-drug comparison is far safer for them, and these blown-out-of-all-proportion comparisons of one ineffective drug versus another ineffective drug will keep the drug wars continuing for pharma while the chronic disease prevalence continues to explode globally.

What matters most is not whether one drug outperforms another but what happens to an individual in the long term, irrespective of ANY drug being used. No drug in existence in over 60 years has stopped the progression of the biological rot produced by metabolic dysfunction and after-eating impacts on chronic disease. No drug puts the brakes on the biological rot generated over time. ***What pharmaceuticals do is merely delay the inevitable or hold off a catastrophic medical event for a SHORT TIME ONLY on an individual-by-individual basis.*** Our focus on drug management individual by individual allows populations to be riddled with disease as biological rot will continue despite any drug or drug combination used in an individual with metabolic dysfunction.

The name of the game with pharmaceuticals is always to hold off an adverse medical outcome for as long as possible. But, as you will see, drug-based management is a high-risk strategy that walks a tightrope between a positive therapeutic response and triggering a medical nightmare as drugs pull the rug from under biomarker adaptations designed to support cells in distress. Shouldn't we have stopped biomarkers from becoming a threat a long time before they create a medical crisis?

Gurus in Pharma's "***speaker programs***" will become programmed like robots to regurgitate what Pharma has trained them to say about this amazing glucose-lowering drug or that LDL-lowering drug or any drug targeting biomarkers of metabolic disease.

Our downfall is that we target the effects and not the causes of these metabolic biomarkers, thus ensuring ongoing failure in metabolic disease management!

A huge deceptive strategy is to introduce novel drugs with new actions where these shiny new drugs do the same thing with regard to any biomarker being targeted by previous pharmaceutical iterations - i.e. to lower glucose or LDL or beat down inflammation or triglycerides, etc. ***Novel drugs are still doing the same old thing but differently***. How insane! These biomarker tricks con us into believing that we will have a different outcome. It cons doctors. Do the same thing and expect a different result? Einstein called this insanity. Decades of this kind of deception have seen populations get sicker, leaving nations to struggle with increasing chronic disease prevalence and soaring costs. On top of this, I have mentioned we are expecting tsunamis of metabolic diseases to emerge in the next two decades. What a charade we allow to continue.

The other massive problem that I see in this failed biomarker warfare using the "***New drug, same biomarker effect approach***" is why this deception cons governments and public health groups and why society is paying for this failed approach.

We have a powerful interplay between insulin resistance causing internal cellular energy and structural chaos with metabolic marker ramifications, but we forget all the direct cellular biochemical and molecular impacts from food, epigenetic and environmental impacts that can then lead to insulin resistance. ***High insulin levels on their own are a generator of insulin resistance.*** This fact is now well recognised, and our staple foods are a "great" generator of high insulin levels that linger on for hours many times a day.

We have this loony desire in medical thinking to choose one factor that triggers this cascade of metabolic changes. We even select obesity as the cause of our metabolic misery and fail to see obesity as merely a metabolic biomarker that is a result of cellular energy and structural failure and the result of ubiquitous fructose inputs adding to our obesity pandemic. When will we adopt a big-picture approach rather than senseless reductionism?

Have you been told you have high glucose, high "bad cholesterol", i.e., LDL or inflammatory markers?

The problem of metabolic disease is so widespread, as discussed under ***Metabolic Singularity,*** that most adults will be showing signs of this problem in blood tests that could be ignored or dismissed as having no meaning by a doctor. Ignoring early metabolic marker abnormalities is a fatal mistake. Biomarkers, as drivers of biological rot, acting as a continuum of risks should never be dismissed, even at the earliest flicker of change.

Most adults will be told they have these biomarkers out of range, and you may even get a label put on these markers, such as "MetS", "prediabetes", or "diabetes", but most will be told not to worry about them as they are perhaps "***just beyond the range***". Always ignore such a statement no matter who says it to you, as you need to be concerned from the very earliest biomarker signal that something is not right in a metabolic sense that flicker will snowball over time.

Also, discard the completely illogical statement that abnormal biomarkers like glucose may not reach the "Mt Everest" of glucose levels, a cut-off we label as Type-2 Diabetes Mellitus (T2DM), as this obsessive and outdated thinking has killed many an individual and will keep on damaging and destroying lives as glucose cut-off points are irrelevant and mindless constructs that don't accept that we have a continuum of risk and damage at ***ANY*** point along our metabolic journey and any glucose level towards chronic disease.

So-called drug management "paradoxes"

We will look at drug management outcomes that have produced so-called dangerous or deadly "paradoxical" results. However, there is no paradox here. Let's look at biomarkers through the lens of the Cell Starvation Model, where biomarkers support energy-stressed cells with structural decline. Therefore, by hammering biomarkers down with drugs, as I have mentioned, we deprive these distressed cells of what they truly need to survive – nutrients for energy and building blocks for maintaining structural integrity.

We have to be extremely careful with drug treatment and tip-toe through dosing because a small dose does nothing for risk, and a high dose will deprive cells of the fuel or structural building blocks needed to reduce this cellular decay. Go higher and higher regarding drug dose, and we then risk a cell decompensating all because clumsy drugs hammer down nutritional resources.

And so we have a ***Goldilocks Zone*** where at least there is some (arguable) moderation of the "bite" of these biomarkers. But modifying this "bite" is all we will ever achieve with drugs. Our drug "victories" are never long-term, only short-term "wins". We never stop the long-term "bite" of biomarkers or the underlying damaging metabolic dysfunction process as they continue to stay abnormal in the background because we do nothing to stop the after-eating post-prandial effects of food on biomarkers.

Insulin resistance is all about a fuel and building block supply crisis, i.e. preventing glucose, amino acids and fatty acids from entering cells. So, what do we do? We target glucose with drugs and decrease glucose availability even further. Shouldn't we support cells that are biological entities with nutrient resource needs rather than threaten those resources through drug means? Why do we wait till glucose or other markers become a major threat to us? Just so we can use a drug and say, "***Look, we can lower the effect of glucose damage by using drug-X or Y?***" If there is logic to this approach, then I don't understand it!

In this chapter, we are going to expose a world of deception with regard to blood biomarkers where this deception is buried under a crushing weight of deceit, downright lies, "speaker program" hocus pocus statistics and complexity designed to confuse everyone for commercial gain. If you don't believe what I have just said, then please read on to see what experts and expert bodies have to say about all of this. I will show you that when we look at all these biomarkers through the lens of the Cell Starvation Model (CSM), we can easily see why drug treatment disasters occur so often and, in many cases, are lethal. After reading what I have to say about these biomarker wars, you be the judge.

Biomarkers: The fall-guys of metabolic dysfunction

So, over decades, a simplistic approach was adopted, and a war was declared on biomarkers. Glucose, cholesterol, and LDL were declared mortal enemies that needed to be crushed by drugs at all costs. How convenient for Pharma. These biomarkers became enemies based on hunches, guesses (hypotheses) and associations but not true and conclusive science. ***If these biomarker wars were based on conclusive science, then our battles with biomarkers would have seen chronic disease prevalence plummet and not "explode".*** All these drug treatments should be halting and reversing metabolic disease. If drugs actually worked, why are we seeing chronic diseases being driven into the stratosphere where healthcare systems struggle to cope anymore?

We discuss these hunches or guesses below. As researchers love to say, correlation does not imply causation. In other words, just because these blood biomarkers change over time during the insulin resistance continuum doesn't mean they are the bad guys. They have, in fact, been the ***fall guys*** for poor medical science.

However, the twist in all of this is that these Janus-faced (two-faced) blood biomarkers do become bad guys or enemies over time. We have failed to see the purpose of these biomarkers in the early stages of metabolic disease as being supportive to cells starving of energy and undergoing structural decay. We have waited and waited for biomarkers to reach magical cut-off points rather than stopping them by dietary and nutrient management.

We always neglect to stop biomarker damage early on this journey and foolishly only want to deal with the end result of this damage – our organs failing. In medical thought, biomarkers are only relevant if they reach dizzying blood levels. Drug-filled medical toolboxes have been totally inadequate for the job at hand for 21st-century diseases that do not respond to silver bullets. We look at this drug-centric madness in the chapter "***Revolution Time***".

It is no mistake that doctors at the undergraduate level are not literate in statistics, as statistically savvy doctors would see through the shonky statistics used by Pharma and medical gurus to convince doctors that drug-based approaches are the only way forward. In this chapter, we will look at the deception of ***Relative Risk Reduction (RRR)***.

So, Pharma took advantage of an emerging chronic disease problem from the 1950s and 60s that accelerated after the Green and Farming revolutions, producing that glut of cheap high-carb grains, a big factor that ignited this chronic disease disaster. If dietary inputs are not the major cause of these horrendous diseases, then what is? Radiation from Mars?

These food revolutions spawned all the horror cereal-based glucose-spiking foods that dominate dietary intakes. From this time on, Pharma has been calling the shots, and like lambs to the slaughter, the medical profession follows their drug lords like a meek and totally dependent profession dependent on the crumbs Pharma throws its way. Right now, the medical profession is on bended knees, begging Pharma to come up with something to stop this embarrassing failure of deadly metabolic diseases, making them look incredibly bad. We naively wait and wait for a wonder drug.

Our only proven strategy to truly stop and reverse this process comes from food and nutrient-based approaches, as shown in the Lyon Diet Heart Study. We have seen a significant reversal of metabolic disease as shown in the MIND study, the PREDIMED Study, the DASH Diet and a plethora of other food and nutrient-based studies, including intermittent or timed fasting. When have you ever seen a claim made that a drug will reverse or cure any of these diseases? As a medical practitioner with decades of experience, I have never heard this declaration.

Evidence-based approaches are not the exclusive domain of drugs. We ignore evidence-based food and nutrient approaches out of conceit and arrogance that drugs are our only answer. In fact, food and nutrient-based approaches are the only answer to this nightmare problem of chronic disease armageddon.

Guesswork – Our hypotheses in action

"For every complex problem, there's a solution that is simple, neat, and wrong." H.L. Mencken

Declaring war on single biomarkers is unbelievable folly. It is naïve, embarrassing and highly amusing. As mentioned, we declared war on biomarkers based on the association between biomarkers and biological damage. We failed to see why biomarkers existed in the first place, and we still don't get that we have allowed biomarkers to damage us throughout our lifetimes by inaction.

Our focus shifted from glucose to LDL cholesterol (LDL-C). Yet, another opportunity for Pharma. It is not total LDL but modified LDL, which is the problem, as many experts note. It is damaged or altered rogue (modified) LDL, which is the problem, as I will highlight. However, attacking total LDL means more people will need treatment, and thus, more money will be made.

So, we developed the ***Glucose Hypothesis*** or ***Lipid Hypothesis***, but these are just guesses, as I have mentioned, dressed up as the more academic-sounding "***hypotheses***". These guesses have backfired spectacularly. Other enemies, such as cholesterol, triglycerides, HDL, and inflammation (inflammatory markers), were also proclaimed "evil". Has this war on biomarkers or inflammation won this metabolic disease war? Of course not. This war rages on irrespective of drug treatment and is about to get far worse.

The mechanism of a drug's actions is redundant. What matters most is whether that drug can reverse and cure the disease. Nothing else matters. We must learn to demand cures, not a stop-gap, temporary modification of the "bite" of biomarkers as drugs do.

For every "victory" at an individual level in a wealthy nation, millions will live miserable lives riddled with disease at the population level in many countries that will see loss of life early, let alone all that misery of a chronic disease before death. We will never win in any individual if we allow this metabolic dysfunction continuum to simmer in the background of anyone affected by this process that exists in most of us now.

Paradox? What Paradox? We only have confused professionals

Many studies have shown negative "paradoxical" outcomes to drug management, like the ACCORD, ADVANCE, or VADT studies. For example, the aggressive blood-glucose-lowering arm of the ACCORD study (and others) revealed a higher death rate in these individuals, resulting in premature termination of this study.

Trying to lower blood pressure too much, for example, can pull the rug from under the microcirculation pressure head, leading to catastrophic medical outcomes like heart attacks or strokes. Try to lower glucose too much, and you may also trigger a deadly cardiovascular event such as a heart attack or stroke. All of these drug-induced catastrophes can be viewed as the result of drug actions that undermine metabolic biomarkers as nutrient resources that cells need and demand to survive. It is a case of already inadequate nutrient resources being even more threatened by drug action. These "paradoxical" damaging and deadly drug treatment outcomes are a step too far. Increasing the dose of a drug or adding other drugs (polypharmacy) to the mix makes matters worse with regard to cell nutrients and energy supply.

How do the medical profession and research bodies face these seemingly paradoxical results? These negative results are justified in one way or the other in subsequent research papers. Can you guess who benefits from gaslighting these results?

Supporting distressed cells through nutrient means is alien to medicine or dietetics. By providing cells with a wealth of nutrients and preventing ongoing damage by adverse food and other inputs, we are actually helping cells fix themselves to optimise energy (ATP) levels, achieve cellular balance and decrease entropy (cellular decay). Fix the cell, and you fix the problem, is the motto we need to adopt. But no, in practice, we want to treat the "cries" of dysfunctional cells by attacking the biomarkers required for survival.

It can take decades for these rising metabolic biomarkers to manifest as a blocked artery or dementia, kidney failure or blindness, peripheral arterial disease, or a mental health disorder. That these metabolic biomarkers cause extensive damage to our cells, tissues, organs, and vascular systems is not in doubt. This damage is the long-term result of these Janus-faced biomarkers in action that we have ignored negligently. We pay the price for not acting early enough to prevent these biomarkers from harming us.

Declaring war on obesity: Let's see what can go wrong with weight loss

There is currently a huge amount of misleading hype about injectables and weight loss. We cling to the notion that if people can only lose weight, then we can eradicate metabolic diseases like diabetes or any acquired chronic metabolic disease. We cling to this utter simplicity of thought. But, if this thinking is correct, then how does weight loss prevent the constant barrage of harmful factors described in the BIG-10 Womb-to-Tomb list? Why, then, is it possible that even a small amount of weight loss can increase the risk of heart failure? We discussed previously how even a small 5% decrease in weight can result in a massive 42% increased risk of heart failure in predisposed individuals (Huang, Guo et al. 2021). This risk of heart failure with weight loss is a worry as heart failure is an emerging epidemic in many countries (Roger 2010).

Aggressive weight loss has another dangerous downside in terms of triggering frank diabetes. Does anyone bother with this potentially drastic outcome with weight loss? We had a warning shot about the possibility of adverse consequences of weight loss and "diabetes" risk in a study of 7 obese individuals where war was declared on their obesity and where there was an aggressive effort to help them lose body weight. These individuals were put on a "strenuous" weight reduction program. None of the seven (7) individuals studied had any history of diabetes. However, out of the 7 individuals in this aggressive weight-lowering program, five (5) developed non-insulin-dependent diabetes mellitus, and 2 required insulin to control their glucose levels (Koffler and Kisch 1996).

Wow! 7 out of 7 in the study ran into metabolic trouble, where weight loss triggered advanced metabolic dysfunction. This outcome is frightening, especially when we have a frenzy of activity with new anti-obesity medications (AOMs) coming out.

If fat is seen as "***energy memory***" monitored by the brain and immune system to tell the body we have enough stored energy onboard in case of a medical emergency, and if fat is a survival adaptation to cells in an energy crisis, then losing this stored energy created for survival purposes will then be seen as a threat to the whole body. Thus, the reason for decompensation to frank diabetes with the loss of energy reserves should be self-evident in my mind. We already have cells in cell starvation mode as most people in populations now have insulin resistance pulling the rug from cell energy supplies and where cells will have significant structural damage. If we then deplete stored fat energy, what can we expect in clinical outcomes as energy reserves for struggling cells will be cut back even further? We have discussed the very high rate of insulin resistance and "diabetes" in those who are obese previously.

With fewer calories being consumed in fat-reducing strict diets, we have far less blood glucose derived from food and on top of this, we are depleting fat stores, so now we can't even produce glucose from the glycerol backbones of triglycerides in that stored fat. We worsen cell starvation and hence the decompensation to "diabetes".

This adverse result of a strict weight loss diet was dramatic and unexpected in the study discussed above. The researchers hoped to see significant fat loss as a benefit to the individuals, but instead, they scratched their heads at this unexpected diabetes outcome. Until then, no one had recorded such an adverse outcome produced by weight loss. Are people warned of this possible outcome?

If obesity were due to an energy surplus, then wouldn't aggressive lowering of energy intake result in dramatic weight loss and fat loss and thus cause a reversal of metabolic dysfunction? One would have thought so, right? However, this aggressive weight loss program pushed them into a metabolic crisis that zoomed them along the insulin resistance metabolic dysfunction continuum to an advanced point of glucose elevation. Totally predictable by the Cell Starvation Model.

Most drug-induced weight loss programs will have pathetic dietary and nutrient support behind them, so all we are doing is creating medical malnutrition, as I have discussed previously, on top of preexisting cell starvation pressures.

This story is a cautionary tale for the new anti-obesity "wonder drugs" - the hyped injectables and oral versions that will be released. There is a lot that can go wrong with significant fat loss. We are headed for a disaster, but we are in the honeymoon gold rush, money-making drug sales phase. Drug gurus hired by Pharma will do their best to stoke this fire and paint these anti-obesity drugs in the best light possible. What can go wrong? There is money to be made, so who cares about lives lost? When has that stopped Pharma?

When things do go wrong, as they have with multiple medications in the past, they will withdraw these drugs, bury the dead, pay a huge fine which will be a fraction of what they have made and banked with interest alone on banked money offsetting the frivolous 1 – 2 billion dollars in fines—a pittance. If fines were tens of billions of dollars, then attitudes may change, but a billion or two are nothing to these companies.

What are lipoproteins?

A little knowledge about lipoproteins at this point will be helpful. These lipoproteins are LDL, a cholesterol carrier (the 'bad' guy), HDL (the 'good' guy, removing cholesterol back to the liver) or VLDL (the high-energy triglyceride carrier), also a "bad" guy.

We await advanced signals like high glucose or lipid levels to raise the alarm but fail to recognise that all our lipid fractions become damaged (modified) over our lifetimes by glucose, inflammation, oxidative stress, postprandial (after-eating) hits, etc., as part of the insulin resistance continuum and daily food intakes.

Cholesterol and triglycerides are needed by cells, as we have discussed, for energy or structural components such as membranes. Lipids or fats are required for various biological tasks, but lipids need a lipoprotein carrier to take them to the cells and tissues that need them. This lipoprotein carrier, like low-density lipoprotein (LDL), is the "ship" carrying the cargo (lipids) in the blood. We need these carriers as lipids are water-hating (hydrophobic), and the lipoprotein carrier (ship) is water-loving (hydrophilic). This hydrophilic characteristic of lipoproteins enables lipids to be carried to other body parts through blood vessels in a watery medium - our blood.

To get this lipid cargo to various cells in the aqueous environment of the bloodstream, they must be transported in the lipoprotein "ship" (Batty, Kivimäki et al.). Please view Appendix-10 for more information about lipoproteins.

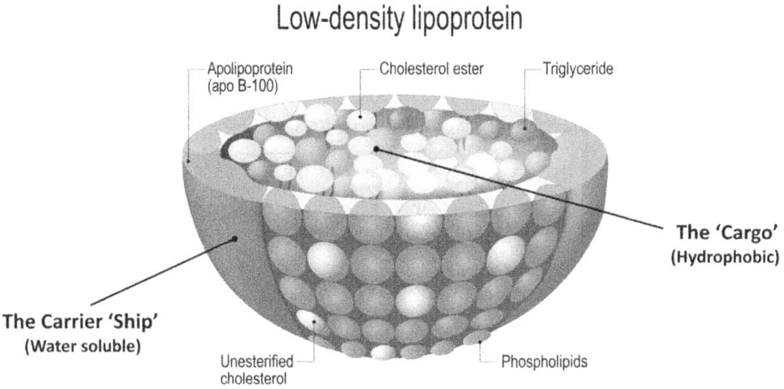

Declaring war on LDL (The "Bad" Cholesterol)

Our attention shifted from glucose to lipids and lipid fractions like LDL as enemies that need to be crushed in a pharmacological battle. LDL will often be referred to as the "bad guy" by your doctor, and like all bad guys, we want to restrain or punish them somehow.
LDL and statins became the new money-making battleground in this biomarker battle to win ground in this metabolic disease war. In the case of LDL, we recruit statins to restrain and lower LDL levels. The use of statins opened up a huge opportunity for Pharma to make a lot of money as statin lipid-lowering medications became a huge seller.

The longitudinal Framingham Study was launched impressively in 1948 to look at cardiovascular risk factors and is still ongoing. The multigenerational Framingham study started in 1948 because the cardiovascular death rate rose steadily in the first half of the 20th Century and started to level off from the 50s to 60s, reaching a peak in 1968 (AIHW 2017). But now, cardiovascular disease today is the biggest killer in populations worldwide.

Changes to the numbers smoking tobacco, blood thinning with aspirin, and control of blood pressure will all have had an impact on decreasing cardiovascular risk, and in high-income countries, coronary artery stenting would have also had an effect in lowering the mortality rate. The benefits of all these measures are short-term and help decrease immediate risk. None of these measures has stopped the prevalence of metabolic chronic disease from skyrocketing out of control or fixed any individual long-term.

There is no cure, and so all we do is delay the inevitable. What we do with drugs is hocus-pocus by preventing short-term lethal heart attacks or strokes by kicking the can down the road to a later date in someone's life. This delay in adverse and lethal effects can make current research look good by not providing these later-date negative outcomes that we know will happen.

We have increasing cardiovascular disease in older age groups, as shown in the quote below. What can be expected when the critical inputs are not changed? Mismanagement of cardiovascular disease is our greatest threat in life, but our medical and dietetic management is all smoke and mirrors, as shown in the prevalence figures below. A European Society of Cardiology Roundtable Report stated that:

> *"The incidence of cardiovascular disease (CVD) increases with age from 40% in adults aged 40–59 years, to 75% in those 60–79 years, and 86% in those >80 years." (Lettino, Mascherbauer et al. 2022)*

Do these figures smell of a continuum of risk? It fits the statement of kicking the can down the road to another older age bracket. It is no surprise that medical research uses individuals at younger ages to skew the results in their favour (Watts 2012).

How can anyone be happy that there is a 40% risk of CVD in 40-somethings? That is, 4 in 10 individuals from 40 years of age are at risk of a deadly heart attack or stroke is deplorable. The fact is that despite a drug or a combination of drug treatments, we still have metabolic dysfunction that continues uninterrupted in the background, as statins, aspirin, antihypertensives, and glucose-lowering agents do absolutely nothing to stop this metabolic dysfunction continuum and the continuum of biological rot. Biological rot just lurks in the background like a hooded creep in a dark alley waiting to strike. This stealthy biological rot, as discussed, causes more and more complicated medical problems as time goes by in these 40-somethings as they get older. Drug management and stenting are unbelievably deceitful. Entropy will continue to reign supreme until that final blow.

That LDL causes atherosclerotic (plaque blockage) and vascular disease is a hotly contested topic. I will outline why I think LDL, as an unchanged (native) molecule (i.e. not modified by glucose or oxidized), is a fall guy for heart and vascular disease. I will explain how I perceive LDL lowering to have some effect on cardiovascular disease. However, putting a huge emphasis on LDL is simply foolish. Who in their right mind would think that by focusing on one biomarker out of so many, we are going to conquer heart and vascular disease? Is decreasing LDL going to stop the after-eating (postprandial) damage to our vascular networks? Is lowering LDL going to stop epigenetic programming or environmental impacts? This book is not about simplistic views or promoting standalone (single) biomarker impacts as if they work in a vacuum to other factors that can change their very nature, as we will look at when I discuss glycated LDL (gLDL) or oxidized LDL (oxLDL)

Big Pharma opportunistically hijacked the studies that came out of the Framingham research along with other lipid studies and then sold this lipid hypothesis (guess) as "evidence-based" lipid management using statins to doctors and the rest of us when the evidence had never been there. ***All the evidence points to LDL as the native and unmodified molecule as being benign unless altered, i.e. modified by inflammation or glucose.***

As stated, it is not the native unmodified LDL that is the problem at all, and yet we are told that LDL is a huge enemy irrespective of modification to sell drugs. As this paper states:

> *"Chemically or biologically modified low-density lipoproteins (LDL) but not native unmodified LDL lead to foam cell*

formation in monocyte-derived macrophages" (Lechleitner, Hoppichler et al. 1994)

Foam cells are fat-laden cells that are critical in plaque formation in atherosclerosis. It is interesting, then, that despite statins being handed out like candy, cardiovascular disease remains the number one killer globally, killing vast millions in populations despite these drugs being used so commonly.

"However, statin trials in the elderly (PROSPER), in patients with heart failure (CORONA, GISSI-HF), and in patients with renal failure (4D, AURORA, SHARP) have all failed to demonstrate a mortality benefit" (DuBroff and de Lorgeril 2015)

Currently, according to the WHO, 16% of deaths worldwide are due to cardiovascular disease. This figure is set to jump to a staggering 31.7% of all deaths in 2030 in less than a decade (Varounis and Beshiri 2021). In fact, almost 1 in 3 individuals affected by cardiovascular disease deaths is only a few years away. So, where are statins in all of this? Why aren't statins and all the other biomarker wars being fought not halting and reversing these damning statistics?

Am I missing something in all of this? Medical gurus bask in the "glory" of drugs like statins, and yet we are seeing carnage in populations and health outcomes deteriorating at a galloping rate. Will gurus next say that we need statins in the water supply globally before we see a lowering of cardiovascular disease? What about treating all babies born with statins at birth? Pharma salivates at this prospect of universal use of statins to fix something caused by dietary inputs (mainly) and other significant insults like food impacts multiple times a day to our cells, depriving them of energy, increasing structural decay and crushing our microvascular networks.

Doctors have been gullible pawns in all of this and still are. They are caught up in the headlights of this complexity and statistical hocus-pocus nonsense. Smoke and mirrors will only hoodwink us for so long until the numbers of diseased become so huge and crushing that there will be nowhere to hide from this disaster.

Crunch time is only around the corner!

Low-density lipoprotein (LDL). Fact or Fiction?

LDL is an important topic for all of us. Many of you may be on a statin or will be on a statin in future as you have nowhere to hide from these chronic diseases where heart and vascular disease is the most likely way you will leave this planet. So, let's look at LDL in more depth.

The mantra is to go lower and lower in terms of LDL levels in the blood. The paradigm of the "***lower the better***" may indeed have a benefit, but not for the reasons we think. It is not the level of normal or unchanged LDL that counts but the underlying metabolic dysfunction process that actually drives changes to the very nature of that LDL molecule, making LDL more dangerous (pathogenic). So, it is the ***quality*** of LDL and ***not the quantity*** that counts?

These altered LDL changes are caused by 1) our metabolic dysfunction continuum and 2) the after-eating (postprandial) impacts resulting in modified LDL molecules. After eating the wrong type of food, our blood glucose levels rise, and the accompanying after-eating inflammation changes the LDL with every meal or snack. Modified LDL should be our absolute focus. Controlling modified LDL means early nutritional interventions to prevent LDL changes. We will discuss oxidized and glycated LDL and the modified versions of LDL shortly.

By asking doctors to push LDL lower and lower, this directive is oblivious to the fact that LDL is the major cholesterol carrier, and we know that cholesterol is a building block for steroids and Vitamin-D, and where cholesterol is vital for cell and organelle membranes. Without a steady supply of cholesterol to cells, they start to undergo major structural decline (increasing entropy). Is it clever then to use statins to lower native (unmodified) LDL that is not a risk to our vascular systems? What do you think is a better strategy? Should we use a drug to lower LDL or prevent LDL from being modified in the first place by a great dietary plan?

Vitamin-D, made from cholesterol, is also vital for oxidative phosphorylation (OXPHOS) and ATP production. So, a lack of cholesterol will also impact Vitamin-D and cell energy production, thus decreasing the chances of lowering entropy through repair and restoration, which requires energy input. Lower cell energy will drive insulin resistance and metabolic dysfunction even further. And so cellular entropy blasts off without adequate energy, nutrient resources or Vitamin-D production.

As you can see by looking through the lens of the Cell Starvation Model, if we unthinkingly lower LDL to cells already suffering from cell energy starvation and structural decline, then cells are not going to fare very well. It becomes a tug-of-war between the body trying to support energy-starved and distressed cells with LDL (cholesterol + triglycerides) versus drugs attempting to do the opposite to this biomarker LDL survival adaptation.

In a letter to the British Journal of Nutrition, the authors stated that "***multiple lines of evidence***" have shown that LDL is a relatively poor marker for cardiovascular disease. In fact, in individuals admitted to hospitals due to an adverse cardiovascular event such as a heart attack, 50% of those affected individuals had LDL in the optimal (normal) range (Wood, Hansen et al. 2016).

> *"Multiple lines of evidence suggest that LDL-cholesterol is a relatively poor marker of CVD risk. This includes one very large study of patients hospitalised with CVD, almost 50% of whom had LDL-cholesterol levels within the 'optimal' range (<100 mg/dl or 2·6 mmol/l)." (Wood, Hansen et al. 2016)*

An impressive list of multiple authors in an expert review published in the journal ***Expert Review of Clinical Pharmacology*** stated in the headline of this paper that "***LDL-C does not cause cardiovascular disease: a comprehensive review of the current literature***". This same expert review pointed out some incredibly important points about total cholesterol (TC) and LDL, considering that LDL is by far the major carrier of cholesterol in the body (Gopalan and Kirk 2022). Let's look at these important points against LDL as the "bad guy" of lipid fractions. There are many contradictions concerning this LDL hypothesis. These contradictions regarding LDL are:

1) **THE LDL PARADOX:** People with the highest LDL level should have shorter lives if LDL were such a bad guy, right? But, the opposite was found in a study of 68,000 older adults over 60 years. Those with the highest LDL levels actually ***lived longer than those on statin drugs*** that were used to lower LDL levels (Ravnskov, de Lorgeril et al. 2020). Who do you believe? The spruikers of drugs or the facts?

2) **PARADOXICALLY:** For each 1 mg/dl ***drop in total cholesterol***, there was actually an ***11% increased risk*** of death from heart and vascular disease and total mortality risk. One study in Hawaii showed a 30% increase in mortality risk with lower cholesterol. (Jeong, Choi et al. 2018). Would this happen if lipid fractions were so dangerous?

3) **THERE SHOULD BE A DOSE-RESPONSE EFFECT:** That should be obvious regarding the reduction in absolute risk, but this dose-response was not shown in studies. So if a drug is increased and LDL and cholesterol are lowered, then the benefit of lipid-lowering should be seen as a proportionate lowering in cardiovascular risk and mortality. ***There is no obvious dose-response effect seen.*** The authors of one expert review paper stated the following about dose-response:

> *"The idea that high cholesterol levels in the blood are the main cause of CVD is impossible because people with low levels become just as atherosclerotic as people with high levels, and their risk of suffering from CVD is the same or higher. The cholesterol hypothesis has been kept alive for decades by reviewers who have used misleading statistics, excluded the results from unsuccessful trials and ignored numerous contradictory observations."* (Ravnskov, de Lorgeril et al. 2018)

Only a forensic examination of the income and association of authors who praise the benefits of statins will show their affiliations with Pharma and, thus, their motives to use shonky statistics to promote statin use. When money is at stake, then who cares?

Of those unfortunate individuals admitted to the hospital with an acute heart attack, 66% had preexisting Metabolic Syndrome (MetS), which is a high cardiovascular-risk prediabetic problem made worse by a high starchy carb diet in many individuals where high carb intake increases damaging small dense LDL (sdLDL) adding greatly to risk. To blast a huge hole in this "cholesterol is bad" motto, 75% of these acute heart attack individuals have normal total cholesterol levels (Malhotra 2013)- so much for this lipid hypothesis (lipid guess). After-eating impacts matter. Dietary impacts matter.

It has become impossible to tease out why statins showed some minor benefit in studies that found risk reduction. Was lowering LDL the actual cause of the cardiovascular risk reduction? Or was it due to the so-called pleiotropic effects of statins? (Ravnskov, de Lorgeril et al. 2018). These pleiotropic effects of statin drugs include decreasing inflammation, improving function in the lining of blood vessels (endothelial function) or decreasing oxidative stress. These pleiotropic effects have nothing to do with cholesterol-lowering.

We miss the point that LDL does not work in isolation from what is happening in the biological world around it. Inflammation drives up oxidized LDL (ox-LDL), and inflammation is increased by increasing metabolic dysfunction and the consumption of so-called "healthy" foods that can increase blood triglycerides to produce a "soaring" inflammatory response, as discussed. Glucose slowly but surely rises from worsening metabolic dysfunction or after-eating (postprandial) effects from high starchy carb intakes. High blood glucose ramps up glycated LDL (gLDL), forming a damaging modified (glycated) LDL rogue form, and to add salt to the wound, we also have a carb-mad world glorified by dietetics, where high carb loads drive up vascular damaging small dense LDL (sdLDL). So, concentrating on just total LDL is nonsense and highly simplistic.

The theme throughout this book is about bioenergetic decline in cells. We use statins to lower risk, but in the end, we damage our mitochondria and ATP production by the use of statins. Statins harm mitochondrial ATP generation by inhibiting the production of critical ETC components – CoQ10 and Heme-A. See Appendix-5. It is no wonder, then, that statins have the potential to induce diabetes as energy levels drop in cells and entropy ramps up, as we have discussed previously.

Interesting how studies that fail to show what we want them to show are excluded

LDL lowering showed a weak association with cardiovascular risk in 26 trials included in a meta-analysis, but importantly, 11 trials that were not included in the meta-analysis showed an ***inverse risk*** response where the higher the LDL, the lower the cardiovascular risk (Ravnskov, de Lorgeril et al. 2018). How incredibly shonky to **exclude** these unsupporting trials in the data that showed better outcomes with higher LDL levels. It shows how statistics can be totally distorted in favour of statins. Statins are a multi-billion dollar business, so fraudulence goes hand in hand in any industry involving vast sums of money being made from drug sales.

So, a higher LDL may be associated with true cardiovascular **health** and not the other way around. We can't get around the fact that LDL is critical to health and is a supplier of cholesterol and triglycerides to cells. This LDL delivery of cholesterol and triglycerides is especially important when cells are undergoing bioenergetic decline and structural decay. In my mind, the answer to why we have conflicting findings is a no-brainer. ***The higher the LDL levels, the more LDL particles will be available for modification by oxidative (inflammatory) processes and glycation.*** In a world of increasing insulin resistance and metabolic dysfunction where inflammation glucose levels start to soar, in this very circumstance, the more LDL around, the more LDL will be modified to more pathogenic (harmful) oxidized forms.

Modified LDL (mLDL), such as glycated LDL (gLDL) or oxidized LDL (oxLDL), are the rogue LDL variants that damage blood vessels and hammer our microcirculation networks. These modified LDL rogue variants will love to take advantage of the glycocalyx damage to blood vessel linings caused by high glucose levels spiking after eating high starchy carb meals.

Why have we ignored this obvious reason for LDL risk? The best way to deal with modified LDL is through a food and nutrient-based approach to control and reverse insulin resistance and metabolic dysfunction, dampen down oxidative stress and inflammation, minimise postprandial (after eating) glucose and glycation impacts and stop this high carb nonsense driving disease. A diet rich in plant-based antioxidants, a high vegetable intake and low-fructose fruit consumption, Vitamin-C and N-Acetylcysteine with meals and nutrient factors that support Glutathione production along with a diversity of fibre (prebiotics) to strengthen our gut microbiome will go a very long way to prevent modification of LDL, thus slashing cardiovascular disease. Simple but true, but who makes money from this simplicity?

The LDL particle: Quality matters greatly

We are also using very outdated tests to stratify cardiovascular risk. We need to assess risk by looking at these lipid markers and then determine the size, density and particle quantity. The Type-B pattern of small dense LDL can penetrate blood vessel walls far more easily than the Type-A pattern of large buoyant fluffy LDL.

The Type-B or small dense LDL (sdLDL) lipid pattern increases significantly with high carbohydrate intake but not fat intake (Malhotra 2013). So, knowing someone has the Type-B LDL pattern, wouldn't it be a no-brainer to stop those unnecessary starchy carbs from increasing this deadly small, dense LDL subtype? Lowering carb intake makes great sense if that individual has had a heart attack, a high coronary calcium score, coronary blockages on an angiogram or has a metabolic disease, putting them at high risk for a deadly cardiovascular event. Dietetics and dietitians will need to decide what is more important: agricultural wealth or the health of individuals, populations and their nations.

A high carbohydrate diet is unequivocally associated with a significant increase in small dense LDL (sdLDL) (Siri-Tarino,

Williams et al. 2009). This sdLDL is highly atherogenic (blood vessel damaging) by itself but is even more dangerous when glycated (damaged by glucose) to form gLDL, which then is oxidized to form oxidised LDL (ox-LDL) (Wood, Hansen et al. 2016).

Small dense LDL can be easily modified by glucose and inflammation to make them even more dangerous. We can test for oxidized LDL (oxLDL), and this warns us of underlying oxidative stress and inflammation modifying the LDL lipid fraction.

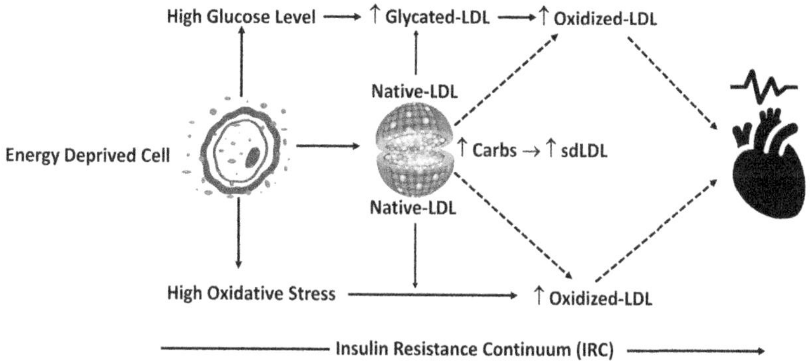

Using a gentle ketosis non-starchy diet as outlined in the final chapter based on a wealth of existing research will significantly impact the formation of the three (x3) highly atherogenic LDL-modified variants below (Wood, Hansen et al. 2016):

1. **Small Dense LDL (sdLDL) – These are strongly associated with high starchy carbohydrate intake (Siri-Tarino, Williams et al. 2009).**
2. **Glycated-LDL (gLDL) and AGE-LDL** - AGEs are Advanced Glycation Endproducts produced by advanced glycation (glucose damage) effects where glucose (or fructose) attaches and modifies LDL and other lipoprotein subfractions. Keeping after-eating glucose levels low is key to helping decrease glycated LDL. Let's not forget that ***fructose is 7 – 10 times more glycating than glucose.***

3. **Oxidized-LDL (OxLDL)** – This is the final modification point in the LDL modification cascade produced by oxidative stress (ROS and inflammation).

Death by Carbs: The madness of diets high in starchy carbs. Our "*Mini diabetic episodes*"

> *"Carbohydrates usually provide between 55 and 75% of daily energy requirements. Although they are not essential nutrients, they substantially impact health maintenance." (Farías, Cisternas et al. 2023)*

Saturated fat and cholesterol were initially targets since the Ancel Keys "seven countries" studies in the 1970s. As a result, fat consumption dramatically declined, but "paradoxically" cardiovascular risk increased significantly (Malhotra 2013). Fatty liver is a major problem now skyrocketing as well in populations in parallel with chronic metabolic diseases. ***Yet, it is not fat that drives fatty liver; it is carbohydrate consumption.*** It is known that a low-carb diet can decrease fatty liver by 32% on MRI studies (Farías, Cisternas et al. 2023).

A high carb load can increase not only glucose levels but also inflammatory blood triglycerides (fat) levels and drive up small dense LDL (sdLDL). The spikes of triglyceride in the blood after eating carbs are called ***carbohydrate-induced hypertriglyceridaemia.*** This postprandial (after-eating) high triglyceride (fat) level is an independent risk factor for heart disease and stroke (Lechleitner, Hoppichler et al. 1994). High triglycerides in the blood are a big inflammatory risk, and we need to keep in mind that LDL can be modified to oxidized-LDL in the after-eating period (ox-LDL) is not in doubt, as shown in the Lechleitner et al. paper. It is interesting, then, that - ***even a small 10% carb increase can cause high blood triglycerides,*** which rise even higher with higher carb intakes (Hellerstein 2002). Raised blood triglycerides also increase triglyceride-rich LDL, which is another modified form of LDL.

We are destroying the lives of our children who develop fatty liver in huge numbers by feeding them massive amounts of grain-based and processed carbs along with high intakes of sugar, dairy and fructose that will drive this fatty liver pandemic along even further. We often think we will harm children long-term by restricting carbohydrates, which are glucose, plain and simple, but this is ridiculous when the body can produce all the glucose it needs without carb consumption. We destroy the lives of our youngest people with staple foods, which is not a good mantra when other food sources will be far better by a long shot. Think twice, starting your child's day with a huge carb and sugar hit from twisted cereals in a colourful box. It's a toxic start to a day.

The term "essential" means that you can only get glucose through starchy carbs, which is 100% incorrect. It is a sobering fact that sugar and other refined carbohydrates can actually cause Type-2 Diabetes Mellitus in the absence of other risk factors (Bhardwaj, O'Keefe et al. 2016).

Ironically, Asian Indians have been credited with creating sugar in 350 BC by crystallising sugar from sugarcane juice. Sugar and sugar-sweetened beverage intake in that country has jumped significantly since 2005. They are paying the price for their discovery. The incidence of diabetes, cardiovascular disease and stroke has soared by 100% in the past 20 years. Developing countries have 7x the number of people disabled by stroke compared to wealthier nations where strokes are a common complication of diabetes (Bhardwaj, O'Keefe et al. 2016).

However, as deadly as sugar is, as we see in countries like Mexico and India, let's not forget the fatal outcomes in wealthy countries where diabetes and stroke are also very common. It is not all about sugar or processed carbs. We now need to think about the amount of carbs being consumed or the ***carbohydrate load*** in any given meal. This carb load will determine how high and for how long glucose and triglycerides or small dense LDL (sdLDL) will stay elevated in our bloodstream.

However, sugar and sugar-sweetened beverages are a definite problem, so don't get me wrong, we should be concerned about sweetened foods and drinks, but we need to focus on the carb load from grains, bread, pasta, etc., as well. For those individuals with insulin resistance, "prediabetes", "MetS", and "diabetes", it is downright negligence and malpractice to use high carb loads in individuals who cannot tolerate high blood glucose levels. We subject ourselves to high glucose levels after we consume mounds of potato, pasta, rice and other grains we throw on our plates. These foods are really mounds of glucose, plain and simple.

High carb loads equal high blood insulin levels after eating

This carb load also determines how high insulin-IgF-1 will increase and stay elevated, which is yet another risk factor that we have discussed to not only trigger insulin resistance but fat gain and is a potent cell multiplication trigger. High energy hits from carbs can also shut off mitochondrial ATP production through disruption of the balance of the NAD^+/NADH redox couple (nutri-stress).

How many times are such carb-riddled, high-energy meals eaten in a day? Each high-carb meal damages us slowly, incrementally and cumulatively, whether wholegrain or not. The wholegrain message is another way to sell more grains to make it sound healthy. The starchy, glucose-spiking carbs are still within whole grains.

A low-carb diet can shift us away from generating small, dense LDL (sdLDL), decrease carb-induced high blood triglyceride (fat) levels and decrease the risk of the LDL modification cascade discussed above. IR in the quote below is Insulin Resistance, and CVD is Cardiovascular Disease. As these authors stated:

> *"... the most robust effect of any single long-term dietary intervention in terms of improvement in parameters of IR, dysglycaemia, atherogenic lipidaemia and CVD risk, is the restriction of carbohydrate intake." (Wood, Hansen et al. 2016)*

High-carb recommendations should now be seen as medical and dietetic malpractice for the vast number of people who can't tolerate the toxic effect of postprandial high blood glucose and triglycerides, along with the risk of beta cell burnout as a result of a constant demand for insulin from struggling beta cells.

That we downplay food as the biggest killer on the planet is simply shocking. If blood glucose is raised because of insulin resistance, then providing more glucose in the form of starchy carbs is breathtakingly ignorant and negligent, putting lives at risk. Only academics want to argue about glycemic index (GI) or glycemic load (GL) to complicate matters and confuse people. In the end, carbs are not essential, they lack multiple nutrients, and are not a brilliant source of fibre. Only gurus in the pocket of corporations will sell the "***grains-are-good***" mantra or the "***sugar-in-moderation***" message irrespective of any existing metabolic dysfunction problem in an individual and regardless of a history of a metabolic chronic illness and ignore the fact someone may have already suffered from a life-threatening cardiovascular event just to sell grains.

Ascorbic acid (Vitamin-C) can markedly lower the risk of LDL modification

Vitamin C consumed with a meal can markedly decrease the risk of LDL modification, so why then aren't we promoting this to individuals with metabolic disease (Lechleitner, Hoppichler et al. 1994)? So why don't we consume an antioxidant-rich tablet with Vitamin-C and N-acetylcysteine (NAC) with each meal?

Most medical and dietetic professionals probably don't know about the HP-2-2 genetic variant so common in populations that can rapidly deplete Vitamin-C in so many people. See Appendix-41. Also, you can't trademark a natural compound like Vitamin-C. So, how do you make money?

Also, having fibre with meals can lower postprandial impacts, and there are highly researched fibre combinations that can do this. Vinegar with your salad (a vinaigrette) can reduce the glycemic index of a meal. So why aren't these strategies mentioned to at-risk metabolically compromised individuals to lower postprandial effects? I discuss alpha lipoic acid, which can help regenerate our Vitamin C and antioxidants and provide ongoing protection against oxidative stress and inflammation.

It is not just LDL that can be glycated or oxidized. We can have glycated VLDL (gVLDL) and glycated HDL (gHDL) and then oxidized versions of these lipid subfractions as well being generated (Lyons 1992). Thus, inflammation caused by insulin resistance or after-eating impacts can damage a range of lipid markers.

The final chapter examines Nutritional Ketosis (NK), which I suggest as our saviour. This diet uses a low starchy carbohydrate diet with abundant dietary antioxidants and phytochemicals, compounds like NAC, and other known antioxidants and anti-inflammatories like Vitamin-C, omega-3s, and Choline, which can make a world of difference to distressed cells that need nutrient resources to recover and to protect us in the after-eating period.

> *"Over the last 30 years, deaths and disability from cardiovascular disease have been steadily rising across the globe. In 2019 alone, the condition, which includes heart disease and stroke, was responsible for a staggering one-third of all deaths worldwide." (NHLBI 2021)*

It is also wonderful to see a government body like the National Heart, Lung and Blood Institute (NHLBI) state the following about cardiovascular health beginning in childhood and start our preventative campaign very early in life. Think of your children:

> *"We also need strategies that promote ideal cardiovascular health beginning in childhood so that we can ensure healthy ageing for all" (NHLBI 2021)*

This letter to the British Journal of Nutrition editors rightly points out that cardiovascular disease is a multifactorial process that starts in the womb and childhood. So logically, any treatment must follow a multifactorial approach (Wood, Hansen et al. 2016).

Declaring war on HDL – Did increasing HDL the "good guy" work?

According to this fantasy of lipids as the enemy, we declare HDL is the good guy, and if we increase the level of this good lipid, then the world will be a wonderful place with regard to metabolic diseases and cardiovascular risk.

As stated, concentrating on one biomarker and ignoring other harmful inputs is naivete in the extreme. So, did increasing HDL produce brilliant results?

HDL usually takes cholesterol back to the liver for processing (**Reverse Cholesterol Transport or RCT**). So, taking cholesterol away from cells using simplistic thinking to guide us sounds like a good thing. Once again, the Cell Starvation Model shows how wrong

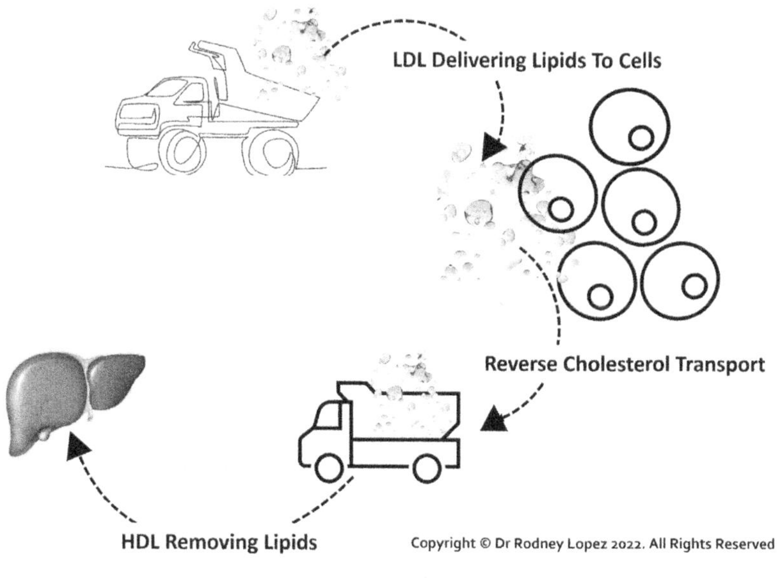

this thinking is, as low HDL has cell survival advantages in metabolic disease.

Suppose we view LDL delivery as a dump truck loaded with cholesterol and triglycerides, moving from the liver to other cells in the body. LDL is a major cholesterol and phospholipid carrier but also transports triglycerides, an energy source for cells. We can then view HDL as a ***lipid "bandit"*** loading up on fat near cells and driving the truck, the other way to transport these lipids back to the liver. This action helps to prevent the unused or excess lipids dumped at cell sites from creating problems like plaque and artery blockages. That is all well and good, but cholesterol and triglycerides are energy or structural sources. So HDL can be seen as a robber of cell lipid resources needed by cells distressed by a bioenergetic and structural decline for reasons discussed.

From the Cell Starvation Model lens, the fact is that all our cells and organelles, like mitochondria, need to be constantly repaired and renewed using cholesterol and phospholipids. If cells were normal (highly unlikely in anyone), then increasing HDL might be of some benefit. But if our cells are struggling with an energy crisis and building block shortages due to insulin resistance, then taking away precious nutritional lipid resources will never be a good thing at a time of cellular stress.

Our Cell Starvation Model (CSM) clearly predicts that increasing HDL will be a disaster. Let's look at this little gem of a treatment approach. If lowering glucose fails and statins are useless, why don't we try to increase HDL? What a great idea. Let's do it!

So, with this rosy thought in mind of raising HDL to prevent cardiovascular disease, ***Cholesteryl Ester Transfer Protein (CETP) Inhibitors*** were developed. CTEPs transfer cholesterol from HDL to other lipid fractions. So, by blocking CTEP, we promote HDL elevation and maintain HDL at higher levels, thus increasing cholesterol transport back to the liver and away from struggling cells. Did CTEP inhibitors decrease cardiovascular risk?

Let's look at how raising HDL levels with CTEP inhibitors went

Torcetrapib was the first CTEP inhibitor developed. This drug's results were "awe-inspiring". Notice the sarcastic inverted commas with a 72.1% increase in HDL levels, a fantastic result to be "celebrated" as it achieved raising HDL levels exceptionally as an endpoint. We also had a "fabulous" 24.9% decrease in LDL to boot –

wow, how brilliant. Results exceeded expectations. So, have we beaten cardiovascular disease by raising HDL? Should we run a victory lap yet?

Sad then that the ILLUMINATE trial designed to test this hypothesis of raising HDL through a CTEP inhibitor like Torcetrapib was terminated prematurely because the trial showed a massive 25% increase in cardiovascular events and a horrific 58% increase in deaths from ANY cause in the torcetrapib treated group (Kosmas, DeJesus et al. 2016). So much for "awe-inspiring" HDL increases.

Interestingly, this article discloses these disastrous cardiovascular events with the following statement - "*Past Failures and Future Hopes*" in the title. Future hopes? Are you kidding? Like all the failures of aggressively lowering blood glucose or blood lipids and now the failed attempt to increase HDL (the good guy), the "hope" part of the title suggests that if we use another drug that does the same thing in raising HDL using a different biochemical or molecular mechanism, that we will get a better result – the ***new drug, novel mechanism but same biomarker effect approach yet expecting a different result***. Insanity right?

If the medical profession and researchers saw HDL lowering from the Cell Starvation Model perspective, they may finally see the light and predict negative outcomes easily. Researchers forget that insulin resistance is the new norm and try to increase HDL when the evolutionary adaptation for starving cells is highly predictable – they need ***LOWER HDL*** to support them. It's an obvious survival mechanism. So, this disastrous effect of raising HDL is 100% predicted by the Cell Starvation Model! If silver bullets are the only way we think and our minds are focused on money-making blockbuster drugs, these drug treatment tragedies will continue.

Roche's dalcetrapib and Ely Lilly's evacetrapib also failed in trials raising HDL, but surely, if Big-Pharma keeps on trying, there will be an eventual success. Researchers see drug failures as a "paradox." Those who understand the Cell Starvation Model see these results as highly predictable 101 events that a child could understand conceptually. Lipid changes produced by cells in energy and structural decline are an evolutionary adaptation. Why do we miss this point? New drugs doing the same thing is a brain-dead concept to me, so why do we allow this and allow people to suffer and die?

Hot off the press: Declaring war on HDL

As I was writing this section, a fascinating study landed in my inbox from Medicine Today, a medical magazine in Australia. This article stated:

> *"A prospective, multicentre cohort study has found a paradoxical association between very high HDL-cholesterol (HDL-C) and all-cause mortality in patients with coronary artery disease (CAD). The study, published in JAMA Cardiology, recruited 14,478 patients with CAD from the UK Biobank and 5467 patients from the US Emory Cardiovascular Biobank in Atlanta, Georgia." (Lathlean 2022)*

It's amazing how these findings seem "paradoxical" to medical gurus and researchers where cell starvation issues go over their heads. It seems stunning to imagine that a high HDL will increase "all-cause mortality", i.e. death from all causes. And yet, we have had this fantasy that a high HDL is a good thing. There is nothing paradoxical in this at all. We are just looking at these findings through a money-distorted lens. There is nothing contradictory in these results because it is the price paid for removing nutrient resources from cells starving of nutrients. Plain and simple!

Another study reinforces the fact that high HDL levels increase mortality. If HDL levels are high and above two (2) mmol/L (80 mg/dL), the following risks apply:

> "...96% higher risk of all-cause mortality and a 71% higher risk of cardiovascular mortality."
> *(Liu, Dhindsa et al. 2022)*

Wow! Go figure. Remember that this result is only "paradoxical" when we view metabolic markers as enemies, not beneficial adaptations for cells in distress. Isn't it time we dumped this thinking that metabolic markers are enemies at all costs and see them finally for what they are – adaptations for cell survival? We wouldn't need drugs if we stopped this Dark Age thinking about biomarkers and simply support cells nutritionally to survive and function normally.

Declaring war on blood lipids: Shonky statistics. The Relative Risk Reduction (RRR) deception

Once again, as stated, this war on lipids is based on a guess – the "Lipid Hypothesis" theory, which proposes that lipids matter in terms of cardiovascular risk. Lipids, in fact, are marginal and become destructive due to factors happening around them. We make them matter due to all the insults that modify them, as we discussed. As usual, we forget about the main causes of risk.

A paper published in the "*Scandinavian Journal of Cardiology*" titled "*The fallacies of the lipid hypothesis*" points out what many in the profession see as gaslighting with downright corrupt research:

> *"The lipid hypothesis has dominated cardiovascular research and prevention for almost half a century, although the number of contradictory studies may exceed those that are supportive." (Ravnskov 2008)*

Why let the truth get in the way of a mega money-making enterprise? Pfizer, the maker of one of the biggest sellers of lipid-lowering medications called Lipitor® had this said about them in a paper:

> *"Pfizer has been a "habitual offender," persistently engaging in illegal and corrupt marketing practices, bribing physicians and suppressing adverse trial results. Since 2002, the company and its subsidiaries have been assessed $3 billion in criminal convictions, civil penalties and jury awards." (Evans 2010)*

If Lipitor®a statin lipid-lowering agent, made around 2 billion a year, what the heck does it matter with one-off fines of a billion dollars or more? Such fines that sound big are minuscule in the scheme of annual ongoing profits.

In statin research, they have almost exclusively used statistical "hocus pocus" by quoting ***Relative Risk Reduction (RRR)*** figures instead of absolute risk reduction (ARR). This statistical illusion means that negligible findings can greatly magnify the benefits, giving the illusion of an amazing outcome, but it is all statistical smoke and mirrors.

This relative risk reduction (RRR) can impress grassroots doctors who are not trained to examine statistics critically. Producing doctors who are unable to evaluate the statistics presented to them critically makes sense if pharmaceutical corporations influence universities and undergraduate training.

Don't you think it is a disgrace that medical undergraduates are only taught about drugs and not nutrition and prevention? Gullible doctors keep on writing scripts, not aware they are being duped as the vast majority don't really understand or question the statistics presented to them; otherwise, they would have woken up to this sleight of hand a long time ago. Relative Risk Reduction (RRR) is described as very deceptive (Diamond and Ravnskov 2015).
If we look at Relative Risk Reductions (RRRs) in comparison to Absolute Risk Reduction (ARR) from the Royal Australian College of General Practitioners (RACGP), the figures in the RACGP paper put this statistical gimmick into sharp focus:

> *"Imagine your chance of dying from a certain condition prematurely is 0.2%, and there's a drug that reduces your chance of dying to 0.1%. In relative terms (relative risk reduction), your chance of dying has been halved or reduced by 50%. But in absolute terms (absolute risk reduction), your chance of dying has only gone down by 0.1%." (RACGP 2022)*

Another example to clarify how misleading RRR can be is the following:

> *"For instance, in a trial where 2 of 100 participants in the control group died but only 1 of 100 in the treatment group died, the absolute risk reduction (ARR) is only a 1% benefit. However, if one reports the RRR, then a 50% benefit can be reported because one is 50% of two." (Ravnskov, de Lorgeril et al. 2018)*

Wow, how corrupt and misleading figures can be. So, a difference of just one life saved is stated as a 50% reduction in mortality risk. It sounds fantastic but distorts the reality, and governments will be conned to pay a huge price for this drug with potentially horrendous side effects, all due to a shonky statistic that pulls the wool over a doctor's (and politician's) eyes. We put nations at great risk.

Where are the government, regulatory bodies, or public health departments involved in all of this? That this is allowed with no one having the authority to shut down this deception is shocking. Imagine representatives seeing GPs in their practices or GPs listening to drug-centric medical gurus thumping their chests at conferences using these RRRs on a gullible medical audience who will be amazed by the huge RRR benefit of Drug-X.

The RACGP article went on to say about RRRs:

> *The relative risk reduction for those taking statins compared with those who did not was 9% for deaths, 29% for heart attacks and 14% for strokes. Yet the absolute risk reduction of dying, having a heart attack or stroke was 0.8%, 1.3% and 0.4%, respectively. (RACGP 2022)*

Using a statin to prevent an adverse heart and vascular event has never prolonged the life of anyone, and in secondary prevention trials, i.e. after someone has had a cardiovascular event, the benefit of statins has been quite small and rarely exceeding two (2) percentage points (Diamond and Ravnskov 2015). Do these drugs deserve subsidies? Why don't we dump statins and subsidize fresh foods or nutrients instead?

The question to statin-loving gurus is, will this statin stop and reverse the underlying insulin resistance metabolic dysfunction process? Will drugs stop the biological rot that worsens slowly in the background to generate complex medical issues eventually? Will this statin completely cure me of vascular disease? Will this statin stop me from having a heart attack or stroke in the near future and prevent heart attacks and strokes long-term? Sure, a statin may have a minor role in preventing an immediate vascular disaster over a very short period, but never long term as the underlying disease-causing biological rot process is never addressed and never halted. This biological rot keeps chugging along in the background of anyone given a statin.

What I am saying is not something that any guru can argue with. Remember the shocking statistic that 1 in 3 deaths will be caused by cardiovascular disease by 2030, a few short years away. Why haven't statins made a dent in these prevalence statistics if they were that amazing? So what's the use of a statin if a comprehensive diet, as shown in the Lyon Diet Heart Study, showed a whopping 70% reduction in all-cause mortality (Leaf 1999), not just from cardiovascular events but all causes and where such a diet can actually prolong life?

Statins, in comparison to a diet, are redundant. But this doesn't stop more and more "research" papers from coming out in favour of statins being used in prevention. Should they be given to children? It may surprise you that statins were recommended for children as young as eight (8) years old by the American Heart Association in 2007 and backed by the American Academy of Paediatrics (O'Gorman, O'Neill et al. 2010). If ever a statin was given to a child, unless in very rare circumstances, it would be deplorable. The article above pointed out how critical diet was for the whole family, which was a saving grace for the paper.

Heart and vascular disease is a childhood problem

Russell Holman, a professor of pathology, described atherosclerosis as a paediatric problem in the 1960s. He stated that fatty streaks began in infancy and accelerated during puberty (HOLMAN 1961). Our 21st-century issues started in the 1960s, and as discussed previously, diabetes was unheard of prior to the 1960s.

Holman pioneered this concept of the early origin of cardiovascular disease without the vast amount of information available currently. A developing baby in the womb and from birth can be exposed to many factors that increase the risk of diabetes, obesity and cardiovascular disease. After-eating impacts are a huge driver of vascular disease, as we have discussed in depth.

In the mother's womb, foetal hypertension, high maternal glucose and raised maternal lipids leading to fatty streaks in the blood vessels of a developing baby all condemn a child to a life of cardiovascular disease (Aaltonen, Ojala et al. 2008). Yet governments waste money on statins despite the poor scientific findings and results. Senseless when you read this quote that should be constantly repeated:

> *"The 4S study employed a cholesterol-lowering statin drug and reported a 30% mortality reduction. The Lyon Diet Heart Study utilized the Mediterranean diet and reported a 70% mortality reduction. Something is very wrong."* (DuBroff and de Lorgeril 2015).

Indeed, something is very wrong when we ignore the huge benefits of a diet like the Mediterranean Diet when it crushes the benefits of a statin. That this is disheartening to researchers is summed up in this quote:

> *"Despite the striking findings in the first report of a 70% reduction in all-cause mortality due to a reduction in coronary heart disease (CHD) mortality and comparable large reductions in nonfatal sequelae, I have encountered few cardiologists here who are aware of that study." (Leaf 1999)*

The PREDIMED study reinforced these primary prevention effects of diet, showing a 30% reduction in cardiovascular events and a 42% reduction in stroke using the Mediterranean Diet (MeDiet) supplemented with Extra Virgin Olive Oil (EVOO) or nuts. The MeDiet + nuts showed a 13.7% reduction in Metabolic Syndrome (MetS) compared to a traditional low-fat control group (Ros, Martínez-González et al. 2014). Yet all diets that have shown considerable benefit can be improved greatly by taking off the shackles of having to include staple foods by governments.

Declaring war on inflammation – how did this go?

If inflammatory processes promote insulin resistance, why have 70% of anti-inflammatory studies failed to improve insulin resistance? (Wang and Ye 2015). Standard laboratory tests that show raised systemic inflammation include a raised hs-CRP (highly sensitive C-Reactive Protein) or ESR (Erythrocyte Sedimentation Rate). Inflammation commonly accompanies insulin resistance. Anyone can purchase over-the-counter anti-inflammatories or get powerful anti-inflammatory medications on a prescription. Such scripts can be given out easily by doctors. We can use numerous anti-inflammatories, whether Celecoxib (COX-2 inhibitor), anti-TNF-α, anti-IL-6 and others, all of which can backfire and induce weight gain and fat accumulation (Wang and Ye 2015).

We need to ask: What adaptation role does inflammation play in energy and nutrient-starved cells?" It is well known that inflammatory cytokines such as TNFα, IL-1, and IL-6 increase lipolysis, which is the release of free fatty acids from the breakdown of stored body fat. Using the Cell Starvation Model, we can predict that releasing free fatty acids to increase energy supplies is a beneficial adaptation of inflammation. So, these inflammatory cytokines are being recruited by the body to help supply energy to energy-starved distressed cells by increasing fatty acids for ATP production. Remember, inflammation also widens blood vessels (vasodilation), as discussed next.

Inflammation increases vasodilation and angiogenesis (new blood vessel formation), thus increasing blood, oxygen and nutrient supply to the cells in tissues and organs undergoing oxidative stress - this essentially includes all the energy-starved cells (Wang and Ye 2015). Suppose our small blood circulation networks, particularly our microcirculation networks, are critical for delivering fuel, oxygen and micronutrient supply to cells and organs. Then, suppose these small blood vessel networks are blocked due to stiffness and loss of vasodilation, leading to a decrease in blood supply. In that case, inflammation will lead to the opening up of these damaged blood vessels, a huge benefit to blood-starved struggling cells and organs. Inflammation that promotes the formation of new blood vessels to boost the vascular network would be a massive bonus.

Once again, the cell starvation model provides an amazing reason why inflammation exists as a necessary adaptation. Many Non-Steroidal Anti-Inflammatory Drugs (NSAIDs) have been withdrawn from the market for cardiovascular deaths in my career. Heart attacks, strokes, and arrhythmias can all occur when NSAIDs are mindlessly used against inflammation as the enemy. When you see the benefits of inflammation, it is no wonder that anti-inflammatories can cause so much harm and death.

However, it is important to note that inflammation, like all the other Janus-faced (two-faced) biomarkers, will cause damage the longer we leave this inflammatory process to run. We need to wake up and see that diet-based, nutrient-based approaches are the perfect way to prevent the long-term damage caused by inflammation.

NAC, Omega-3s, Magnesium, Choline, phytochemicals, diversity of fibre for the gut microbiome, and many other nutrients can help dampen inflammation. Once in that normal state, inflammation is no longer needed to support cells as they have resumed a state of energy and structural balance. Inflammation becomes redundant in this circumstance. It seems like a no-brainer approach to me!

Pro-Inflammatory versus Anti-Inflammatory Cytokines in MetS (Srikanthan, Feyh et al. 2016)	
RAISED Pro-Inflammatory Cytokines	IL-6, TNF- α , markers of pro-oxidant status Ox-LDL, & uric acid, prothrombic factors (PAI-1)
DECREASED Anti-Inflammatory Cytokines	(IL-10), ghrelin, adiponectin, and antioxidant factors (PON-1)

Why are pro-inflammatory cytokines raised while anti-inflammatory cytokines are decreased in Metabolic Syndrome (MetS)

Cytokines are small protein molecules released for cell-to-cell signalling that impact our immune systems. So, why are proinflammatory markers raised while anti-inflammatory markers decreased in Metabolic Syndrome (MetS), an advanced insulin-resistant and metabolic dysfunction state? To think these cytokine changes happen randomly in a body created by evolution over millions of years is just absurd. There is no way to answer this imbalance using the current standard metabolic dysfunction model that treats all biomarkers or adaptations, including inflammation, as enemies. Suffice it to say that inflammation serves a purpose early in the piece in metabolic dysfunction, as discussed above.

Humiliation for Public Health

When you review the literature littered with what is essentially nonsense, you sometimes come across an honest statement that stuns you. It is because there is no hidden agenda, no rubbish about relative vs. absolute values, NNTs, P-Values, Hazard-Ratios or statistical parameters used to mislead and confuse.

The refreshingly honest statement is as follows:

> *"The huge toll of death and disability caused each year by cardiovascular disease (CVD) continues to represent a great humiliation for public health. More people die annually from CVDs than from any other cause, and global projections are somber, with a projected increase from 17 million to more than 24 million yearly CVD deaths in 2030. Not a minor part of this humiliation comes from the knowledge that CVD can largely be prevented by timely population changes in metabolic risk factors, including obesity, hypertension, dyslipidemia, and diabetes. This unambiguously indicates the need to address unhealthy lifestyles and replace unhealthy food patterns with their healthiest alternatives." (Martínez-González 2016)*

It is important to remember that anyone reading this book is at high risk of a cardiovascular event such as a heart attack or stroke. We used statins to lower lipids when the Lyon Diet Heart Study showed that diet had a:

> *"dramatic mortality benefit"... without a reduction in cholesterol" (DuBroff and de Lorgeril 2015)*

Diabetes and high blood pressure go hand in hand.

"Dangers of Overly Aggressive Blood Pressure Control"

This title is from a paper on aggressively lowering blood pressure (Rahman and McEvoy 2018). 90-95% of hypertension cases are called "essential" or primary, meaning there is no obvious cause (Sur 2017). To me, this is not the case. Hypertension, as I have discussed, is simply an adaptation to increasing obstruction of microcirculation networks. It is a survival mechanism trying to "push" blood to our cells; otherwise, how can those cells and organs survive?

If we try to decrease blood pressure too much, we pull the rug from under this vital microcirculation network blood supply.

Around 66% or 2/3's of people with diabetes have hypertension, and for every 20 mmHg increase in systolic blood pressure (the top number), there is a 77% increased risk of Type-2 Diabetes Mellitus (Nazarzadeh and Rahimi 2020). So, we have a huge bidirectional component with hypertension and diabetes. ***However, we should consider this connection as just one process that causes both problems.*** Diabetes and high blood pressure are just branches of one metabolic dysfunction process – our "mother" of chronic metabolic diseases.

Hypertension is a continuum, and we don't recognise the slow slide upwards, so this statistic of 2/3s is a gross underestimation of this problem. Blood pressure on the slide upwards could be an early warning sign rather than high blood pressure cut-off points. Drugs are a knee-jerk reaction when diets like the DASH diet are amazing at lowering blood pressure.

Around 60% of those with insulin resistance are non-dippers, i.e. where the blood pressure does not drop during sleep. This pattern predicts cardiovascular risk and is an early warning sign for those with Metabolic Syndrome (MetS) (Tartan, Uyarel et al. 2006).

A 24-hour blood pressure monitor can show non-dippers. Why would you be a non-dipper? Normally, blood pressure drops at night to decrease the pressure load on blood vessels and protect them. However, when microcirculation network systems are damaged, we do need a higher blood pressure head 24/7 to "push" blood to organ systems, even during sleep. Thus, lowering blood pressure at night may be a big risk for organ perfusion, like in the brain. Many strokes occur in sleep or the early hours of the morning. Being a non-dipper is a warning sign of underlying microcirculation compromise. Causing a significant drop in blood pressure with drugs used overnight may be a big risk for a stroke unless the drug dose is carefully considered. A 24-hour blood pressure monitor can determine if you are a dipper or non-dipper.

Dietary Approaches to Stop Hypertension (The DASH Diet)

Instead of using drugs to declare war on hypertension, we should be looking at our diets instead. In a paper published with the title "The hypertension pandemic: An evolutionary perspective", it was stated that:

> *"Only very recently (12,000 years ago), plant and animal domestication led to the introduction of a monotonous but energy-rich neolithic diet ...Human beings were genetically set up to survive and reproduce under conditions of low Na (sodium) and high K (potassium) dietary intakes, which sharply contrast with modern diets that are rich in Na and poor in K." (Rossier, Bochud et al. 2017)*
>
> "Na" is Sodium, and "K" is Potassium.

For those with high blood pressure, keeping salt intake down is vital. However, increasing potassium intake from dark green leafy vegetables is a smart move, and if salt is required, then "lite" salt that has a high potassium content is also a smart move, as shown in the China Salt Substitute and Stroke Study (SSaSS) to decrease the risk of stroke, heart disease and death.

Dark green leafy vegetables are rich in Potassium and Magnesium, which are beneficial for lowering blood pressure. Up to 99% of populations may not get anywhere near their recommended vegetable and fruit intakes (AIHW 2018).

These two minerals are highly interdependent—lower Magnesium levels will trigger kidney Potassium loss (Wu and Carter 2007). Depletion of both Potassium and Magnesium is a risk to life due to abnormal heart rhythms (arrhythmias). Is it any wonder that the health of populations is going down the gurgler with miserable intakes of fresh food and low dark green vegetable intakes? Governments should wake up and subsidise this fresh food intake heavily and stop killing us with grain-based products.

In Appendix-21, you can see the wealth of nutrients supplied by fruits and vegetables and how cell energy can be compromised when energy pathways don't have adequate coenzymes (vitamins) and cofactors (minerals).

We recommend five servings or around 5 cups of veggies when, in fact, we need 10 servings (800 grams) for optimal nutrient intake.

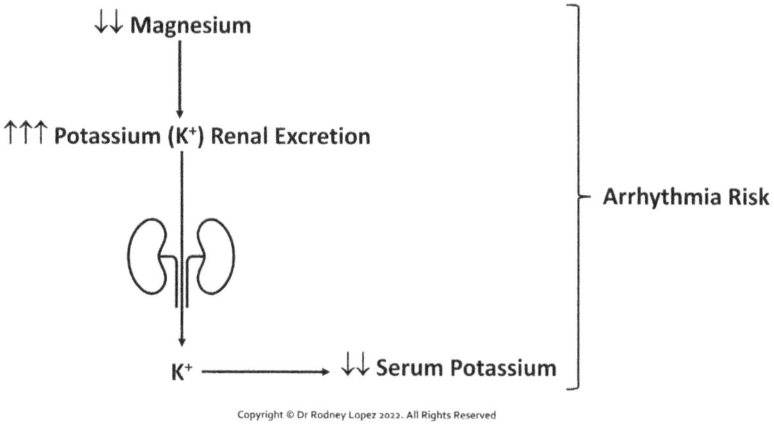

Comparing blood pressure lowering between drugs and diet

I will discuss the blood pressure lowering of the DASH diet below as a diet formulated by the US government's National Heart, Lung and Blood Institute (NHLBI) to help lower blood pressure in the US population. To compare drugs vs. diet, you need to know the average blood pressure lowering of various classes of blood pressure drugs.

A meta-analysis of 354 randomised, double-blind, placebo-controlled trials of 5 classes of drugs: 1) Thiazides, 2) Beta-blockers, 3) Angiotensin-converting enzyme (ACE) inhibitors, 4) Angiotensin II receptor antagonists, 5) Calcium Channel Blockers.

These drugs at a standard dose showed an average blood pressure lowering of (Law, Wald et al. 2003):

- 9.1 mmHg Systolic and
- 5.5 mmHg Diastolic

In comparison to the drugs discussed above, the DASH diet produced a drop of 11.4 mm Hg systolic and 5.5 mm Hg diastolic blood pressure. Is this good? It is wonderful! As you can see in the table below, diets are more than a match for or exceed any of the common antihypertensive classes.

Please do not underestimate the power of food-based approaches, as our minds have been distorted by drug barons who cannot think beyond a drug approach.

Comparing 5 drug categories to the DASH diet for blood pressure		
	5 Drug Categories	DASH Diet
Drop in Systolic Pressure	9.1	11.4
Drop in Diastolic Pressure	5.5	5.5

DASH + Low Sodium Intakes: Produced outstanding results

For those with systolic blood pressure readings of 150 mmHg or greater, there was a "striking" 21 mmHg drop in systolic blood pressure (SBP) in individuals who adopted both the DASH style of eating and low sodium intakes (Juraschek, Miller et al. 2017). Imagine a lower sodium intake but a higher intake of potassium, and what would this do for lower blood pressure results? The authors of this study stated with regard to a DASH diet + lower sodium intake:

"Among persons with baseline SBP ≥150 mm Hg, mean SBP reduction was striking (i.e., >20 mm Hg)" (Juraschek, Miller et al. 2017)

Diets can always be improved

Revered diets can be modified to improve them greatly. Martha Clare Morris, Professor of Epidemiology at Rush University Medical Centre in Chicago, and her team set about redesigning the Mediterranean diet to develop the MIND diet, emphasising dark green leafy vegetables, berries, and wine but limited dairy, sweets and fried food. The result of reversing cognitive decline was amazing, taking back memory to a younger age by 7.5 years (Morris, Tangney et al. 2015).

We can do so much good through food-based approaches, and yet we waste massive sums of money targeting a marker like beta-amyloid in the brain, which is so costly that only a minute fraction of the world's population will be able to afford it. However, targeting beta-amyloid has been a complete failure.

Appendix-39 shows what is involved in the DASH diet, which is far better than a diet of ultra-processed foods but still riddled with vested interests. We know we can prevent high blood pressure by 36% by adopting the Mediterranean Diet (MeDiet) (Magriplis, Panagiotakos et al. 2020). However, the Mediterranean Diet (MeDiet) is also imperfect. This MeDiet can be improved with targeted supplementation and excluding some components; for example, the Mediterranean diet includes whole grains, potatoes, and legumes, which are not exactly low-carb.

If we look at the Mediterranean Diet that restricts red meat, processed meats, simple carbohydrates, refined grains, and unhealthy fats such as vegetable oils, then how many food corporations and food boards do you cheese off? Is it any wonder that an amazing dietary plan, although one that could be improved, was not adopted despite the striking results shown in the Lyon Diet Heart Study or PREDIMED studies?

The restrictions of all these diets of staples or processed foods are a threat to vested interests who will protect their turf at any cost, irrespective of the huge toll on lives destroyed.

CHAPTER 6

Revolution Time

"The way to get started is to quit talking and begin doing." Walt Disney

One thing is certain: a revolution will come, but sadly, this will happen after a monumental healthcare disaster overwhelms us.

Tony Abbott, a former Prime Minister of Australia, said when he was the Minister for Health in 2006 that "***The only person responsible for what goes into my mouth is me" "...and the only people who are responsible for what goes into kids' mouths are the parents***". If only food consumption were this simple.

Think of all the road and driving rules: wear seatbelts, don't use your mobile phone while driving, don't drive under the influence of alcohol or drugs to protect the individual and others, but where are the rules about food consumption with deadly outcomes and where society as a whole picks up the healthcare tab for poor dietary choices?

Road rules save a fraction of lives in comparison to the tens of millions lost every year from preventable metabolic diseases. The sad fact is that when this careless consumption of food leads to a heart attack, stroke, vascular dementia, kidney failure and so on, the reality is that the healthcare burden falls on all of us in society. These individuals don't just say, "***Oh well, I ate one too many family-sized pizzas in my lifetime***", and then accept their fate. Once they get angina, suffer a heart attack or get that sinking feeling they are suffering a stroke, they will then want the best medical care that ***OUR*** money (the taxpayers) can buy to prolong the lives that they put at risk by dumb food choices. Should we turn them away?

But foolishly, we patch them up, maybe with an expensive stent procedure that re-establishes blood flow to the heart or brain, but then what? They will order a family-sized pizza delivered to them via the gig economy and consume this dreadful food post-surgery in their hospital recovery beds. I don't know what you think, but when medicine has such a disregard for preventative healthcare, then it is money down the drain. Those drugs given or those stents inserted won't stop biological rot, and so they wait for the next potentially deadly event around the corner that will cost us even more money.

As far as what goes into a kid's mouth being determined by a parent, who is teaching the parents what is right or wrong in terms of food inputs? Just look at what parents allow their children to eat in food malls, restaurants, etc. Who is changing the nature of foods in supermarkets that are supposed to be "healthy" for their kids? Some parents think fast food or sugary foods are fine for children on a daily basis. If cardiovascular and other chronic diseases are set in this early childhood period, then what are we doing but creating the next few generations to become riddled with chronic disease? Shouldn't we start to change the perception of food by mandating ugly images of disease be placed on fast and processed food choices as we do with tobacco products to get people thinking about dreadful food inputs? Such images showing the outcomes of bad food choices will inform the ignorant, and we may just save generations to come.

We desperately need a Future Generations Healthcare Commissioner (FGHC)

In 2016, Sophie Howe was appointed as the future generations commissioner in Wales, UK, and this was a world first. This position is important as it oversees government decisions and intends for this commissioner to assess how those political decisions will impact the welfare of future generations. How incredibly brilliant and important this appointment is! I think Wales has taken a great leap forward and proven to be a forward-thinking leader in governance matters. As a result, many countries are now thinking of having a commissioner for future generations, and many organizations are taking up this model because the worth of doing so is obvious.

With no CEO to guide the medical profession, this profession sails on like a ship set to autonomous mode. But this profession, without deep oversight, can be highly dangerous to society. The medical profession makes decisions as a fragmented group driven by self-interest and vested interests. We fund the medical profession, and so shouldn't we demand that the medical ship be steered by responsible individuals who focus on health and not wealth? How unbelievable we have a group given so much privilege and autonomy when just one profession can bring a nation to its knees with horrendous healthcare expenditures. Why is this the case?

We urgently need an independent and objective FGHC to deal with the gigantic "prediabetes" and chronic disease problem that will engulf populations sooner or later as we reach the universality of the "***Metabolic Singularity***".

A motto for the future generation's commissioner could be as simple as: ***"Striving for population health now and into the future."*** This FGHC can't just be a think tank and a "toothless tiger". This FGHC needs teeth for real change. Governments hindered by fear and a lack of knowledge can execute healthcare change through this department, where doctors and medical gurus will fear a polymath from this department. Medical and dietetic gurus wouldn't dare try to deceive an FGHC polymath for fear of looking like fools.

Doctors and medical gurus bully politicians through medical complexity, bad statistics, or bad logic. A politician with no medical qualifications will be intimidated by that medical background and complex arguments. What could be more appealing to the public than to have a department like the FGHC with a mandate to ensure the health of future generations - their children, grandchildren and great-grandchildren? We have to remember that through gestational diabetes and epigenetic programming, we affect a whopping four (4) generations (mother included) due to our incompetence at the medical and dietetic levels. This is not acceptable in the least.

With 90% of total deaths in 2020 related to the top 10 chronic diseases, taking action to save current populations and future generations is imperative. The medical, dietetic, public health, and regulatory bodies seem witless and powerless in controlling what is a highly preventable medical disaster. The medical and dietetic professional autonomy must end.

Only a polymath with multiple qualifications and experience beyond medicine and dietetics should apply for an FGHC role

This FGHC department must be full of polymath specialists, from the department head to the workforce. All medical and dietetic gurus should be humbled in front of a polymath expert and fear trying to pull the wool over their eyes. A polymath is someone with a formidable academic background in multiple fields. For example, these well-rounded polymath employees could be doctors or specialists with qualifications well beyond a medical degree or a fellowship. So, they are masters of many academic disciplines that can have implications for population health.

These polymaths must be squeaky clean and have no Pharma, agricultural or food interest affiliations at all. If we drew a team member from medicine, this polymath could hold a medical degree and perhaps a farming qualification or food production and manufacturing qualification. Importantly, these polymaths may have a computer programming background and an understanding of AI.

Dietitians in the FGHC may be chosen because they have food engineering qualifications or skills with artificial intelligence (AI) in food production and manufacturing or experience in genetically modifying foods to produce foods fit for consumption, altering food composition that promotes health and not disease.

The overarching idea is to have such polymath individuals act as a cohesive team with extensive big-picture knowledge that works towards the ideals of the motto of the commission - ***"Striving for population health now and into the future."***.

With a broad understanding of healthcare and a focus on population and intergenerational and transgenerational health, this team will go a long way towards removing the self-interest and vested interests that currently corrupt and drive so much damage in professions like medicine or dietetics. Politicians need to keep their grubby hands off these polymath experts who need to do what is right for population health and not what is right for politicians or professionals on the take or somehow influenced by money or jobs.

We need teams like this to change the composition of food and food recommendations forever and shape the medical and dietetic professions to be fit for 21st-century diseases. This FGHC team will help promote new food technologies, such as the 3D printing of food. What was seen as a "replicator" in Star Trek and science fiction is now becoming reality. This food printing machine can produce any food item in a small machine similar to a microwave, seemingly out of thin air. It is now becoming a reality and moving at "warp speed" to a kitchen near you. But this replicator can be so much more. This FGHC could use its polymath experts to combine AI and computer technologies to integrate blood test results into this machine to fine-tune nutrients such as iron, magnesium, omega-3's and a range of vitamins, minerals and trace elements to ensure our cells have all the nutrient power to produce ATP, decrease entropy and repair themselves.

Technology does not move at the pace of an impaired snail, as we see with professional bodies. Even more sluggish are governments in effecting change. Technology moves at a rapid pace, and we need to keep up. We cannot crawl anymore. We need to run.

Big data will drive a new revolution in food as we move into the ***Fourth Agricultural Revolution*** or ***Agriculture 4.0.*** Big data and AI will propel this food revolution. We will need a wealth of data specialists and specialists in artificial intelligence (AI) who can view the data through the lens of AI, which could be designed in-house to look for trends, inappropriate practices, and pointless and harmful medical or dietetic policies driven by self and vested interests.

Remember what I said about a quote in the book ***Hippocrasy***: 30% of what medicine does is of "no value", and 10% is harmful. Is this acceptable? So, 40% at least of our expenditure on healthcare is useless and going down the drain. But also remember what I said earlier that, in my opinion, the vast majority of what doctors see and work on is useless or harmful all because their appointment schedulers are crammed with individuals suffering chronic metabolic diseases that are never cured. The huge bulk of what GPs see is made up of those with insulin resistance-based chronic metabolic diseases. Those in line to see a doctor are given one script after another but do nothing to stem the prevalence of chronic metabolic disease exploding globally. Money for nothing.

Medicine does do some very good things, but all these good things pale into insignificance when we look at the overwhelming prevalence statistics of these deadly chronic diseases that medicine has no answer for and the whopping mortality figures in excess of 40 million deaths in any given year and the loss of 100s of millions of lives over six decades.

All of this data gathering by the proposed FGHC and data analysis will point the way towards paths that have true positive outcomes for the population and nation. We focus on individuals when our focus should be on population health, which ultimately means we don't have to waste time and money on individuals riddled with diseases.

This FGHC team can become the referee that can end the false and endless medical reductionist approach and say enough is enough to pointless research – the FGHC can state no more research. We will call it now. Reductionism stalls progress and drives the drug-centric system that has failed all of us. Whatever happened to reasoning, observation, deduction and plain common sense?

Rotten to the core: The proposed FGHC can help stamp out vested interests that drive population disease prevalence

Getting into this medical and dietetic corruption in detail is beyond the scope of this book, but the Guardian Media Group's exposé will open your eyes and will be a good introduction to the nature of corruption in these professions (Perkins 2022).

Humanity has paid the ultimate price for their health due to this corruption, whether overt or covert, due to academic control, postgraduate education or the meddling of agricultural corporations and food boards and lobbyists influencing dietetic dogma and how a dietitian thinks and acts with regard to dietary advice.

A recent 2022 paper titled "***The corporate capture of the nutrition profession in the USA***" will further open your eyes as to how rotten the medical and dietetic industry can be. Society has allowed this to happen by stealth. This paper stated:

"The involvement of unhealthy commodity corporations in health policy and research has been identified as an important commercial determinant contributing to the rise of non-communicable diseases." (Carriedo, Pinsky et al. 2022).

Chronic diseases are also called non-communicable diseases (NCDs). To think that this only happens in the USA is laughable. This paper by Carriedo et al. was an important exposé of big corporations' deep influence on the huge and highly influential Academy of Nutrition and Dietetics (AND) in the USA. This very recent paper went on to say that:

"AND acts as a reference for dietetics curricula accreditation and as an authority in US food policy making." (Carriedo, Pinsky et al. 2022)

The fact that the medical and dietetic professions can be so influenced is of monumental concern. Our academic gurus can be controlled in many ways, consciously or subconsciously. However, many good gurus of medicine and dietetics see through this corruption and fight against it in academic papers or editorials. The problem is that the bad guys make a lot more noise and gaslight. This situation is where the FGHC with polymaths can be of great value.

Corporations can influence the design of undergraduate courses through the lens of their vested interests. This highly objectionable influence is deplorable. To think that the Academy of Nutrition and Dietetics (AND) is any different from dietetic associations worldwide is implausible and dangerous. Only a forensic examination of how entrenched all these influences are will expose the depth and breadth of corrupt teaching and corrupted mandatory continuing education, which becomes an extension of the indoctrination received at university.

As the saying goes, "***Follow the money***". An FGHC should have the power to authoritatively examine the corporate influences, including financial kickbacks, to any individual, academic or professional group and then impose truly stiff fines or expel them from their lofty positions and, in their place, add a polymath with a clean record of influence that will have a focus on population and future generation health. Is this draconian? What punishment should individuals get if what they have done has created the worst medical disaster in the history of humankind over decades despite compelling evidence that what they were doing was wrong and where this pandemic has killed 100s of millions of people?

According to the WHO, 41 million deaths occur yearly due to chronic disease (WHO 2022). Extrapolate that now to over 60 years of past harm and then into the future but at the accelerated pace of doubling and tripling rates, and you will see billions have or will die due to this blatant corruption. So, should we be soft on the medical and dietetic professionals doing the wrong thing?

So, knowing this, how many of these professionals and gurus have lived magnificent lives spruiking drugs and changing curricula at universities due to corporate directives and financing? Should these professionals and academic gurus enjoy nice homes, nice cars, children educated in private schools, rorts like trips overseas on a corporate bill, meetings in expensive restaurants and hotels, and perhaps staying in a penthouse suite paid for by food corporations or Pharma running their "Speaker Programs? All of this is at the expense of lives and the health of nations. Should the FGHC tackle these rorts? What do you think? What hope do people have when these corrupt practices entangle themselves in all aspects of training and government policy?

Sponsorship advertising, once foolishly but proudly and blatantly displayed on dietetic association websites, has now gone. However, there are many hidden ways to benefit from corporations. For example, the Carriedo et al. paper above describes how dietetic associations secretly benefit through food boards, corporate alliances, and even investing in food companies, creating a conflict of interest.

A highly respected crusader for transparency in all things dietetics is Prof. Marion Nestle, who wrote a book titled "***Food Politics: How the Food Industry Influences Nutrition and Health***" (Nestle 2019). Prof. Nestle describes the "finesse" used by corporations and outlines the detailed thought processes regarding corporate influence on dietetic experts and practice. She tells how the industry can hire dietitians or dietetic academics as "advisers" or "consultants" and perhaps give them research grants but, in the process, never make these professionals feel they have lost their objectivity.

However, you can see how diabolically subtle and pernicious this process can be in this statement made by Marion Nestle in her book mentioned above: ***"At a minimum, a programme of this kind reduces the threat that the leading experts will be available to testify or write against the interests of the regulated firms."*** (Nestle 2019), (Dixon, Sindall et al. 2004). How clever is it then to use ***conflict of interest*** as a tool against using these same researchers or experts to expose corrupt behaviour?

The fact that we have a neverending and ever-expanding pool of individuals with "prediabetes", all predisposed to deadly chronic diseases, is a testament to the power of vested interests and professions that look away. When will the public, public health advocates and governments wake up to this deceit and corruption?

And now a word from our sponsors – Australian Edition

Just like there are mavericks in the medical profession, so too do they exist in the dietetic industry. These medical and dietetic practitioners are shocked, embarrassed and disillusioned by what their industry is doing. An excellent public health exposé on the

Dietitians Association (DA)/Dietitians Association of Australia (DAA) can be found online by the public health watchdog ***Croakey Health Media***. This exposé is an excellent but shocking review of the vested interest-riddled DAA. This webpage shows an exceptionally brave and personal view of a dietitian disillusioned by her profession and how food interests and money are placed above health. This courageous dietitian stated on Croakey's website:

> *"As a dietitian, I feel like I'm forced to be a mouthpiece for the food industry. I object to being fed masses of industry-funded 'research updates' with messages that I am supposed to work into my practice, such as eat red meat 3 times a week from Meat and Livestock Australia or consume 3 servings of dairy per day from Dairy Australia. The worst is from the food companies themselves, like Coca-Cola telling me how wonderful their calorie-controlled smaller cans are." (Sweet 2015)*

We need more brave dietitians like the one above and more doctors with the courage to say enough is enough in their field. How can change ever start, and how can we save future generations if no one dares to speak up? Governments can rip apart trillion-dollar companies, so minnows like dietetic associations need to be very careful. The more they draw attention to themselves, the more they risk scrutiny or even a Royal Commission. However, perhaps weak souls full of hubris in these dietetic associations may want to wield what they see as "power" and then find out how powerless they are when the population they represent turns on them. I feel this will happen in the not-too-distant future as the health of nations is being ripped apart as health takes second place to self and vested interests.

A report titled "***And Now a Word From Our Sponsors – Australian Edition***" and available as a PDF by EatDrinkPolitics (see reference for the URL) exposes the huge conflict of interest within the Dietitians Association of Australia (DAA). Their sponsors are Meat and Livestock, Dairy Australia, the Egg Nutrition Council, Nestlé, and many others, which you will see in this report (Simon 2015).

The Dietitians Association of Australia (DAA) runs the Dietitians Association (DA) and has thousands of members. The DA/DAA accredits the dietitian courses run at universities. With such vested interests embedded in everything they do, how can any undergraduate course accredited by them ever be objective? How can any postgraduate education program be accurate and aim objectively to embrace and nurture individual and population health? How dare we allow groups like this to determine undergraduate education and then enable them to have the power to dismiss dietitians if they presume to disagree with their accreditation body?

How foolish that regulatory bodies have allowed this gross injustice to not only hand out credentials but also to divest professionals of their professional rights if they speak out against their association out of concern for individual and population health. This situation is a professional dictatorship and an absurdity that has to end. Dietitians should not answer to their associations but only to an objective group like the FGHC structure that I recommend, where a professional and their grievance can be evaluated independently and objectively.

We have unbelievably and foolishly allowed groups like medical and dietetic associations to be deeply affiliated with corporations and yet also have the power to decide who they will accept as a professional under their purview. This ability to accept or exclude a professional means that mavericks who drive change in professions by questioning their ethics can be threatened by expulsion, as professionals must have compulsory registration and accreditation under these groups who will decide the best practice where "best practice" is determined by self and vested interests. Conflict of interest reigns supreme in both the medical and dietetic accreditation bodies. So, in essence, professionals must keep on following corrupt practices driven by vested interests to maintain their registration. Tell me, what is wrong with this scenario?

So, how do you create a professional "robot"? You train future professionals at that undergraduate university level and then keep feeding them propaganda at the postgraduate level. You then use ploys, gaslighting and threats to keep everyone in line. We need to keep that corporate gravy train chugging along, and professions feed these corporations, whether they are pharmaceutical or food. A Royal Commission is required in order to root out corruption in the medical and dietetic hierarchy. This Royal Commission will happen when healthcare systems implode, as they are about to do in the next decade or so. Any dietetic or medical group that sticks their heads out now by showing indignation at these accusations will have their heads cut off when this disaster reaches monumental proportions and where legal class actions galore will emerge against associations, professions and the leaders of professional groups who turned a blind eye to a disgusting medical disaster that could have been avoided.

Our politicians are weak and won't do anything that angers Pharma or a food lobby or threatens jobs in agriculture or the food industry, as that will be political death. And so this sorry saga of exploding population sickness continues until there is *"hardly a healthy human left"*.

The DA/DAA mission statement on their website states:

> *"Our mission is to champion the professional nutrition and dietetic workforce to empower people and communities. We help build healthier communities by communicating credible and timely nutrition messages to the public."*

Really? So why are chronic metabolic diseases exploding under your dietary guidance? Journalist Peter FitzSimons excellent article in the Sydney Morning Herald made this statement about the Dietitians Association Australia (DAA):

> *"Do you find it, perchance, weird, and even troubling, that just last month the DAA held a seminar for its dietitians on "The Future of Foods" within the offices of Coca-Cola in North Sydney"? (FitzSimons 2017).*

With the huge damage caused by fructose-rich, sugar-sweetened beverages, how could any self-respecting dietitian attend such a meeting at the offices of a company associated with sugar-sweetened drinks? Sugar-drenched foods and beverages have caused so much misery, disease and death over decades worldwide. How humans can sell their souls for a dollar at the expense of other people's lives is beyond me, but humans can also be corrupted due to their naivety and ignorance – they don't think twice about the "optics" and are then taken advantage of by their associations, who should know better. Pharma and food corporations are incredibly good at taking advantage of bad situations and naïve professionals.

Pain Hustlers, Speaker Programs, Pharma Greed, and an Opioid Epidemic

"***Pain Hustlers***" is a movie about how corrupt Pharma can be. It is based on the true story of a company called ***Insys*** and its founder, Dr. John Kapoor. The FBI monitored those involved, and ultimately, all faced prison time.

The movie made me cringe as a medical practitioner. In my working life, we had many reps come to my clinic during that period, bringing lunch for the clinic doctors and spruiking opioids. My concern was always the addictive nature of opioids, and I would only use them in cancer cases, post-op and for short periods. You can't let people suffer from painful conditions, but you can't make them drug addicts, either. We have to look at the toll of the Fentanyl epidemic in the USA to see how devastating these drugs can be to lives and the number of lives lost from opioid addiction and overdoses.

The fact that prescribing doctors played such a large part in this drug epidemic is truly shocking and deplorable. Doctors are not above self-interest or immune to the charms of a rep. That doctors do not question drug peddlers in their practices is also startling and not acceptable. Are governments so naïve to think our universities, professions, and professionals are squeaky clean?

The speaker programs involved are at the heart of the movie mentioned above, which is truly embarrassing for the medical profession. Speaker programs are where doctors may be wined, dined or flown to wonderful locations while being primed (pimped) to become salespeople for a drug company. That this happens is undeniable, and we allow Pharma to have this influence on doctors.

We need to look at every specialist that dominates medical meetings and conferences and all the medical gurus strutting stages like Jagger to convince doctors that a particular drug is indispensable in their medical toolbox.

According to a paper by New York University's School of Law, in 2019, Teva Pharmaceuticals was fined $54 million for "sham speaker programs and events" (NYU 2020). As this NYU paper stated, the Teva settlement was followed by a "wave of settlements". This corrupt behaviour by Pharma shows the extent of such influence in the medical profession.

The only "speaker programs" that should be allowed should come from medical gurus trained by a government body like the Future Generations Healthcare Commissioner (FGHC). Medical gurus strutting stages will often receive honorariums and be paid for "their views" by Pharma. That they should be paid for their time and effort is not in question, but payment should be for objective talks and not for marketing drugs for Pharma. Meetings should never be purely for the promotion of drugs as the only game in town in managing disease. No drug presentation should ever occur without alternative drug-free dietary management possibilities being discussed by non-drug gurus. The ignorance of the concept of "food as medicine" is shocking in both the medical and dietetic professions.

A noble profession goes down the gurgler for the privileged lives of a few who corrupt a profession and bring this profession into disrepute. Doctors need to wake up before it is too late. Corrupt individuals beware, as Freedom of Information (FOI) laws make it easy to find you. We now have a powerful social media presence with people who seek justice against corrupt behaviour and professional bullies. Let's not forget tech-savvy individuals who can and will hunt corrupt individuals down. Many corporations have felt the full force of the power of social media. All it takes is a social media post or an article to bring down a corporation or a corrupt individual or professional. People are much smarter now, and the zeitgeist has changed dramatically against professions corrupt corporations and corrupt professionals. You can't hide!

Technology is now keeping the bastards honest and not allowing their privilege to harm others. The privileged lives of corrupted academics should never be at the loss of someone else's life.

University education. Doctors and dietitians are not fit for purpose for chronic diseases. What needs to be done?

The FGHC needs the power to deal with undergraduate curricula and rid the educational institutions of vested interests that drive what is being taught at universities that distort the minds of future doctors with drug-only solutions or encourage dietitians to become salespeople for staple foods, causing so much harm. Get rid of Pharma, food corporation interests and government influence on what is taught at this important undergraduate level. Governments need to wake up to their impact on undergraduate teaching because of their vested interests in agriculture, food and farming export taxes.

How do you wipe away indoctrination at that young age in a university setting? That doctors come out of a university as script-writing robots beggars belief. That dietitians are churned out without a firm understanding of food's pathophysiological and medical impacts is also beyond belief. Doctors prescribe drugs, while dietitians are the salespeople for agriculture, staple foods, and food and beverage corporations that drive population disease.

Dietitians need to question why disease prevalence is exploding on the planet despite their food recommendations. You never hear about dietetics wanting to change or challenge what we feed babies or question the effects of staple foods on everyone. There is a deafening silence coming from that profession. Why bite the hand/s that feeds dietetics, right?

If universities receive billions of dollars in funding from government support, then they are not autonomous institutions. A paper discussing university funding stated that 35.6 billion dollars was spent on research and development in Australia in 2019-2020 (Australia 2023). Universities have a finger in many project pies through businesses that get tax offsets and benefits and where there is a collaboration between universities and private research groups. A lot of this research is looking for drug targets as silver bullets. Is this money well spent? Will the underlying tainted academic practices discussed above influence these research projects? It is easy enough to see how the dice are loaded to keep the status quo in play and to keep populations teeming with disease.

Universities cannot expect a handout from the public on the one hand and then harm them on the other by producing professionals or research that is not fit for deadly 21st-century diseases.

We are producing doctors clueless about nutrition and dietitians ignorant about the medical impacts of their advice.

The FGHC, if created, should ensure the education of doctors and dietetics are entwined and not taught as separate undergraduate degrees that don't overlap. Instead, we should be churning out doctors with a powerful understanding of nutritional principles and dietitians with a solid understanding of medical issues that can be impacted by poor dietary advice honeycombed with vested interests. Having these two professions swimming in their respective lanes has been an unmitigated healthcare disaster.

Food is not just an amalgam of nutrients or energy. Food is far more than the sum of its parts. We ignore the powerful impacts of food components like fructose or carbohydrate loads or the negative effects of food staples on disease causation.

Individual foods can have significant biochemical, molecular and physiological impacts with vastly different postprandial (after-eating) effects on blood glucose and lipids and unique food impacts on the gut microbiome, oxidative stress and systemic inflammation. See Appendix-18. All of these matter in our lifetime, increasing the risk for negative health outcomes ***slowly, incrementally, and cumulatively.*** This *SIC* process continues throughout our lives, meal by meal and snack by snack, as you are now well aware of.

Continuing Professional Development (CPD). Throwing doctors into the arms of drug corporations and dietitians into the arms of food corporations

We need to change the face of continuing professional development (CPD/CME) rather than push medical professionals into the arms of the pharmaceutical industry and dietitians into the arms of food corporations to get points. We must create independent educational avenues for doctors and dietitians to learn how to deal with chronic diseases effectively and embrace technological advances.

We have allowed this area of ongoing postgraduate education to be captured by vested interests. For example, the pharmaceutical or medical device industry provides vast educational programs that generate CPD points that doctors must acquire. We need to remember that from a metabolic perspective, any surgical procedure like bariatric surgery or a stent in a blocked artery is a stopgap measure with minimal long-term impact on an individual, but the cost of surgical procedures is astronomical. The medical device industry benefits from these marginally beneficial surgical procedures. The following quote relates to Canada but reflects what happens elsewhere concerning devices or pharmaceuticals:

"***The pharmaceutical and medical device industries fund a substantial portion of the continuing medical education (CME) of physicians in Canada. Along with this financial support come avenues for industry influence. Continuing medical education organizers are often under overt pressure to design sessions and choose faculty to attract industry funding. Organizers might also be affected by more subtle tactics. Research in social science demonstrates that the recipient of a gift feels a sense of obligation that is often subconscious.***" *(Spithoff 2014)*

So, if you get a free lunch delivered to your practice by a rep or attend a dinner in an expensive restaurant, or if medical gurus are treated like rock stars and sent to overseas conferences and recruited into “speaker programs”, put up in expensive hotel rooms, all to be trained in what to say about particular drugs to indoctrinate grassroots GPs and specialists, would these chosen doctors and medical gurus feel privileged and obliged if they received travel, food, drinks and accommodation as gifts all paid for by Pharma? Of course, they would. Who doesn’t like feeling special and wanted and made to feel as if they have superpowers even though this is all grooming by an industry that knows psychology 101?

Most GPs can attend an evening meeting held most nights of the week that provides fine wine and meals. If you attend an evening meeting even infrequently, you often see the same faces and wonder if they do this most nights of the week. Loneliness? Attending due to rep “friends”, the lure of free meals and wine? Don’t you think these evening meetings in a nice restaurant are a perfect avenue to “educate” a needy and gullible audience that drugs are the answer to a complicated problem? Would they feel a sense of obligation?

To be fair to doctors, getting independent and objective academic CPD points untainted by commercial interests is almost non-existent. Yet ongoing education is vital. Other than corporate CPD points, I know very few academic bodies that have provided independent and objective avenues for CPD/CME points that are convenient for doctors and not riddled by vested interests. Yes, some independent CPDs exist, but how do you compete with fine wine and food? How do you compete with just signing in at a nice restaurant, giving your CPD ID and CPD Home, and then leaving everything up to a pharma company to deal with the points you need? Wow, it's so much less hassle. So enticing!

So, doctors are thrown into the arms of pharmaceutical corporations as they are very slick at getting CPD points for doctors to meet their educational points targets. So, as mentioned above, getting CPD points becomes a seamless and effortless exercise for the GP when CPD comes through Pharma. Going to these drug-focused “educational” programs is easily attractive but crawling with corporate interests, thus keeping drug-centric views and failed chronic disease pharmacological management front and centre.

We force CPD/CME on doctors, and ostensibly, it seems like a good idea to have ongoing education to keep doctors up to date. But look under the surface to see how CPD falls into the laps of pharmaceutical and food companies when the only viable game in town is CPD/CME provided by them. This situation is crazy to me.

Is it any wonder that doctors have a drug-centric view of medical management and are so conceited and arrogant towards preventative and nutrient-based treatments? Where do doctors learn about nutritional modalities of clinical management? Do they know when to use particular nutrients or when not to? Is it any wonder they have such insular minds, especially when university training on food-based and nutrient-based approaches is incredibly limited? Nutritional training threatens drug-centric views. Doctors are embarrassingly inept at nutrition-based strategies? How do we fit nutritional-based processes into a 6-minute consultation that earns money rapidly for GPs? Scripts are a rapid-fire solution that fits beautifully within a quick 6-minute consultation. Is it any wonder healthcare is going over a cliff?

No drug-centric meeting should ever occur without a talk on unbiased food-based and nutrient-based approaches. How many doctors or drug-centric gurus of medicine would even know about the landmark Lyon Diet Heart Study that used the Mediterranean diet compared to the findings of the Scandinavian Simvastatin Survival Study (4S) showing "striking" positive benefits of that diet? We discussed these findings earlier. If medical gurus are aware of this diet-based study, then they would never discuss the superiority of diet over any drug in a meeting. Why would they? They have been hired to sell drugs and not promote diets that would crush the effects of any drug/s! Their Pharma masters would not approve.

We need to look at how to fund independent meetings, and professionals need to understand that there is no free lunch. Governments can help with tax incentives and help subsidise unbiased educational programmes free of vested interests. This ongoing education can all be done through a Future Generations Healthcare Commissioner's department. After all, it is in their interest and the interest of the nation that they are responsible for focusing on individual and population health.

Emerging technologies. Adapt or perish. How technological advances can crush professions that are unprepared for change

The internet, Artificial Intelligence (AI) and ChatGPT, as a version of generative AI, seem to have fallen from out of nowhere into our laps. We know what disruptive technologies can do to unprepared individuals and professions. You either adapt or perish! The emergence of the internet has taught us this and caught many businesses off guard. With this in mind, it would be rare to find any current doctor or dietitian able to talk with any authority about the emerging disruptive technologies in nutrition that continue to develop rapidly around them, threatening to crush them.

These emerging technologies are metagenomics and the gut microbiome, nutrigenomics (nutritional genetics), and nutritional and functional laboratory testing. Is ignorance of these new technologies acceptable? These technologies mentioned above are already here, but you would think they don't exist when you visit a doctor or a dietitian. With so much access to leading nutritional knowledge, those in the lay community with a deeper understanding of food and nutrient-based health will make doctors or dietitians look foolish and backward in this respect. How embarrassing.

Doctors only have drug options to offer individuals becoming more and more sceptical of pharmaceutical interventions. Dietitians will look inept with eyes glazing over as a clever layperson questions every word they say with a deeper knowledge of available paradigms in nutrition. Remember, the public has the most amazing encyclopedia of knowledge in the palms of their hands – their smartphones.

We must change our food composition along with changes in the fast food and beverage industry

Here is a huge opportunity for innovation and long-term economic benefit. We are not going to destroy the agricultural economy. We can't, can we? We are just going to change the nature of what this economy produces as food. We need to declare war on dangerous food composition that promotes disease. The fundamental nature of food needs to change to put a halt to metabolic disease. It starts with the very essence of food grown and its composition. Why do we allow "bliss points" that can addict someone to food or allow foods like pizzas, bread, or buns created by nutrient-poor and fibre-deficient flour? We can demand the use of modified flour with far more nutrients and fibre and far lower carb loads. By engineering flour, we change the foundation of a multitude of foods being served in a takeaway, restaurant, café or food mall. Can this be done? Absolutely. We are not primitive hominins or Neolithic creatures. We can engineer food grown, but what about the seed banks that house far better grain options? We worship yield at the expense of health. Foods must change; otherwise, we will be a very sick species in just a few decades.

Where is the diversity of fibre or micronutrient content in ultra-processed foods and grains? Where are the critical phytochemicals and plant antioxidants? We seem ignorant of postprandial (after-eating) damage to our cells, tissues, organs, and vascular systems that persist for hours after eating those meals high in starchy carbs that increase insulin and glucose levels that linger in our bloodstream, damaging our bodies - this is gross negligence. Genetic modification of plants can see foods that are nutrient-dense with minimal postprandial (after-eating) impacts.

Australia leads the way in many things, and changes in food composition should be a challenge we should take on and show the world what can be done. This change in food composition could be a priority for the FGHC department. We don't dismantle but modify agriculture or food corporations. We must demand change in the composition of foods being offered.

Imagine a world hungry for such amazing health-promoting foods. Imagine how much more money agriculture can produce for this nation and the world. It is agriculture and food corporations reimagined. For food corporations, we need to use a carrot-and-stick approach and force them to change from damaging all of us to creating foods that have a health benefit. This change should be non-negotiable but a do-or-die ultimatum.

Dedicated preconception & pregnancy care

Here is another piece of low-hanging fruit we can easily tackle to stop damage to future generations that drive this pandemic even further. We let health opportunities slip by so easily. Epigenetic programming affects many generations from just one pregnancy, as I have discussed earlier. This pregnancy programming is a disaster for humanity due to the disease-amplifying effect as a result of the intergenerational and transgenerational risk for metabolic disorders, with four (x4) generations affected, including the mother. Our metabolic disease problem is set to explode exponentially due to the magnifying effect of epigenetic programming.

Each of those children born to a mother with gestational diabetes (GDM) has the potential to transfer metabolic risk to their children, who will themselves increase metabolic risk in another three (x3) generations and so on. With a tripling of gestational diabetes in the past two decades, why are we tolerating this? This issue should be a huge priority for the proposed FGHC. We must act now!

We should make it a priority to look for early markers of metabolic disease in women who are planning pregnancy and to do this long before conception. We should not use crude pregnancy Glucose Tolerance Tests (GTTs) that discover way too late that a woman has gestational diabetes risk, especially when epigenetic programming may have already occurred long before those fake GTT glucose cut-off results at 24-28 weeks in pregnancy. How dumb!

We should never miss iron deficiency before or during pregnancy, and we need to warn women about gaining weight before and during pregnancy and the dangers of ultra-processed foods consumed during pregnancy. Telling a pregnant woman to eat a "healthy diet" is vague and not acceptable – where is the detail? Please provide details, not vested interest and staple food-riddled details! Diets as optimal as possible should commence long before falling pregnant, with pregnancy supplementation a must. It is a medicolegal risk for any professional not to inform a woman about the critical nature of supplements before and during pregnancy to prevent negative pregnancy and negative baby outcomes, which are now well-established in the literature. Any guru or medical practitioner with conceited and arrogant views of nutrients will now face medicolegal action if a mother suffers a preventable pregnancy complication that could have been prevented with a pregnancy supplement that includes Omega-3s and Choline.

Supplementation is vital pre-pregnancy, during pregnancy and postnatally. These supplements should include, at a minimum, a pregnancy-designed multivitamin with the recommended amount of folic acid, iodine and all the vitamins, minerals and trace elements vital for optimal pregnancy and foetal outcomes, and we need to include Omega-3s, in particular, ones rich in DHA with added Choline.

Governments must subsidize essential supplements in pregnancy and early childhood. Investing in the health of future generations is not just wise—it's imperative. By preventing metabolic and mental health issues from the start, we can save our nations from immense suffering and economic burden. Is there a more crucial investment? Choline has every chance of preventing mental health diseases in future generations, and issues with mental health are a huge burden on society (Ross, Hunter et al. 2013). Omega-3s can significantly decrease the risk of premature birth (Middleton, Gomersall et al. 2018). Premature birth is another burden on hospitals and healthcare expenditures and a common cause of neonatal death. Isn't it foolish then not to subsidize Omega-3s in the prepregnancy and pregnancy period? It's a no-brainer to me!

These new findings make it a huge medicolegal risk for doctors who do not become engaged in supplementation information and nutrition adequacy for positive pregnancy outcomes. Conceit and arrogance against supplements need to now die in the minds of drug-centric medical practitioners and dietitians who have brought healthcare systems to the brink of disaster with their biases.

Many diseases can be linked to poor nutritional support that could have been avoided by supplementation. It is well within the realms of possibility that legal action could be brought upon medical and dietetic groups if a child is born with well-known complications beyond spina bifida caused by nutritional neglect, which now includes premature birth, schizophrenia or a range of other mental health and behavioural problems, along with cardiovascular disease all avoided in the womb through timely dietary and nutrient supplement advice. Legal eagles will be sharpening their knives as this knowledge about preventable mental health issues becomes known far and wide. The medical and dietetic professions should be very careful now about their nutritional biases as this will come to prey on them as chronic diseases continue to soar and healthcare systems go over a cliff.

Laboratory Results: Early recognition of a metabolic disaster ahead. Understanding Quintiles and the Quintile-Climb

An FGHC can ensure that doctors know about early red flags. Discussing early metabolic signatures at meetings and conferences should be compulsory to prevent future diseases in individuals. Compounds like ***α-Hydroxybutyrate*** can be used in the non-diabetic population to detect insulin resistance and glucose intolerance. Many early markers exist, so why aren't we using these to detect a devastating disease process that is now becoming the norm – as we approach our ***Metabolic Singularity***? Just because we don't have a drug is a poor excuse for not checking if someone is at risk, as we do not need a prescription to stop this process. I list the many early markers of insulin resistance in Appendix-31.

Like all markers or red flags, they need to be viewed in a clinical context and the presence of other risk factors. My medical teaching has been to view not just one marker but numerous markers in the context of family history, medical history and physical characteristics such as hypertension, central adiposity, etc.

We discussed Quintile-Climb in the prediabetes chapter, and this Quintile-Climb can easily be generated as a graph or percentage in laboratory results. So this is yet something else the FGHC can ensure concerning how laboratory results are presented to doctors and specialists to bring their attention to a developing metabolic problem. A quintile climb for all the metabolic dysfunction biomarkers should be looked for in prospective mothers. Not doing this is negligence, pure and simple.

So, as you can see, continuing medical education to gain CPD points can be so much more than a sales pitch for pharmaceuticals for doctors or the "staple foods are good" dogma pitched to dietitians.

Continuums: We must recognise that disease processes are continuums that begin in pregnancy and accelerate after birth

Claiming ignorance is not a valid defence in legal proceedings. Our ignorance that metabolic dysfunction acts as a continuum throughout our lives is not acceptable and is dangerous and anachronistic. Our medical and dietetic revolution must ensure doctors, dietitians, and the lay public view these disease processes as continuums that can be halted and reversed. The earlier, the better.

Every scientific paper, expert report, and textbook now defines chronic metabolically based problems, from hypertension to blood glucose or vascular disease, as continuums. The fact we don't have a department like the Future Generations Healthcare Commissioner (FGHC) leaves it to chance that doctors will recognise these problems as continuums. Who tells them? Is Pharma interested in conveying this continuum knowledge to people? Why would they, as it is not in their interest to turn off the tap of diseases they depend upon? The medical profession is embedded in self-interest and vested interests even to consider preventing disease by informing people they have a continuum of risk and that it can be reversed. Drugs are simple tools that can be quickly dispensed to individuals but ultimately fail to halt this singular insulin resistance–metabolic dysfunction continuum, leading to multiple continuums, as I have discussed. Understanding a process as an elastic continuum that can stopped to prevent disease is vital. Most doctors see chronic metabolic diseases as an accomplished fact, so they don't bother. Doctors don't have a drug tool that does anything to stop the biological rot, and so no drug tool exists to put an end to a 6-minute consultation to keep the money flowing from a long line of individuals affected by chronic metabolic disease waiting to see them, but for what? Ineffective drug scripts?

It can be decades before this thinking of continuums and reversibility filters through to grassroots practitioners, just like the aspirin story I discussed. This sluggishness is not acceptable for a profession like medicine but fosters ignorance in clinical management. The FGHC could easily mandate that there is a discussion of continuums in metabolic disease at all medical conferences or meetings and that continuums can be halted and reversed. After all, these meetings should not be about drug sales.

Allostatic Load – What is this?

Our revolution should target our overly simplistic view of single-impact factors and understand our diseases are due to multiple factors (cell shocks) all acting simultaneously. Each factor damages an individual to a lesser or greater extent at any given moment in time. If an FGHC is appointed, we can target a wide range of inputs (allostatic load) that have been ignored in the causation of cell starvation and, hence, all these insulin resistance-related diseases.

We can see allostatic load as all our energy-damaging inputs in that acute phase of biological rot. For example, I discuss the modifiable BIG-10 Womb to Tomb list in chapter one, and all these inputs are known as the allostatic load that cumulatively disrupts cell function over time. We allow these loads to cause damage to cells throughout our lives, causing cells to become energy-deprived and riddled with increasing entropy. Such allostatic loads affect pregnancy and the baby through epigenetic mechanisms, as I have discussed. These factors are, for the most part, highly adjustable, and we also need to target the 350,000 environmental chemicals by banning any new, untested chemicals from entering our environment and getting rid of as many of the existing environmental toxicities as soon as possible.

Targeting these toxic loads will make a world of difference to all of us and future generations. It is truly naïve to think that pharmaceutical drugs can decrease any of these inputs or even touch allostatic loading. It is laughable to believe that any drug we use will somehow overcome any environmental toxic impact! A "switch" is turned on in cells if these allostatic loads impact our cells continuously. This "switch" is linked to cellular ATP (energy) (Leist, Single et al. 1997). This "switch" results in irreversible cell changes with knock-on effects on tissues, organ systems and vascular networks that house those cells.

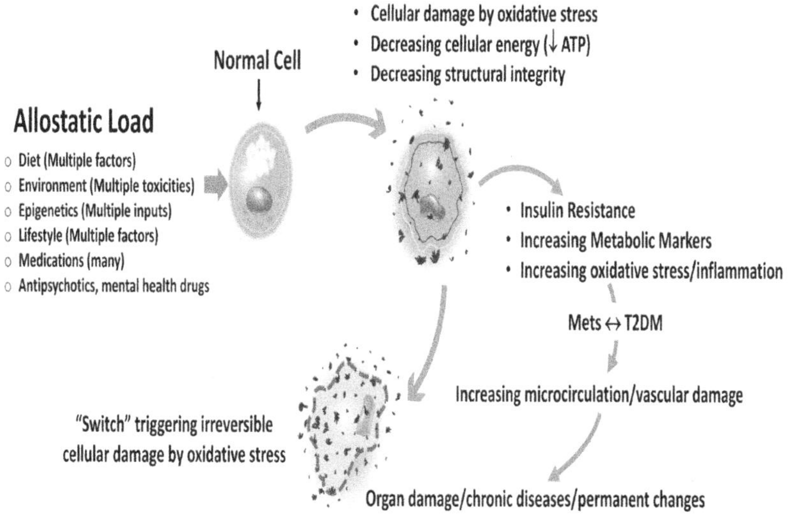

Affected cells become increasingly impaired and will die or become senescent cells, producing the ***Senescence-Associated Secretory Phenotype (SASP),*** which is persistent inflammatory signalling from "zombie" cells that are almost dead but not quite dead. At this switching point, nothing will help, as we know from a similar endpoint in small vessel damage - our discussions on "metabolic memory" that we reach a threshold of damage that we can't reverse.

One certainty exists: Drug management becomes futile when we reach advanced stages of cell damage. The only hope will be a food-based, nutrient-based approach using ketone bodies through gentle and timed ketosis to replenish cell energy and reconstruct damaged cellular components. Drugs are pointless and useless in a nutritional sense, so why bother? If you have advanced metabolic disease, drugs will never be your saviour. Only a strategy, as I outline in the final chapter, will offer you any hope.

After a lifetime of damaging effects from multiple inputs, your damaged and distressed cells must be rescued. Nutrient rescue through a food-based and supplement-based approach takes time, unlike magic bullets like drugs that work fast and cause huge collateral damage. We should train our future doctors to become warriors of disease prevention (metabolic health warriors) and, provide script-based nutraceuticals and supplements subsidized by governments and turn their backs on drug-only solutions to a vast pool of diseases not responding to any drug.

CHAPTER 7

Nutritional Ketosis (NK)

THE R.M.LOPEZ NUTRITIONAL RESOURCE PROTOCOL

Dietary approach to halting and reversing diabetes and chronic diseases of the body and brain, including mental health disorders

As I have mentioned, a food-based, nutrition-based approach is our only way out of this chronic metabolic disease nightmare. Nutrient resources for our struggling cells must be our focus, but this does not mean supplements without a meaningful dietary plan. My protocol will use both diet plus supplementation.

We have discussed how our cells have been under siege from the womb to the tomb by multiple, simultaneously acting 21st-century factors acting as "energy bandits' or from various food impacts. With glucose entry into cells being denied by an ultra-common problem in populations, our insulin resistance pandemic, our only hope for survival then is to bypass this glucose blockade with ketones.

Ketones will provide that "spark" of energy for cell survival, helping them repair, recover, and thrive after decades of neglect that led to impaired cells and chronic illness. We tend to forget that individuals will need far more nutrient support due to their genetic makeup, lifestyle, age, gut microbiome issues, food allergies, coeliac status, medications, mental health issues, gender, and chronic illnesses—the ketosis plan to be outlined aims to fill in all the gaps in nutrition and provide insulin resistant cells with a boost of energy from ketones because how will cells generate energy if their primary fuel source that is glucose is being denied entry into cells?

The term diet needs to be ditched, and instead, we need to think about a ***targeted nutritional protocol*** based on the cellular defects we want to target, such as the ubiquitous insulin resistance problem and the after-eating (postprandial) impacts. Therefore, the range of nutritional inputs that need to be considered is vast and includes all our micronutrients, vitamins, minerals, trace elements, phytochemicals, antioxidants, fibre diversity and essential fatty acids (Omega-3s, Omega-6s) that are required to keep the energy-producing engine fired up in cells. It is farcical that medical research has always cherrypicked nutrients or dietary approaches but never used a comprehensive nutritional strategy to provide all the nutrients needed for health. The macronutrient wars that are based on fat, protein and carbs are a redundant concept. The needs of cells are the absolute focus. This section is not about a diet as such; it is about a protocol to ensure cells get the wealth of nutrients needed for health.

Conceit and arrogance towards supplementation is a dangerous bias now. Please view Appendices 25 and 26 and compare this nutrient risk to Adverse Drug Reactions (ADRs) in Appendix-35. Cell energy production and repair depend entirely on adequate nutritional support that is often totally lacking in whole foods or where food choice is horrendous. Cells become more and more damaged over our lifetimes because of arrogance against nutritional support. This thinking makes the medical and dietetic professions look very small, incompetent and powerless to stop this juggernaut of deadly chronic metabolic diseases due to anachronistic thinking.

Supplementation is never about mega-doses; it is about RDAs at the upper level to support cellular repair mechanisms and cellular health after years to decades of nutrient neglect. We must move beyond the concept of dieting and see food inputs through the lens of a ***Metabolic Impact Reduction Strategy (MIRS),*** as I discuss in this ***RMLopez Nutritional Resource Protocol.*** A diet without rhyme or reason makes no sense. I don't target fatness but support cells so that losing fat becomes a natural process through timed fasting.

Reversing diabetes in 6 days after bariatric surgery

That insulin resistance and diabetes can be reversed is not challenged anymore as the evidence is in and undeniable. If research, as discussed previously, shows almost 100% of our elderly have diabetes and 100% of those 90 and over have microvascular disease, we must assume this will be our destiny; should we not?

Those who are obese and undergo bariatric surgery have been shown to have an improvement in insulin sensitivity within six days post-op (Dixon 2009), and 50% will be in remission within only 2 to 4 months from the time of the surgery (Conte, Lapeyre-Mestre et al. 2020). Not that I am advocating the use of drastic surgery to reverse diabetes, but it may be lifesaving for some people, buying them that little more time on the planet. It is not a cure. Nothing medicine does is a cure for metabolic diseases. These are all piecemeal, bandaid treatments of short-term benefit only.

Of interest from a dietary perspective is the fact that Intermittent Fasting (IF), a far less drastic intervention than surgery, produced a 47.2% remission of diabetes in comparison to a paltry 2.8% in the control group (Yang, Zhou et al. 2023). If diabetes is pushed back towards a normal state, then so too is the insulin resistance process that leads to diabetes and the chronic metabolic diseases we all fear. As you can see from the figures above, the intermittent fasting group produced a remission rate close to that produced by a drastic surgical procedure. There is nothing magical about the surgery that caused this remission of diabetes; it was a surgically enforced change in dietary caloric intake – decreased food energy and nutri-stress.

Surgery is not foolproof by any means and can be a dangerous undertaking. You can still put a cheeseburger in a blender and then suck it up through a straw. What bariatric surgery will do is limit the intake of food calories, which, as you know, is "nutri-stress" that can choke off cell energy production through the NAD^+/NADH redox couple with high food energy intake and this, in turn, can trigger insulin resistance or worsen diabetes due to cell energy impacts. So taking away this nutri-stress allows cells to produce ATP again in the amounts needed to reverse insulin resistance and all that entropy (decay) caused by poor food choices and disease processes.

Not that research papers talk about things like nutri-stress, micronutrient deficiencies, fructose impacts and the many factors we have discussed that can inflict cell energy starvation. By ignoring these factors, we condemn anyone who has undergone bariatric surgery to a life of ill health, as all these energy-robbing factors need to be addressed post-surgery. Surgery doesn't stop these cell shocks!

What follows is a dietary framework that healthcare professionals or anyone can use even after bariatric surgery with modification. It is a protocol that is based on the predominant hormonal problem of insulin resistance, which is overwhelming populations worldwide. It aims to restore cells to normal function by providing them with an energy "spark" in ketones as an alternative to glucose and to ensure not even one micronutrient is lacking through supplementation. To have the dietetic profession mislead people into thinking that they can get all the nutrients they need from "whole" foods is highly dangerous. Has this message prevented chronic disease? Has it stopped Scurvy in children and adults from making a comeback in the 21st-century? Has this message stopped the massive problem of hidden hunger?

The bonus of creating ketones is fat loss as fat is burnt to produce ketone bodies. Such a framework aims to provide ALL nutrient resources, as even one deficiency can cause dramatic cellular impacts. By shifting to ketosis and the production of ketone bodies, we shift cells to this alternative fuel source, enabling energy-starved cells to begin the repair process, decrease entropy and nudge them back to a normal state while at the same time, we lose body fat stores. Without the need for insulin to assist ketone entry into cells, gentle ketosis becomes a very smart move in all these energy-deficient diseases.

Right now, medicine is not even engaged in a conversation to move to another source of fuel for the 100s of millions of people with insulin resistance and T2DM. They are more concerned about supporting Pharma with drug sales and quick 6-minute consultations ended by a script. As a society, we must put an end to this way of treating disease and demand a far more enlightened approach to supporting cells nutritionally. Drugs are now a brain-dead approach to managing chronic metabolic diseases as their failure is obvious when we look at the prevalence figures of disease globally soaring upwards and not affected one bit by any drug being used.

The ketosis strategy I propose is not the fad high fat, high protein dietary principles being promoted in many books to create ketone bodies, as this can be deadly through cardiovascular complications. This strategy I suggest is no race but a slow and steady process that takes advantage of a time in the day when we produce ketones naturally, and that is during sleep. We take advantage of this normal fasting period in sleep but extend it.

I will discuss the use of MCT oil and Beta-hydroxybutyrate (BHB) to help boost ketones available for struggling energy-starved cells. BHB is a ***ready-made ketone***, whereas MCT has to be converted to ketones in the liver. Thus, BHB is an immediate "spark" for cells in distress to begin the repair process towards normality.

So, we have a safe replacement of glucose as fuel that provides ketones as an energy spark for a cell to repair itself as long as we also ensure a rich supply of critical nutrients to produce that energy. Ketones still need to be converted to ATP energy, and thus, all the enzymes involved must have the necessary nutrients (mineral cofactors and vitamin coenzymes) for these enzymes to function, enabling ketones to be converted to ATP.

The ***RMLopez Nutritional Resource Protocol*** focuses on the vital after-eating (postprandial) impacts through meal composition. Without a well-structured diet to stop those damaging after-eating impacts, then why even bother with such a ketosis strategy as the staple foods consumed will keep driving the biological rot onward? So, why are we waiting for a drug to do what we can do naturally and easily without Pharma and the risk of horrendous side effects of drugs?

Time Restricted Fasting & Ketosis

We will use time restriction and our period of fasting in sleep to help us create and boost the production of ketone bodies. We can extend the fasting period of sleep to at least 12 hours and, if possible, 16 hours 2 – 3 times a week or more once used to it.

This ***time-restricted fasting*** can be increased gradually. We can boost ketone body formation by adding C8:10 MCT oils and even adding beta-hydroxybutyrate (BHB), a preformed ketone body mentioned above that is the most abundant ketone in mammals (Newman and Verdin 2017). MCT and BHB can be used at the start and end of the fasting period 2 hours before breakfast.

Let's look at how we can achieve cell support and ATP restoration through some food-based, nutrient-based principles.

Pillar-1: Nutrient-Rescue & Maintenance: Cells that have undergone so much damage over time need to be rescued, as mentioned above. I have discussed nutrient rescue principles above. Cells have been tremendously damaged over time due to nutrient resource neglect by our professions. Supplement arrogance in this setting puts lives at risk and drives drug-centric madness.

Pillar-2: Nutritional Ketosis using Chrononutrition (food timing) to guide us:

We have studied the effects of timing of food consumption on adverse health effects over time. What follows is a guide based on thorough research that tells us the best time to consume food. This timing of food intake is discussed below.

Timing, Timing, Timing: Chrononutrition matters. Overnight fasting, carb cheating and ketone supplements will help us achieve sustainable ketosis

We often ignore the fact that the timing of our meals can make a big difference to the cardiovascular risk we all face later in our lives. The connection between the timing of meals and the risk of cardiovascular disease (heart attacks, strokes, transient ischaemic attacks (TIAs) and others) has been studied for decades now as we wanted to know why shift workers had such an increased risk for adverse medical outcomes. Dietary advice should be far more than calories or nutrients. A paper published in Medscape 2024 was based on this published study - (Palomar-Cros, Andreeva et al. 2023).

The take-home message about meal timing is the following:

1. Delaying the first meal of the day increases your risk of overall cardiovascular disease (CVD). Aim to have breakfast between 8 - 9 am or after a long overnight fast. Have a dose of C8:C10 MCT with beta-hydroxybutyrate 2 hours before the low-carb breakfast. A brisk walk during this fasting period before breakfast will help boost ketones exp if you have taken your MCT/BHB before your low-carb breakfast full of veggies, some low fructose fruit, and some protein such as salmon, turkey, sardines and, better still plant-based protein along with Essential Amino Acids (EAAs) where these essential amino acids offer a huge benefit for struggling cells. Eating after 9 am increases cardiovascular risk.
2. Eating a meal after 9 PM was associated with a 28% increase in cerebrovascular (brain vascular) disease than eating a meal before 8 PM.
3. Every hour that you increase in fasting before you go to sleep will mean a 7% reduction in cerebrovascular (brain vascular) disease. How amazing it is when stroke risk is so high in populations.

4. Make lunch the main meal to decrease the risk of increasing body fat.
5. Have an antioxidant plate around 3 pm. Appendix-37 gives you an idea of what I mean. Vary this plate and use seasonal foods to add diversity. Limited food diversity is not conducive to good health.
6. Start your fast from 4 pm, so by 8 am, you will have fasted for 16 hours if you are medically able to do so. Even if you fast from 6 pm, it will be 14 hours of fasting. A dose of the C8:C10 MCT oil + beta-hydroxybutyrate before the fast and in the morning after the fast, hopefully 2 hours before breakfast, will boost ketone body formation and provide that greatly needed energy "spark" for repair.

Eating after 9 am	Eating after 9 pm	Lunch	Fasting at night
Eating after 9 am increases cardiovascular risk, esp. for women[2].	A 28% increased risk for cerebrovascular risk, e.g., stroke[2].	Lunch as the main meal is protective against fat gain[1].	For every hour you increase fasting, there is a 7% reduction in brain blood vessel injury[2].

References:

1. Longo-Silva, G., de Oliveira Lima, M., Pedrosa, A.K.P., Serenini, R., de Menezes Marinho, P. and de Menezes, R.C.E., 2024. Association of largest meal timing and eating frequency with body mass index and obesity. Clinical Nutrition ESPEN, 60, pp.179-186.

2. Palomar-Cros, A., Andreeva, V.A., Fezeu, L.K., Julia, C., Bellicha, A., Kesse-Guyot, E., Hercberg, S., Romaguera, D., Kogevinas, M., Touvier, M. and Srour, B., 2023. Dietary circadian rhythms and cardiovascular disease risk in the prospective NutriNet-Santé cohort. Nature Communications, 14(1), pp.1-12.

3. Sonnier, T., Rood, J., Gimble, J. M., & Peterson, C. M. (2014). Glycemic control is impaired in the evening in prediabetes through multiple diurnal rhythms. Journal of Diabetes and its Complications, 28(6), 836-843.

4. St-Onge, M.-P., Ard, J., Baskin, M. L., Chiuve, S. E., Johnson, H. M., Kris-Etherton, P., & Varady, K. (2017). Meal timing and frequency: implications for cardiovascular disease prevention: a scientific statement from the American Heart Association. Circulation, 135(9), e96-e121.

If you want more information on meal timing and adverse vascular outcomes, then read an excellent review by St-Onge et al. (St-Onge, Ard et al. 2017). These profound meal-timing risks for cardiovascular and cerebrovascular events make a mockery of the dietetic food salesperson model that thinks about food as calories and nutrients only and never about the immense pathophysiological impacts of food and our circadian rhythms that determine the negative effects of food eaten at the wrong time.

Ketone bodies and ATP production

It is important to remember that we all produce ketone bodies constantly, especially while asleep and that ketone bodies can make 22 ATP each in a cell (Dhillon and Gupta 2022). By following carb-cheating principles, using C8:C10 MCT and beta-hydroxybutyrate (BHB) and using the golden rules regarding the consumption of quality ***non-starchy carbs***, we will trigger ketosis and truly nourish our bodies without the constant consumption of damaging grain products and staples.

The C8:C10 MCT oil stimulates the production of ketone bodies in our liver, whereas the Beta-Hydroxybuturate is a ready-made ketone body, as mentioned, that a cell can use immediately by energy-deprived cells to create ATP, enabling cells to lower the disorder and decay (high entropy state) in cells.

Starchy high-carb consumption – our bread, pasta, potatoes, fries, sweet potato, yams, beans, chickpeas, lentils, pastries, sugar, honey, agave, and grains (rice, wheat, barley, millet, oats) and other legumes will shut off ketone body production as you will have a huge supply of glucose from these high-carb foods, and your body will want to use glucose as the primary fuel. Your body will not need to tap into fat stores for energy if your diet is rich in starchy carbs, providing a ton of glucose as fuel. A high blood glucose level after starchy carbs will cause insulin levels to surge, and insulin will put an abrupt halt to the use of fat as an energy source. Insulin will shut off ketone body formation. The carbs are good mantra has been a healthcare disaster.

Your brain will love this boost of ketone bodies. It is important to remember that insulin resistance is a major driver of pathology in Alzheimer's Disease (AD). AD makes up 50% to 70% of all dementia cases, and the incidence increases rapidly in those from 70 years and beyond (Park, Zhang et al. 2020). Women run a very high risk for Alzheimer's when they hit perimenopause/menopause as a ***metabolic switch*** is flicked, turning off glucose utilization in the brain by up to 30% - yikes! It is a pity and, in fact, quite sad that women are not told they can overcome this metabolic switch by simply changing the fuel being used by brain cells from glucose to ketones as a source of energy (ATP) in the brain. We condemn many women to dementia and other diseases through this neglect to inform.

Our bodies have been designed throughout evolution to cope with long periods of famine. We have had millions of years of safety trials for ketones over millennia, during which ketosis was quite normal in the lives of our human ancestors, who produced copious amounts of ketone bodies out of necessity during periods of famine or long periods of hunting and gathering as a survival mechanism.

Carb cheating: Shifting from glycolysis to ketosis.

The Glycolysis pathway, which uses glucose as the main fuel, has its own set of genes that need to be activated, which happens when you consume a lot of starchy carbs in your diet. However, we want to shift from glycolysis or glucose-burning to fat-burning and ketosis, which uses a different set of activated genes and enzymes.

PPAR-α (Peroxisome Proliferator-Activated Receptor Alpha) is a transcription factor also required to activate those fat-burning genes. PPAR-α is regulated by free fatty acids becoming increasingly available in a restricted carb and low glucose environment.

Carb cheating: A great strategy for inducing and maintaining ketosis

The table below helps you to understand carb cheating. Taste is highly subjective and can change over time. All the meals you enjoy can be created using a low-carb approach. You must check the labelling if you want gluten-free (GF), dairy-free (DF), or egg-free (EF) options. But remember, just because it is GF or DF or anything "free" doesn't mean these are healthy options, but where possible, always go for GF and DF and EF options.

Check energy, salt, trans fats and level of processing if possible. Although a huge step in the right direction, plant-based foods can be highly processed and lack nutrients and fibre density. So caveat emptor – buyer beware! Check labels thoroughly and research that product. A least-worst approach is wise, as nothing is perfect.

Slash your starchy carb intake. Remember, increasing fibre may cause bloating, but this happens because you have made your gut organisms very "happy", so they produce gas. Gradually increasing vegetable intake will help to decrease bloating. No matter which culture you come from and which dish you love, you can use the low-carb substitutes mentioned below to create that dish using all the herbs and spices you love.

From Asian, Indian, Italian or Middle Eastern cuisines, you can create culinary delights using this strategy. You will be doing your body a favour by restricting unnecessary and highly damaging carbs that spike blood glucose and avoiding harmful effects in the postprandial period.

Carb choices that you love:	Carb-Cheating Substitutes: Bulk-up or substitute with the following.	Comment: Use the following to ease your way by combining with carb cheating options.
Rice	✓ Veggie Rice ✓ Cauliflower Rice	✓ Instead of regular rice, use

	✓ Konjac Rice	Clever Rice, normal rice but lower in GI ✓ Basmati and Wild Rice are better options with lower GI
Pasta	✓ Konjac Angel Hair, Fettucini, Spaghetti ✓ Konjac Lazangne ✓ Zucchini Noodles ✓ Spaghetti Squash ✓ Turnip Noodles Use a Spiralizer to create vegetable noodles or purchase them from supermarkets.	✓ Slendier brand options and low-carb sauces are available in many supermarkets. ✓Use low-carb real pasta options
Potatoes/Mash	✓ Cauliflower mash ✓ SNAXX Keto Cauli Mash 4-pack ✓ Rutabaga (Swede) + Cauliflower mash. Rutabaga is a good substitute for potatoes, but adding cauliflower mash will decrease the carbs further.	✓ Spud Lite has 25% less carbs. ✓ Carisma potatoes have 25% less carb. ✓ Other varieties available ✓ Try to wean yourself off potatoes, which are mainly starch and water.
Bread/Wraps	✓ Keto low-carb bread ✓ "No Grainer" bread ✓ Buns, pizza bases	Search online

Pizza Bases	✓ Cauliflower pizza bases ✓ Low-carb pizza bases ✓ Use low-carb Pita bread	Most supermarkets now have these low-carb options.

With these combinations, you can recreate any recipe that your Mama, Nana, Papa, Nonno or Nonna used to make. For a low-carb seafood risotto or curry and rice, use a combination of a low GI form of rice like ***Clever Rice*** and mix with the carb-cheating low-carb rice substitutes, or create a Shepherd's Pie, using the cauliflower mash mixed with a low-carb mashed potato from ***Spud Lite*** potatoes.

However, it will be best if you move onto the very low-carb options most of the time when you are ready. You will not die as starchy carbs = glucose, remember, and your body can produce all the glucose it needs from fats (the glycerol backbone of triglycerides) or many amino acids. Fear-mongering helps dietetics to drive more cereal and staple food sales. Don't be conned.

Your tastebuds and mouthfeel will change, and hopefully, you will love this new healthy person you have become due to these simple hacks to cut down on carbs and pump up vegetable intake.
You can blend and add more multicoloured vegetables to a bolognese sauce with a plant-based mince, or add them as toppings on your low-carb pizza, or San Choy Boy pumped up with these veggies using a meat-free mince for a low-carb veggie and phytochemical-rich meal. It is up to your imagination and taste preferences. Carb-cheating is highly adaptable to any culinary preference.

I say we have dinner for breakfast instead of cereal. So, you can have anything you eat at lunch or dinner for breakfast. Keep it low-carb, full of multicoloured veggies and low-carb fruits. Don't be conned into something created from grains and poured out of a box.

Think twice about using staples such as dairy, meat, eggs and grains, potatoes, sugar, and honey or agave and think outside the square. Plant-based egg substitutes now exist. All staple foods have their own specific risk. We discussed these risks in Chapter-1.

We are nudging our cells to health

None of this is a race. Every time our body enters ketosis, we provide struggling cells with a fuel lifeline to boost their ATP levels and strengthen them. Each nudge towards effective ATP production from ketones will help anabolic processes and support repair mechanisms. Our mitochondria and other organelle numbers will increase. Over time, we will produce cellular balance and homeostasis. Remember, no matter what stage you are in your life, it is a balance between cellular energy and entropy (cellular decay) that matters. This tug-of-war is a lifelong problem.

Keep portion size the same with carb cheating

Ideally, you want to use all non-starchy veggies and low-fructose fruit or carb-cheating substitutes. However, if this is too daunting, you can mix starchy and carb-cheating substitutes as mentioned above and gradually decrease the starchy component over time. For example, you could start with ½ and ½ of each, and then, if you are comfortable enough, slowly lower the starchy carb-rich option to, say, 1/3 and 2/3's non-starchy substitutes, then 25% carb to 75% non-starchy and then 10% carb option to non-starchy option then zero starchy carbs. As you can see, the switch will be gradual, but even at 50:50, you have slashed your starchy carbs by half!

Always go back to basics in that starchy carbs = high postprandial glucose = high insulin/IgF-1 = shutting off fat burning = glucotoxicity = increased brain fructose production from high blood glucose. Supermarkets now have many low-carb options, so you should have no trouble finding these bulking-up carb-cheating options.

Meet the ketone family

We see that ketone bodies (acetoacetate, beta-hydroxybutyrate, and acetone) can be converted to acetyl-CoA except for Acetone. Acety-Co A can enter the Krebs cycle for ATP production through the Electron Transport Chain of the Mitochondria. Acetone is useless in cellular energy (ATP) production as it can't readily convert to acetyl-CoA. However, the acetyl-CoA from acetoacetate and beta-hydroxybutyrate can enter the Krebs Cycle (Citric Acid Cycle) and generate 22 – 24 ATP each (Dhillon and Gupta 2022). This point of entry into the Krebs Cycle can be seen in Appendix-7.

Beta-hydroxybutyrate (BHB) is the most common form of ketones in mammals and can be used to boost ATP production for an immediate energy "spark" for struggling cells. This is a compound that our bodies can naturally produce when fasting. In terms of BHB safety, as I have mentioned, we have had millions of years of safety trials, as starvation has been the norm in our evolutionary history. In my mind, we need to do all that we can to provide an alternative fuel source for cells in starvation mode caused by insulin resistance.

The MCT1 cell membrane transporter for ketone bodies is present in virtually every cell. A paper published in the International Journal of Molecular Sciences stated:

> *"Ketone bodies (bHB and acetoacetate) are avidly absorbed from blood by the peripheral tissues by monocarboxylate transporter 1 (MCT1), which is expressed in virtually every cell" (Grabacka, Pierzchalska et al. 2016)*
> *bHB = Beta-Hydroxybutyrate.*

So ketone bodies are the perfect candidates to enter all our cells without any help from insulin and provide a lifeline for mitochondria that are starving of energy. Many people have an abundance of body fat that we can call upon for this ketosis process. Fat resources for ketosis are not exactly in short supply in human beings. Lean individuals with insulin resistance often have abundant intraabdominal (visceral) fat to draw upon for ketone body formation. Fat can also be used to create glucose, as I have mentioned a few times in this book for those "experts" who may be clueless that the body can produce an abundant amount of glucose from other molecules where we don't need starchy carbs. See Appendix-9.

Ketones are our *Guardian Angels*: Everyone benefits, but who specifically will benefit from ketosis and ketone bodies?

1. **INSULIN RESISTANCE, TYPE-2 DIABETES MELLITUS:** Ketosis and Ketone Bodies (KBs), if done safely, offer tremendous benefits in insulin-resistant states and Type-2 Diabetes Mellitus. A scientific paper indicates that Ketone Bodies (KBs) act as "***Guardian Angels***" for cells in distress (Kolb, Kempf et al. 2021). This same paper points out that ketone bodies can trigger several gene sets that dampen inflammation. Ketone bodies are regarded as signals for starving cells to tell the body they need fuel and nutrient resources and to make adjustments for famine pressures. KBs also improve the NAD^+/NADH redox ratios to help boost mitochondrial function for ATP production to help cells restore energy (Kolb, Kempf et al. 2021). Remember that high-energy food intakes decrease this NAD^+/NADH redox couple and put the brakes on ATP production.

2. **CHRONIC DISEASE STATES:** Ketosis is for anyone with one or more of a vast array of chronic diseases, the majority of which are caused by insulin resistance (IR), which seems to be a default problem in humans. Ketone bodies are an effective fuel source for body and brain cells and so will be helpful for all the chronic diseases listed on the back cover where glucose entry into cells is blocked. Insulin resistance is a huge component of the bioenergetic deterioration in body and brain cells over our lifetime. Alzheimer's Disease is called Type-3 Diabetes due to brain IR. Let's rescue these cells through ketone bodies and allow cells to become functional again.

3. **OBESITY AND WEIGHT MANAGEMENT:**
   A peer-reviewed website called MEDSCAPE published an article titled "*Intermittent Fasting Wins." (Larkin 2024) (Zhou, Wu et al. 2023).* This article outlined the tight connection between the gut and the brain and the importance of this connection for weight management. Gut microbial diversity increases with these fasting periods. Obesity and fat loss are dealt with very simplistically using injections like GLP-1s, which decrease appetite but do nothing to help underlying cells struggling with energy and structural decay. The dietary suggestions following the ***RMLopez Nutritional Resource Protocol*** look at what cells need from all nutritionally-based angles, including the huge benefit to our gut microbiome, which is a contributor to fat gain.

4. **MENOPAUSAL TRANSITION (The *Metabolic Switch*)**:
   With estrogen decreasing during menopause, we have an uncoupling between estrogen and brain bioenergetics, which declines over time (Scheyer, Rahman et al. 2018). Alzheimer's markers can manifest decades before onset. Estrogen deficits can begin in the 40s and, more likely, in their 50s (Scheyer, Rahman et al. 2018). Along with other risk factors for Alzheimer's disease (AD) like age or APOE4, it is also gender that matters, with the female sex at high risk for Alzheimer's.

   It is not just a woman's longevity advantage as a risk factor for AD prevalence. It is now well-recognised that in the menopausal transition state, these women's brain cells do not utilize glucose as they once did. Remember, brain cells normally use glucose avidly for energy (ATP) production. Half the population, as females, could benefit from nutritional ketosis and ketone bodies in this peri and menopausal period of their lives, which decreases estrogen and glucose brain utilization. Glucose use as fuel can be reduced by up to 30%, meaning we have slashed our glucose to ATP potential by up to 1/3 of these women who are undergoing hormonal changes.

Ketone bodies can take over the energy resources of cells suffering from this abrupt hormonal effect in women. Imagine protecting women from dementia by simply shifting from decreased glucose utilization in this transition phase to ketones as an energy source in the brain. Nutritionally inept medical and dietary professionals put women at huge risk by not informing them of the benefits of ketones. What is the alternative? Use drugs that have failed dismally to protect anyone from Alzheimer's? Or should we wait for a few more decades of research that will see millions die of dementia in the interim? How foolish to not provide a potentially life-saving, incredibly safe dietary intervention and instead use drugs that are thousands of times more dangerous than any dietary intervention.

We could use body-identical hormones in the perimenopausal (not menopausal) period to help delay this ***metabolic switch***, and while in this transition period, we can also use ketosis to protect a woman's brain. Using hormones in the perimenopausal period and not beyond five years of onset of menopause and also not in people with diabetes may offer an advantage (Scheyer, Rahman et al. 2018). Always use hormones for a short period of 1 – 2 years in conjunction with a ketosis diet to protect the brain. Ensure that there are no hormone-sensitive tumours in the breast or pelvis before commencing any hormone therapy, and seek specialist advice if there are any clotting concerns.

5. **MENTAL HEALTH DISORDERS:** All our mental health disorders can result from bioenergetic decline due to impaired biochemical energy-producing pathways and

mitochondrial impairment (Palmer 2022). The same continuums that drive chronic diseases in our body organs result in brain defects leading to mental health disorders. Insulin resistance is strongly associated with all our mental health disorders. Ketone bodies can offer a great advantage to brain cells deprived of their preferred energy source as glucose utilization declines due to insulin resistance in the brain. On top of this is cell deterioration because medicine ignores the need for cellular nutrient resources in our rush to drugs. This nutrient deprivation worsens insulin resistance and cell function even further. Professions need to focus now on the nutrient needs of cells. With so much mental health misery out there, why aren't we using nutritional approaches?

Stanford University is adopting the concept of ***Metabolic Psychiatry*** (Sethi 2022). Stanford University and many others embrace the use of ketosis to help those suffering from debilitating mental health problems made far worse by poor dietary choices and where mental health issues are strongly driven by insulin resistance, fuel (glucose) restriction and metabolic decline. How sad then that we use primitive drugs in these individuals that cure not one mental health problem but can trigger overt diabetes and worsen energy-depleted brains. What a disaster.

6. **KETONE BODY VASODILATION, HEART AND CARDIOVASCULAR DISEASE:** Remember that heart and vascular disease in the form of heart attacks and strokes is a major risk for anyone with insulin resistance. Heart and vascular disease are the number one killers on the planet. Many individuals with chronic disease or mental health disorders have a very high risk of underlying heart or vascular disease that can lead to death. For example, those with Schizophrenia have a 20% reduced life expectancy,

and 67% will die of heart disease (Hennekens, Hennekens et al. 2005). This high risk of cardiovascular disease is also for those suffering from manic-depression or depression and, in fact, all mental health disorders.

That we have such high vascular/microvascular risk in mental health disorders is not a mystery, as we have discussed. The body and brain are subject to the insulin resistance metabolic dysfunction continuum. Ketosis, then, through ketone bodies, can help by opening up blood vessels (vasodilation), thus improving blood supply to cells and tissues (Matsuura, Puchalska et al. 2023). Remember that an efficient microcirculation delivers precious oxygen, micronutrients, amino acids and fatty acids that cells need and removes toxic waste products produced by brain metabolism. An improved blood flow is critical for all disease states, including our mental health disorders.

7. **KETONE BODIES DECREASE INFLAMMATION, IMPROVE IMMUNITY AND HEART HEALTH:** Ketone bodies profoundly benefit tissues and organ systems to remain resilient and survive the insulin resistance continuum process. With ketosis, we see a decrease in inflammation, oxidative stress, decreased systemic vascular resistance, increased blood supply, immune cell modulation, and an energy resource in the form of ketone bodies to increase ATP production. Through ketosis, we can activate the Nrf2 pathway and sirtuins. In doing so, we can dampen inflammation, improve mitochondrial function and increase DNA repair (Kolb, Kempf et al. 2021). By inducing ketosis, we can reduce body weight, increase heart blood flow, decrease heart hypertrophy (increased heart size) and scarring, and positively affect epigenetic modulation to lessen the effects of inflammation and oxidative genes being triggered

(Matsuura, Puchalska et al. 2023). This vasodilating effect of ketones is a godsend for our damaged microcirculation networks, assassinating our organ systems.

8. **ENDOMETRIOSIS & PCOS:** Women with severe endometriosis have a three (x3) times increased likelihood of developing gestational diabetes (GDM) (Salmeri, Li Piani et al. 2023). If populations worldwide are riddled with insulin resistance, obesity and diabetes, then so too will our future mothers also be riddled with the same diseases and predisposition for gestational diabetes as the rest of the population they come from. But endometriosis magnifies this risk. The inflammation produced by endometriosis is a plausible driver of gestational diabetes, made worse by the increasing oxidative stress and inflammation from an insulin-resistant state. Those with endometriosis or PCOS will benefit from all the anti-inflammatory effects of a ketogenic diet. PCOS is another condition highly associated with insulin resistance. The incidence of insulin resistance in PCOS is anywhere from 50% to 80% (Teede, Deeks et al. 2010). Women with PCOS are twice as likely to have a heart attack or stroke than women without this problem (De Groot, Dekkers et al. 2011). Inflammatory processes drive heart and vascular disease and even metastatic cancer – a "***malignant flame***".

9. **AGEING:** If we are guided by the Oxford Community Diabetes Study, showing over 95% of our seniors have Type-2 Diabetes Mellitus, and if we accept that diabetes is a continuum, then we don't need 1000 years of senseless arguing and reductionism to admit that this is the destiny for all of us. Suppose you now see how cellular bioenergetic decline can easily occur from ultra-common everyday factors. In that case, it is easy to see how the

body will deteriorate over time, including loss of muscle mass (sarcopenia). Skeletal muscle is a huge "glucose sink" as muscle is a very active tissue that avidly consumes glucose as the preferred fuel for energy. Losing muscle will make it harder to clear glucose after eating, making postprandial (after eating) glucose spikes all the worse after high-starchy carb meals. Many damaging postprandial (after-eating) effects are described in Appendix-18. Beware of high-carb loads.

Multiple medications given to our senior population can hammer cell energy production in skeletal muscle and other cells. Just think of foods provided in aged care facilities with high-carb, low-fibre, low-nutrient foods and obligatory desserts that drive up glucose levels (our mini diabetes episodes after eating) to make matters worse. All these cells in the aged individual need nutrient rescue and a boost of energy-producing ketone bodies. We always put the cart before the horse, and with ageing, increased body weight is thought to cause insulin resistance in seniors instead of thinking it is the insulin resistance and fructose loads that create increased body fatness in the first place as an adaptation to a perceived famine in cells (cell energy starvation) created artificially by insulin resistance. Increased body fat is a defensive mechanism caused by the Insulin Resistance Continuum.

Ketone body levels: Safe Nutritional Ketosis: Gain without pain

Any dietary approach will be pointless if it cannot be continued in the long term. A gung-ho ketogenic diet requires 50 grams of starchy carbs or less. I don't suggest such a rigid therapeutic ketogenic diet that is used medically for drug-resistant epilepsy or fitness enthusiasts. I recommend a far gentler ketosis diet for the metabolically damaged people who are now the norm in the world.

Remember, we nudge cells back to health. We don't need a sledgehammer approach, as cells need to adjust and repair gradually.

Getting cells back to a functional state is not a race. By using MCT C8:C10 oil +/- beta=hydroxybutyrate during periods of timed fasting, we provide "bursts" of ketone bodies to nudge cellular repair and restoration. The human body will produce 0.1 – 0.4 mM/L of ketone bodies in the normal state (Kolb, Kempf et al. 2021). The MCT C8:C10 blend can then increase this circadian level to 0.6 mM/L (Jensen, Wodschow et al. 2020). It is interesting that a drug class for diabetes, the Sodium-glucose cotransporter-2 (SGLT2) inhibitors, can increase ketone levels to 1 mmol/L, which is equivalent to the levels seen after 1 – 2 days of fasting (Kolb, Kempf et al. 2021).

Check with your doctor if you have diabetes and can use SGLT2's to boost your ketone levels. The problem with drugs is that they are often used with pathetic dietetic advice or dietary advice riddled with vested interests. Always check to see if fasting for prolonged periods is safe for you on any medications you have been given.

Even a mild to moderate exercise routine in the morning at the end of the 14 - 16 hours of fasting overnight will boost KBs even higher, thus tapping into your fat stores for energy to produce the KB fuel for the exercised muscle cells. The benefit of the exercise after fasting overnight is that the fat-blasting (lipolytic) enzymes are already high and active from the overnight fast and ready to create even more ketone bodies from your body fat during even mild exercise. This strategy is fat-blasting in action.

From as early as 6 – 8 hours of fasting, ketone bodies become detectable and signal that fat burning has started. Even at this early point in fasting, LDL levels decrease, and HDL levels increase (Dong, Sandesara et al. 2020). From 12 hours of fasting, your ketone bodies start to rise well and truly, and by 16 hours, significant ketosis is underway, providing struggling cells with an energy resource to begin rebuilding and restoring their energy levels, powering structural repair and decreasing cellular entropy.

Using our sleep time is a huge advantage in ketosis formation. We are just extending the fasting period beyond sleep, thus using sleep as a stepping stone to get to meaningful ketosis. Extending that sleep-fasting time is a smart move. Nutrient rescue and nutritional ketosis's benefits need to be a slow, steady, sustainable process.

With a ketogenic diet, we want to be able to produce ketone bodies, but to do this, we need to limit carbohydrate intake because if we consume a lot of carbs, we increase blood glucose levels and raise insulin levels, and in doing so, this shuts off fat burning and prevents the production of ketone bodies.

We can compare the Standard American Diet (SAD) or Standard Australian Diet (SAD) killing so many and then compare this diet to:

1. Therapeutic Ketosis
2. Nutritional Ketosis

Diet	% Carbs	% Fat	% Protein
SAD	55%	30%	15%
Therapeutic Ketosis	5%	90%	20%
Standard Ketogenic Diet	5%	75%	20%

Long-term high-fat, high-protein diets are never safe; we know this. Such a gung-ho ketosis diet as Therapeutic Ketosis or Standard Ketogenic Diets that involve a lot of fat and protein intake is a recipe for a cardiovascular disaster, doubling the risk of a cardiovascular event (Hughes 2023). High-fat, high-protein diets cause a huge nutrient overload on our cells, which can diminish the NAD+/NADH ratio, leading to a crash in mitochondrial production of ATP energy. We have discussed this ratio previously. Is it any wonder that such a diet worsens cell bioenergetics, thus leading to cardiovascular complications? Anything that leads to cell energy compromise will lead to deadly complications.

A keto diet has many forms, such as the 5:2 diet, where you eat a normal diet for five (5) days and then fast for the remaining two (2) days or time-based fasting, like an overnight fast – this is what I suggest. Time-based intermittent fasting will be much easier to start and stick to. The 5:2 fasting diet, in my mind, seems illogical as any good we do in the fasting moments is reversed when we consume a

Standard American (or Australian) diet in those 5 days, which most people will do, thus doing nothing for biological rot driven by staple food consumption in the non-fasting period.

The fact that insulin resistance in skeletal muscle is seen early with a high-fat diet is now well recognised (Lark, Fisher-Wellman et al. 2012).

What are the risks of a ketogenic diet?

It is important to remember that intermittent or any fasting induces malnutrition. Don't eat, and you run the risk of malnutrition, which can result in sarcopenia (muscle mass loss) and even organ size loss. We want the benefits of fasting but not the potential malnutrition. The body needs to get nutrients from somewhere if you are not consuming them by fasting. If you are not taking in the amounts of nutrients needed by cells, the ***Triage Mechanism*** kicks in, robbing nutrients from tissues, organs and skeletal muscle, which is robbing Peter to pay Paul.

It is for this triage mechanism reason that we need an adequate intake of Essential Amino Acids (EAAs), omega-3s, and a full complement of vitamins, minerals and trace elements so the body doesn't raid its organs, including brain and skeletal muscle, which ultimately weakens the whole body. The body protects organs that can take us out faster, like the heart, kidneys, and brain. Please don't buy into the anti-supplement message promoted by medicine and dietetics, as their failure over six decades should be making us all deaf now to what these failed professions are saying regarding nutrient support, which can be life-saving to cells.

Medication doses may need to be adjusted, however. Discuss all of this with your doctors, who are sympathetic to what you are doing. We don't abandon an incredibly important strategy out of medical or dietetic ignorance.

We don't need Therapeutic Ketosis because long-term use of this type of ketogenic diet may be a cardiovascular risk, as I have mentioned. Malnutrition will increase heart and vascular risk. My ***RML Nutritional Resource Protocol*** is a gentle time-based ketosis and ensures no nutrient is lacking. Medscape is a peer-reviewed website for doctors, and it is interesting to see a headline such as this: *"'Keto-like' Diet Linked to Doubling of Heart Disease Risk." (Hughes 2023)*

Avoid excessive fat intake through eggs, dairy, meat, oils, butter and "fat bombs" such as unsweetened chocolate, coconut oil, or medium chain triglycerides (MCT) apart from the MCT C8:C10 +/- beta-hydroxybutyrate supplements I recommend during your timed fasting used at standard and never mega doses. We need oils in our diets, but not excessively so. All fats contain inflammatory omega-6s, but we can concentrate on Extra Virgin Olive Oil (EVOO) and flaxseed meal sprinkled on salads or smoothies rather than flaxseed oil. Use ½ an avocado rich in monounsaturated oil in your salad or ¼ to ½ an avocado in a smoothie, as the oil will help absorb carotenoids and fat-soluble vitamins in that smoothie.

We need a rich supply of Omega-3 oils (EPA, DHA) through supplementation and oily fish. Hemp Oil and hemp seeds contain GLA and ALA, both beneficial anti-inflammatory compounds. For those with inflammatory bowel disease, it is best to avoid seeds and use the meal (crushed, flour) form instead, as whole seeds may embed themselves in damaged bowel lining.

Oils should always be mixed with lemon juice or a dash of vinegar as a vinaigrette and added to salads to increase the absorption of fat-soluble carotenoids and vitamins. Lemon will add Vitamin-C and vinegar, which can decrease the glucose-spiking effects of many foods. The trick with oils is to achieve a good balance of Omega-6s and Omega-3s to dampen inflammation. Our diet also needs to concentrate on a high intake of the 1000s of phytochemicals in brightly coloured fruit and veggies and to get a great diversity of fibre and carotenoid intake.

Ketosis and Deprescribing: Decreasing drug doses or eliminating drugs.

Remember, you must monitor your biomarkers and blood pressure, as this food-based, nutrient-based strategy is about halting and reversing the disease processes. So many medical problems will, in fact, start to reverse. It is not good for pharma or a doctor's bottom line, but it is brilliant for you in terms of health outcomes.

Monitoring your glucose levels and HbA1c will indicate if you can decrease your drug doses or even deprescribe them. Check these biomarkers, say every three months or sooner, if you think there may be hypoglycaemia (low glucose levels), which may cause you to feel weak or dizzy. Blood pressure needs to be monitored. Your drug doses may need to decrease or be ceased. So please work with your doctor, but don't allow them to dissuade you from adopting such an amazing dietary protocol. A ketosis and nutrient-rich diet can do what doctors and dietitians have failed to do. As long as we provide every nutrient possible through diet and supplementation, you will help fix your health problem.

Supplementation Schedule: Let's look at my recommendations for nutrient rescue

The medical profession has chosen an incredibly illogical and narrow-minded attitude to manage metabolic disease. By the time an individual shows signs or symptoms, they are at huge risk for a deadly cardiovascular event. It is foolish then for this profession to think of critical supplements in this circumstance as a safety risk when drugs themselves will put these individuals at massive risk of an adverse drug reaction.

What I recommend here is backed by decades of research to be used as support for diseases that will take their toll in a relatively short space of time. You be the judge and don't be guided by medical sentiments shaped by Pharma to drive all management towards drugs, which we know has failed dismally for all these diseases.

Decades of cellular damage due to neglect by our medical and dietetic professions will require significant but gentle nutrient resource support for a long time. Don't use mega doses of anything I recommend, and stick to the guidelines. Mega doses are the domain of the medical profession that only knows how to use sledgehammer treatments and doses for immediate responses. Damaged cells cannot ramp up repair and use these nutrient resources instantly by trying to slap them with high doses.

In my mind, nutrient adequacy is one of the most difficult things to achieve. Only a few supplements need to be used to provide huge amounts of nutrient support. Unlike medical researchers who cherry-pick certain supplements or a group of supplements in disease states or who use one supplement at a high dose, trying to achieve a pharmaceutical therapeutic effect is something I avoid, as this is a naïve dangerous approach that has distorted a large amount of nutrient-based research. Nutrients ***work in synergy*** and require all nutrients present in the doses needed for optimal cellular function and for synergistic effect. Massively loading up on one or a few nutrients will impair the function of other nutrients. High doses of supplement treatments are how drug-centric practitioners think.

The table below is just a guide. The philosophy is to ensure the cells have all the nutrients necessary for optimal biochemical and molecular function. Herbal treatments are just like drug treatments in my mind. Using herbal preparations to fix a problem rather than prevent one is no different to drug strategies. My goal is to achieve nutrient adequacy to produce cell self-sufficiency and repair. I want to fix cells in distress and not try to overcome their pleas for help.

It is far better to use practitioner-only products as it is the Wild West out there with regard to supplementation. Doses may need to be adjusted over time. There are many shonky manufacturers of supplements produced in countries with lax quality controls. If the product does not provide the nutrient at the dose required or in the right bioavailable form, then what's the point in taking supplements? Many omega-3 capsules do not have the EPA/DHA values stated on their labels, and damage may occur to these vulnerable omega-3s if they are not created or stored correctly (Albert, Derraik et al. 2015). Please keep all supplements in the fridge, not the freezer, to prevent deterioration. Darkness in the refrigerator also protects many nutrients.

The following regimen will provide a wealth of nutrients to help cells rebuild themselves or build resilience to avoid disease. The broad nutrient adequacy of every micronutrient possible is what I am stating here with energy-supportive nutrients. It is providing all the essential nutrients for cells to function normally. It is not about nutrient pharmacotherapy!

Caution: Consuming multiple supplements increases the risk of overdosing on important and risky nutrients. Please check.

Nutrient/Nutrients	Rescue/Maintenance
Multivitamin + Mineral	1 – 2 daily. You can build a strong case for the use of a twice-a-day multivitamin regimen for at least a few months for cells to establish balance, as a lot of these nutrient resources will be lost initially as cells are too damaged and weak to even use them effectively until the cellular machinery gears up for more and more anabolic action. In standard multivitamins, even two a day will never increase toxicity risk as I will show.
Vitamin-C Vitamin-C 50 mg- 100 mg and NAC with each meal have a protective effect in the after-eating (postprandial) state. Alpha-Lipoic-Acid (ALA) can help regenerate Vitamin-C for ongoing antioxidant activity.	It has been shown that Vitamin-C can markedly reduce modified LDL in the postprandial (after-eating) period. (Lechleitner, Hoppichler et al. 1994). 900 children were tested at the Royal Children's Hospital Melbourne; a whopping 31% were deficient in Vit-C, and 5% had scurvy. With increasing body weight, Vit-C decreased significantly (Van Heerden, Cheng et al. 2024). Consider Vitamin-C in anyone with a chronic leg ulcer instead of primitive superficial lotions, potions and dressings. Ulcers will heal only if the body as a whole is well nourished for collagen synthesis. Numerous nutrients are

	involved in collagen synthesis needed to heal ulcers. Having a small amount of Vitamin-C (100 – 250 mg) with each meal and a multifibre supplement may be a great idea to dampen postprandial damage by lowering the glucose response and the potential to modify LDL.
Essential Amino Acids (EAAs) Use EAAs as a protein-sparing strategy.	Please see "Protein Leverage" mentioned after this table. 1 Teaspoon (5 grams) with each meal initially. Build up to fifteen (15) grams or three (3) teaspoons, which is the maximum amount beyond which anabolic power decreases (Church, Hirsch et al. 2020). Using EAAs is "meat sparing," and you will need to cut back as your body can use EAAs highly effectively without all the fat or risk of heme in red meat, as we have discussed. Why do we eat animal flesh and other proteins? It is for the amino acids they contain. An amino acid is an amino acid, whether it comes from a pea or animal flesh. Only commercial interests will want you to believe anything different. Following these guidelines, you will not miss out on nutrients. Consider adding marine collagen for the glycine, which will be discussed later. The hydrolysed peptide form of marine collagen is even better for bowel health, especially if you have inflammatory bowel disease.

	Consider HMB in seniors to conserve muscle mass.
L-Citrulline Malate	A non-essential amino acid that can boost L-arginine availability and, hence, Nitric Oxide (NO) production is critical for vascular health—dose as per preparation. Opening up blood vessels (vasodilation), which L-Citrulline helps, is vital for damaged microcirculation networks. Citrulline may be of benefit for those with erectile dysfunction (ED) that often accompanies insulin-resistant illnesses and may help ED medications work better (Pizzorno 2010).
DHA (450 mg) + EPA	2 – 3 Caps per day (In the morning). DHA is vital to produce anti-inflammatory compounds and for cell membranes of the body and brain. DHA is important for cell signalling functions, including cell membrane fluidity that impacts receptor functioning. DHA can be metabolized to specialized pro-resolving mediators (SPMs) – Protectins and Resolvins to dampen down inflammatory processes in chronic disease. EPA produces anti-inflammatory eicosanoids and also SPMs. It is best if you can use a combination of DHA, EPA, Choline, GLA, and ALA for a powerful anti-inflammatory effect. DHA and other Omega-3s should be ceased around four (4)weeks before delivery or a surgical procedure, as there is no definitive consensus on bleeding risk. Discuss when to recommence with

	the specialist involved when bleeding risk diminishes.
Choline Bitartrate 349 mg (Equiv Choline 143.5 mg)	3 caps for women (425 mg/d) 4 caps for men (550 mg/d) NB: DHA & Choline combinations exist. There are many critical functions for choline that I have discussed in this book. DHA and Choline should be a must for prospective mothers through pregnancy and breastfeeding. See the potential bleeding risk above.
Vitamin-D3 + K2 Research shows with mixed results that Vitamin-K2 may reverse or prevent calcium buildup in arteries. It is important to know if you have a high Coronary Calcium Score.	Because vast numbers do not get anywhere near their intakes for dark green leafy vegetables, their Vitamin-K1 levels will be affected, and this, in turn, affects Vitamin-K2 formed from K1 by the gut microbiome. What's the use of having calcium absorbed by Vitamin-D3 and then not knowing which tissues calcium should be directed to? Vitamin-K2 is the "cop" that directs calcium to where it needs to go. It is no wonder, then, that our arteries are often riddled with calcium deposits, increasing the risk for deadly heart attacks or strokes.
N-Acetyl Cysteine (NAC)	600 mg/day. In smoothies or water. NAC supports the formation of Glutathione as a ubiquitous but powerful antioxidant used by cells to offset inflammatory processes. All chronic diseases can be helped by boosting antioxidant levels from NAC, plus a wealth of multicoloured vegetables and low-fructose fruits. NAC is a known protector of the glycocalyx, which lines our endothelium.

	NAC with meals can profoundly decrease the thinning of the glycocalyx when blood glucose rises after eating and can also prevent the shedding of the glycocalyx into the bloodstream with high glucose levels (Nieuwdorp, van Haeften et al. 2006). The biggest impact on our blood vessels comes from after-eating impacts such as high glucose levels. It is absolutely shameful we don't tell people to have NAC with meals to protect our blood vessels in the heart and elsewhere. Heart disease is the biggest killer on the planet. I guess you can't put a registered trademark on a natural compound. NAC and Alpha Lipoic Acid are synergistic in keeping glutathione levels up.
Magnesium Combo: Threonate, Citrate, Orotate; Glycinate	400 mg once only at night, 1 hour before bed. I have discussed the critical role of magnesium in ATP formation. Consumption of magnesium-rich vegetables and fruits is pathetically low in populations due to pathetic intakes of fresh foods. Multiple forms of magnesium have an advantage. For example, the Magnesium Threonate form researched at MIT is said to cross the blood-brain barrier, an obvious benefit for highly predominant insulin resistance diseases of the brain where magnesium is critical for insulin to work as it should and for ATP production as ATP-Synthase in mitochondria requires magnesium to function.

Caprylic (C8) and Capric (C10) Medium Chain Triglycerides (MCT)	C8:C10 in a ratio of 60%:40% can significantly boost the production of ketone bodies, enhancing our overnight fasting to produce meaningful ketosis and thus supply struggling cells with ketone bodies to produce ATP. Start with one teaspoon when you begin your fast and then at the 12-hour point of fasting to carry you to the 16-hour mark if you can get there. Increase to 2 teaspoons, then one tablespoon if tolerated as recommended above. Gastrointestinal side effects like diarrhoea and nausea may occur. In Australia, four teaspoons equals one tablespoon, each teaspoon being 5 ml. So you can start with one teaspoon and slowly build to four teaspoons (1 Tablespoon) at the start of fasting and on awakening or at the 12-hour mark. MCT should only be used with a ketosis diet like the one suggested and not with a normal diet. You will be adding unnecessary calories if you are not following a ketosis diet.
Beta Hydroxy Butyrate (BHB) – a Ketone Body	BHB is the most common ketone in mammals. Our need for an alternative fuel source in a world riddled with insulin resistance is real and urgent. BHB can give damaged cells denied glucose (fuel) entry due to insulin resistance, which is a jump-start in ATP production. Doctors have an unnecessary and irrational fear of ketosis and can't seem to separate ketoacidosis, a potentially lethal problem

	in diabetes, in comparison to mild ketosis. As this paper states: *"Although much feared by physicians, mild ketosis can have therapeutic potential in a variety of disparate disease states." (White and Venkatesh 2011)* It is ridiculous to compare ketoacidosis, a pathological condition, to mild ketosis. It is also a pity that evidence-based approaches like mild ketosis, which I promote in this book, are avoided due to senseless, irrational thinking by doctors who confuse ketoacidosis with ketosis just because the names sound similar. Ketones are a lifeline to our brains and other cells affected by insulin resistance. BHB can be used along with MCT to help boost ketone bodies, which are desperately needed by energy-starved cells and organs like the brain. Use BHB in conjunction with the MCT C8:C10 oil at the beginning and end of a fasting period.
Energy Support Boosting fat-burning and ATP production Some multivitamins may have these compounds as components.	1. **CoQ10 (Ubiquinol)** – is a part of the Electron Transport Chain in mitochondria and is vital for energy (ATP) production. 2. **Alpha-lipoic acid (ALA)** – is a compound made in mitochondria and a powerful antioxidant that supports energy production. Alpha-lipoic acid is a cofactor in many of the

Please remember these compounds need all the necessary vitamins and minerals to support enzyme activity.	multienzyme complexes of the Electron Transport Chains (ETCs) of mitochondria to produce ATP energy. ALA has powerful antioxidant properties on its own but powerfully regenerates Vitamin-C, CoQ10 and Gluatatione, making it a powerhouse of antioxidant activity, which is exactly what is needed for damaged cells that have occurred over decades as occurs in chronic disease. 3. **Acetyl** -L-**Carnitine (ALCAR)** has a higher bioavailability than L-Carnitine. This compound plays a crucial role in ATP production by burning long-chain fats in the mitochondria. So fat burning is what we are after to produce ketone bodies as an alternative fuel to glucose being denied entry into cells due to insulin resistance. Research has shown improvements in endothelial function and microcirculation blood supply (De Marchi, Zecchetto et al. 2012).
Diversity of food fibre: Supplement along with food-based food fibre.	Alginate-Konjac-Xanthan can be purchased as a practitioner-only product. These soluble fibres can be used with each meal to increase satiety, decrease postprandial glucose surges and help with weight loss. These are prebiotics that help

	with gut health. This combination of fibre can help with hunger pangs and make time-based fasting easier. When used along with non-starchy vegetables and fruit, it adds diversity to food fibre intake. Your diet will provide a range of soluble and insoluble fibres for gut health as well.
Iron BisGlycinate ***Warning:*** *Do not take iron unless you have had a blood test. Some people can store iron (haemochromatosis). Others may need a lot more iron and even an iron infusion to get their iron levels to normal.*	Iron deficiency is a huge problem worldwide and thus may be needed. Levels should be checked before any treatment is commenced. Iron deficiency can lead to horrendous cellular energy depletion and cell structural damage. Iron sufficiency should not be left to chance, with 1/3 of the world population affected. The right form of iron is vital due to constipation that can occur. Iron deficiency is a disaster in pregnancy for both the mum and the developing baby, who may suffer ongoing brain-related problems.
Animal Flesh Nutrients A good supplementation schedule will ensure adequacy on a plant-based diet.	There is nothing in animal flesh regarding nutrients you cannot get from supplements or other foods. This thinking that animal flesh is the only way to get certain nutrients is just gaslighting. This thinking promotes staple food madness that keeps the sales of farming products in motion and satisfies food boards. The human body can also produce some of the nutrients required. The micronutrients in animal flesh that we need to ensure we have enough of are:

	Vitamin-A**, Vitamin-B12**, Vitamin, D**, Omega-3s (DHA, EPA)**, Heme Iron, Carnitine**, Carnosine**, Creatine**, Taurine**. For adequacy, zinc must come from dietary sources other than meat. Supplementation is fine. A mineral is a mineral irrespective of where we obtain it. Anti-supplement campaigners put people in harm's way and push them towards drug-based approaches that are far more deadly. **- Can be created in the body. However, it is a question of adequacy. Vitamin-A should not be used in pregnancy but beta carotene is safe and can be converted to Vitamin-A in the body.
Endothelial Cells, Glycocalyx Support	The glycocalyx becomes damaged meal-by-meal and by metabolic biomarkers such as glucose. The glycocalyx is rich in proteoglycans, glycoproteins and glycolipids. There are supplement combinations with added hyaluronic acid—Chondroitin sulphate, and other compounds that support this important glycocalyx lining on the surface of the endothelium facing the bloodstream. NAC with each meal can help prevent fragmentation of the glycocalyx. Vitamin-C with a meal can help decrease the risk of modified LDL, which can take advantage of a damaged glycocalyx.

Nutrients you do need to care about

Are there any risks to using multivitamins on a twice-a-day dose regimen? First, a serious threat to our bodies by a vitamin or mineral combination is 62,000 times less likely than any drug (ANH 2012). Appendices 25 and 26 will show this risk comparison to drugs. Don't let ignorant medical or dietetic gurus con you of the "dangers" of supplements and then guide you to a drug that has huge potential to harm. Yet, there are risks with supplementation you need to be aware of. Importantly, don't take multiple supplements with a nutrient profile that can amplify the dose of many nutrients by using a variety of supplements. Get a guided regimen of high-quality critical nutrients through professional guidance, and don't add to them.

So, ideally, nutrient guidance should be under the care of someone who knows the pros and cons of nutrient management. If only doctors and the dietetic profession woke up to themselves, they could be these practitioners guiding nutrient intakes. The risk of single nutrient harm is often overblown by talking head "experts". We do need to be concerned about the following nutrients, however:

1. **Vitamin-B6 (Pyroxidine).** It is important to state that both a Vit-B6 deficiency and excess Vit-B6 can cause neuropathy (Muhamad, Akrivaki et al. 2023). It is rare, but if someone has decreased excretion of B6 due to kidney disease or if used in a very high dose by taking multiple supplements with Vitamin-B6 long term, the B6 can cause nerve damage (neuropathy). Ultra-processing of foods can deplete foods of Vit-B6, and if up to 90% of foods consumed are ultra-processed foods devoid of nutrients, then there is a risk of multiple micronutrient deficiencies, including a risk of Vitamin-B6 deficiency.

   Many drugs can deplete the body of B6. Even commonly used corticosteroids can do this. According to the highly respected Linus Pauling Institute (LPI) at Oregon State University, no study has shown neurological damage at doses less than 200 milligrams daily, and most cases of nerve damage occur at doses between 500 mg to 1000 mg daily used for many months. Most commonly used multivitamins may have an amount of B6 around 2.1 mg and 6.7 mg, which works out to be 95 times (95x) and 30 times (30x) less, respectively, than even the lower dose of 200 mg mentioned. These multivitamin doses of B6 are from two of Australia's most common over-the-counter (OTC) multivitamins. A better option is a practitioner-only formulation, and even then, the B6 level will be far lower than doses that lead to the rare occurrence of neuropathy—scaremongering by "gurus" or other nutrition talking-heads are pointless as they seem clueless about these doses and safety concerns.

It is important to mention that the LPI states that growing evidence shows systemic inflammation from our numerous chronic diseases will degrade Vitamin-B6, and so lower doses in OTC preparations may be next to useless in a therapeutic sense in this nutrient-rescue period as inflammation almost always accompanies metabolic dysfunction, especially in the advanced stages of cellular degeneration that will "chew up" Vitamin-B6 making doses inadequate if we don't consider this inflammation. The risk of Vitamin-B6 deficiency in populations riddled with disease is far greater than an overdose that will cause problems.

We need higher RDA doses of all micronutrients. Apart from the fat-soluble vitamins A, D, E, and K., many vitamins are water-soluble and excreted if not used. Only Vit-B12 and folate are stored in the liver, but you often hear from ill-informed nutritionists that B6 is stored in the body, and this is definitely not the case. B6 is water soluble and excreted from the kidneys. Vitamin-B6 is "***rapidly eliminated in the urine***" (Simpson, Bailey et al. 2010). So, you can see depending on when another dose is taken, most of the B6 has already been eliminated, making an overdose incredibly unlikely. We put lives at risk if we highlight the odd case of irresponsible use of Vitamin-B6 when these cases are entirely irrelevant to the common risk of nutrient deficiencies in populations and where chronic disease dominates populations.

I recommend a twice-daily multivitamin, especially in the nutrient-rescue phase, for a few months to overcome the almost always-present systemic inflammation that can hammer B6 levels, including the need to overcome the rapid excretion of B6 in the urine. Protein Energy Malnutrition (PEM), as discussed, is common in many groups and can make micronutrient adequacy worse in many ways. The medical profession contributes to this problem of PEM with their beloved Proton Pump Inhibitors (PPIs). Also keep in mind metabolic disease is a huge cause for kidney disease and inflammation.

2. **Vitamins A, D, E, and K** are fat-soluble and can be stored in our body fat and accumulated in the body. Thus, these fat-soluble vitamins can become toxic at high doses. Pre-formed Vitamin-A should never be used in pre-pregnancy or pregnancy, but beta-carotene, a provitamin-A carotenoid, is safe as plant carotenoids are generally non-toxic.

   So, Vitamin-A can be made from beta-carotene, and there is a "braking" mechanism for production, as the body will only convert carotenoids to Vitamin-A as it needs it. It is said that *"No nutritional deficiency is more synergistic with infection than vitamin A."* (McCullough, Northrop-Clewes et al. 1999). This protection against infection is at the mucosal surfaces found in our eyes, skin, nose, mouth, throat, the lining of the lungs, ears, gastrointestinal tract, urethra, vagina and bladder. All these surfaces need Vitamin-A to stay healthy and fight off infection.

   Ignoring Vitamin-A in infectious diseases results in millions of unnecessary antibiotic scripts for recurrent ear infections in kids, recurrent tonsillitis or recurrent urinary tract infections, chronic lung and eye problems and pneumonia. We fail to give our kids something like Cod Liver Oil, which has omega-3s and preformed Vitamin-A, which was once used widely in days gone by in children. Extraction methods can eliminate heavy metal concerns now, so not thinking of Vitamin-A in these circumstances is negligence to me.

   Medicine and dietetics ignore a critical vitamin in favour of the recurrent use of antibiotics, which increases the risk of antibiotic-resistant strains and deadly reactions. Is this logical? Let's not forget that antibiotics can destroy the balance of the microbiome everywhere. We are now discovering that the brain and renal tract have their specific microbiomes we can destroy with antibiotics. Infections could have been avoided if we had strengthened our mucosal surface in the first place as the first line of defence by ensuring an adequate amount of provitamin-A carotenoids and/or preformed Vitamin-A.

Dreadful outcomes occur from a medical profession that only thinks of drugs and more drugs and a dietetic profession too blind to see food in a therapeutic and preventative sense. Our twice-daily multivitamin regimen will not cause toxicity of fat-soluble vitamins. Imagine all those pointless courses of antibiotics that could be avoided by preventing disease and preventing gut microbiome damage by unnecessary antibiotic use. This negligence is a shame for the medical profession, ignoring what matters most.

3. **Vitamin-A dosages**. Use a multivitamin with pre-formed Vitamin A, often called retinol, retinyl acetate, or **palmitate**. But don't do this if you are planning a pregnancy or are pregnant. There are specific prepregnancy and pregnancy multivitamins with beta-carotene that the body converts safely to Vitamin-A as needed.

   Why aren't children with severe eczema or asthma told to take high-quality molecularly distilled Cod Liver Oil for omega-3s and preformed Vitamin-A to help their skin, ears, and lungs? How many adults land in an intensive care unit (ICU) because of severe infectious diseases like influenza or COVID-19 or any number of dangerous infections of the ears, throat, lungs, bowel, and bladder, all because of horrifically inadequate diets woefully devoid of precious nutrients like Vitamin-A?

   Where is the vegetable intake to provide the carotenoids that can be converted to Vitamin-A in children and adults? Let's not forget that insulin-resistant states like MetS and diabetes are associated with many infectious diseases like pneumonia. If not trying to conceive and not pregnant, then the pre-formed Vitamin-A multi can be used. These fat-soluble vitamins in a

Multivitamin will never reach toxic doses even if used twice daily.

From the same two common multivitamin examples I used for Vitamin-B6 that are TGA approved for general use and readily available over the counter, one had 750 micrograms and the other 225 micrograms of Vitamin-A (Retinol Acetate). The agreed upper tolerable limit for retinol is 3000 mcg. Even for babies, it is 600 micrograms (mcg). So, a high RDA of 700 mcg to 900 mcg is often used to formulate a multivitamin. So, a twice-a-day dosing is well short of the 3000 mg upper tolerable limit for Vitamin-A toxicity in adults.

It is important to remember that people are more likely to suffer insufficiencies or gross deficiencies rather than overdose on vitamins or minerals. Think of the disaster ahead with the new anti-obesity injectables that can decrease appetite and lead to medically induced malnutrition. What needs to be remembered is that all these micronutrients don't just sit there in our bodies but are consumed in trillions of biochemical or molecular processes in our 37.2 trillion cells every second and thus need to be replaced rapidly. We have been pushed more and more into the arms of Pharma by avoiding hugely beneficial supplementation for the sake of highly risky drug-centric treatments.

4. **Selenium.** Selenium is a trace element that can be toxic in high doses. One or two Brazil Nuts can provide the RDA for selenium; thus, eating a handful of these nuts is asking for trouble. Selenium is critical for our primary antioxidant defence and is incorporated in the glutathione peroxidase (GPX) enzyme family. Selenium is crucial for thyroid hormone conversion from T4 (inactive) → T3 (active thyroid hormone). The enzyme involved in this conversion is a selenoenzyme and, as the name suggests, needs selenium. You may be tired because you lack selenium, which essentially produces a functional hypothyroid state. So we need this vital trace element.

The safe upper limit for selenium intake from food and supplements is 400 mcg daily. As with the supplements above, the two common multivitamins available over the counter for individuals to purchase without any guidance from a professional and with TGA approval had 55 micrograms and the other 65 micrograms. So, a twice-a-day professional multivitamin will get nowhere near this safe upper limit of 400 mcg. So unless you eat handfuls of Brazil Nuts, you will not suffer toxicity. As you can see, whole food itself, rather than a supplement, can be a risk for nutrient toxicity. Twice daily dosing with RDA levels is not a risk for selenium toxicity. Check the ingredients.

5. **Choline.** It is a vitamin-like essential nutrient. I have described how critical this nutrient is in pregnancy, holding so much hope in preventing serious mental health problems if taken throughout pregnancy to ensure adequate choline is available when GABA is "switched" from excitatory to inhibitory – see Appendix-19.

   However, choline is a double-edged sword. If you consume copious amounts of meat, eggs, dairy, liver and peanuts, you may add to the burden of a compound called TMAO, which is toxic to many cells. The gut microbiota creates TMAO from choline, and there is a strong correlation between the TMAO level and cardiovascular disease (Rappaport 2016). In saying this, the dietary intake of choline in the US is well below the recommended intake (LPI 2023).

   The risk, however, is far greater for not getting enough choline for optimal health. Not getting enough choline during pregnancy is a disaster. So even though Choline is so critical for health and may even prevent mental health disorders like Schizophrenia if used in pregnancy, there was zero (0) choline in both the common over-the-counter multivitamins.

   Adults need 425 mg (females) to 550 mg (males) daily. You risk overdosing on choline from staple foods rather than supplementation, but check the label. Choline is essential, so it is not negotiable that you need to consume adequate amounts.

Hence, I recommend choline as part of my recommended supplement regimen.

Antidepressant failures, Tryptophan and Serotonin

We always seem to think that drugs work in a vacuum to the nutrient resources a cell needs. Our major medications used in depression are called Selective Serotonin Reuptake Inhibitors or SSRIs. This name is not important, but for the vast millions out there with depression, what doctors and psychiatrists forget is that serotonin is a neurotransmitter that is created from Tryptophan, an essential amino acid (EAA).

We have discussed why people may be deficient in protein intake and, thus, Tryptophan intake. Many with depression have poor appetites and so can suffer malnutrition; therefore, protein intake and, hence, tryptophan intake will suffer. So, without enough tryptophan, how will an SSRI work? With low tryptophan available, SSRI action is impaired as the drug needs to block the reuptake of serotonin in the synapse, thus increasing serotonin within the synapse. So you see a Catch-22 all because we don't have enough of the precursor amino acid tryptophan to create Serotonin. EAA supplementation can ensure adequate Tryptophan intake.

This low tryptophan/serotonin availability is a factor in the difficulty of controlling depression, but this may not be how serotonin actually works to decrease depression. Serotonin is strongly linked to mitochondrial biogenesis (increasing mitochondrial numbers and hence energy), and serotonin alters brain energy through genes involved in energy production (Cardon, Grobecker et al. 2024).

Serotonin deficiency as a cause of depression is a guess – the ***Serotonin Hypothesis***. There are many holes in this guess, and many anti-depressants have almost no effect on many individuals given them. Serotonin by supporting brain energy is a far more plausible explanation, but we need to ensure adequate tryptophan in the first place. It's better to support brain bioenergetics and avoid damaging the brain with glucose spikes, which can convert to harmful brain energy-depleting fructose after eating. Instead, ensure you use ketones for ATP production and provide the brain with a wealth of micronutrients and amino acids that are needed for a constantly active brain hungry for nutrient resources.

Essential Amino Acids (EAAs), Protein Leverage, Glycine-Rich Marine Collagen

An amino acid is an amino acid, so it does not have to come from a lump of animal flesh on a plate, as vested interests would love you to think. A nutrient is a nutrient, and vested interests will love you to believe as well that you can only get certain nutrients in the amounts you need through consuming the flesh of a dead animal or a staple fold when nothing can be further from the truth. Nutrients and not foods are essential, and if you can't get them from one food, you will find them in another. Let's not forget that we can supplement. Perhaps beyond Pharma and medicine, we need to blame the agricultural and food industries for the contempt shown against supplementation to make us believe we can get everything we need from "whole foods".

Amino acid intake is critical due to the enormous impact a deficiency of even a single amino acid deficiency will have on protein synthesis needed to build proteins, structural components, organelles, receptors, etc. Just because you eat a lump of animal flesh doesn't mean you will absorb all the amino acids in this meat well. It is well known that meat is "energetically expensive" to digest and is associated with poor nutrient absorption or can increase demand for more nutrient resources for digestive purposes, which is a problem, especially if the gut is compromised.

So, how does medicine make things worse with meat digestion? Medicine puts people in harm's way through the use of medications such as powerful antacids called Proton Pump Inhibitors (PPIs) we discussed previously that can pull the rug from under the digestion of animal flesh. The first phase of protein digestion starts with the acid in our stomachs. Our seniors may not produce enough stomach acid or enzymes to absorb protein and may need higher nutrient intakes.

So, is it clever to give our older individuals something energy-intensive to digest where the first acid phase is impaired and where nutrients could be diverted for digestive purposes? Children need far more amino acids for growth, as do older people. The fact that stomach acid can decrease in the older groups and that animal flesh may not be completely digested for various reasons as we age can explain the need for a higher protein intake in this group.

A problem with our gut microbiomes (dysbiosis) may also impair the digestion or absorption of amino acids from the gut lining. Many factors, from anti-inflammatories to antibiotics to inflammatory bowel disease and other factors, can interfere with protein absorption. This issue of getting enough amino acids, in particular essential amino acids, cannot be a hit-and-miss strategy. We cannot consume lumps of animal flesh just to make meat and livestock corporations happy.

Why do we put our children and older groups at risk? Essential amino acids (EAAs) are the perfect solution. Why do we play off animal versus plant EAA availability and simply go directly to the EAAs themselves that are easily created to use as a supplement to ensure we have all the essential amino acids that the human body cannot manufacture? Our bodies can manufacture all the non-essential amino acids (NEAAs), and these NEAAs are plentiful in a plant-rich dietary plan, I suggest anyway. Our free-form EAAs will be far more bioavailable than animal or plant proteins, and these contain all the BCAAs where absorption will not be affected by stomach acid concerns, bowel problems or medication effects.

What has been found is ***PER MEAL PROTEIN*** is vital because if you don't meet your amino acid requirements in any given meal, muscle protein synthesis (MPS) will be affected for the whole day (Weiler, Hertzler et al. 2023). Free-form EAAs included in every meal will ensure we meet our per-meal targets for amino acids, and this is critical in insulin resistance and chronic diseases where there will be tremendous structural damage over the years to decades before we even discover something is wrong.

Not getting enough protein (amino acids) can undermine weight loss and health goals and increase the risk of muscle loss (sarcopenia). Two Oxford and Sydney University professors have thoroughly researched protein as a potent food consumption driver (Simpson and Raubenheimer 2005). Consuming food until you reach the required protein (amino acid) intake threshold for health and survival is the basis for the ***Protein Leverage*** model.

A farmer's nightmare is a swarm of locusts over their grain fields, voraciously consuming all those grains in a frenzy. Grains can lack Lysine, an Essential Amino Acid. Lacking even one amino acid will severely limit protein synthesis, so locusts will eat and eat plant matter like grains in vast amounts to get the right balance of the amino acids required for protein synthesis, health and survival. So do other animals and us as humans.

Professor Stephen Simpson, one of the protein leverage authors of "***Eat Like the Animals.",*** discussed a recent finding where if you consume a low-protein diet, such as a 10% limited protein diet, your liver will produce a hormone labelled ***FGF21.*** This hormone switches on savoury-seeking behaviour (Vernimmen 2023). So now imagine "***protein decoys***" such as BBQ-flavoured carbs like crisps that taste as if they are protein-rich but lack amino acids or nutrients. How will these protein decoys drive food consumption, in particular, and how will these protein decoys drive the protein leverage mechanism? The body thinks these decoys are protein-rich when they are not, thus tricking the body into thinking they are full of amino acids. These decoys are only carb-rich, spiking glucose and insulin levels after eating, leaving the cells craving the amino acid content they need to survive. This situation will drive food-seeking behaviour and worsen our overfat, overweight and obesity problems through protein leverage. Fatness is another pandemic on the planet.

Such foods abound in supermarkets and convenience stores that are low in protein (amino acids), thus driving eating behaviours and pushing more and more food consumption to meet those amino acid thresholds required for cell function and survival. Will you become obese if this is kept up? Without doubt!

If we look at the stunning findings on ultra-processed food intakes in the UK, US and Australia, Professor Simpson made the following statement:

> *"Over the last couple of years, population survey data have shown that the average person in the US, Australia or the UK gets more than half their calories from highly processed foods — in some cases it's 90 percent or more."* (Vernimmen 2023)

With intakes of such horrific (bad) foods lacking in micronutrients and protein (amino acids), please think of how this will hammer our energy pathways and devastate cell structure and function. Without an adequate intake of critical amino acids, how can cells build the cell machinery, i.e. all the enzymes, protein complexes, mitochondria, membranes, etc? Remember, insulin resistance magnifies this problem, as insulin is needed to get amino acids into cells. Yet the myth of an optimal diet being possible in populations riddled with insulin resistance, an ageing population and a population full of medication use that can impair nutrient sufficiency still lingers in the minds of dietitians and doctors.

To reach an optimal diet, you must examine an individual's clinical problem/s, lifestyle factors, environmental toxicity exposures, and microbiome, and also provide a full dietary analysis, blood workup and genetics (nutrigenomics) to come even near to an optimal diet. ***Understanding and* o *vercoming these nutritional variables is precision nutrition in action.*** To think we can eat an optimal diet with foods riddled with inadequacies from suboptimal farming practices, soil inadequacy, dietary guidelines driven by vested interests, loss of nutrients in transit and storage, loss of nutrients by UV light damage or heat degradation through cooking and nutrient depletions due to medications is extremely naïve and yet dietetics promotes this myth. I discuss how we can get close to optimum nutrient rescue and nutrient management by using the ***RML Nutrional Resource Protocol.*** We can't achieve this without nutrient support through supplementation and a best-case food-based diet that doesn't damage us in the after-eating period.

If we do not have a full complement of all our essential amino acids (EAAs), it is hugely damaging to our cells, tissues and organ systems. You will get plenty of non-essential amino acids (NEAAs) in your diet from vegetables, fruit, nuts, and seeds. Remember, being non-essential, our bodies can produce them. Don't be conned by those who want you to believe that animal flesh is the only way to get certain nutrients. This thinking keeps Meat & Livestock boards and corporations happy.

Interestingly, in animal studies, using 100% Non-Essential Amino Acids (NEAAs) as the only source of amino acids in the diet resulted in early death (Romano, Corsetti et al. 2019). It is also important to dispel some myths about EAAs versus balanced amino acid blends containing all the essential ***and*** non-essential amino acids. It was found that the anabolic (protein synthesis effect) per unit of amino nitrogen and energy in just the EAA blend alone was DOUBLE that of the balanced amino acid blend that contained both EAAs and NEAAs (Volpi, Kobayashi et al. 2003).

Even at high doses, non-essential amino acids were ineffective at increasing protein synthesis, but a flooding dose of even a single essential amino acid DOUBLED skeletal muscle protein synthesis.

On top of this, it was shown that EAAs had little to no effect on insulin release from the pancreas or blood insulin levels compared to the Non-Essential Amino Acids or a balanced blend of all the EAAs and NEAAs.

And so we can meet all our essential amino acid needs through an EAA supplement without affecting insulin levels in the least. This fact alone is extremely important in insulin-resistant chronic metabolic disease (the majority of chronic diseases) as whole protein can drive insulin levels through the roof, let alone all that fat and food energy in animal flesh to increase body fat. So, EAAs have an amazing role in the chronic illnesses we all face.

It was shown that adding a carbohydrate source such as glucose to the EAAs was counterproductive, especially in the exercise setting.

This effect prompted the authors to state, ***"...an effective supplement should contain essential amino acids and no carbohydrates"*** (Volpi, Kobayashi et al. 2003).

It is saddening that doctors or dietitians know so little about the critical nature of EAAs, especially when surrounded by individuals metabolically unwell with insulin resistance that prevents amino acids from entering cells for anabolic (protein-building) functions. Insulin resistance chokes off amino acids entering cells, and without an adequate supply of essential amino acids, how can cells build anything? Can a drug help build proteins, enzymes, receptors, signalling molecules, etc., like amino acids do? Absolutely not.

High-energy foods like animal flesh or carbs drive increases in insulin in the after-eating (postprandial) period, pushing an individual towards horrendous long-term complications when so many have insulin resistance and are on the verge of beta-cell burnout. Beta-cell burnout is where no insulin is produced, and thus, insulin injections are needed to survive. The insulin-independent nature of EAAs is a critical positive point for using free-form essential amino acids in insulin resistance-related chronic diseases as EAAs do not demand a lot of insulin from beta cells, but chewing on animal flesh with all that fat and calories will ensure the insulin-spiking effects will occur, putting a struggling beta cells in the pancreas at risk. Ultra-processed foods can significantly dilute the more expensive protein component with cheap carbohydrates and vegetable fats. This protein dilution is a protein leverage driver.

Don't think protein can't create fat. In a famous biochemistry study aid for university students stated the following about protein being converted to fat:

> *"In spite of the exhortation by some popular weight-reducing diets to eat large quantities of protein, it should be remembered that surplus dietary protein can be converted to fat. For protein to be converted to fatty acids and triacylglycerols, the essential precursors for fatty acid synthesis, namely a carbon source, acetyl CoA, and biosynthetic reducing power as NADPH, must be formed." (Salway and Granner 2004)*
> *Triacylglycerols is another term for triglycerides.*

So, too little protein and you are in trouble; too much protein and you will add to body fat. The solution is to get enough of the EAAs in the diet through a pharmaceutical-grade EAA powder that we can have with our meals, thus reducing the need for the consumption of whole protein. Just 2 heaped teaspoons of EAAs three times a day and small amounts of plant-based protein are all you will need.

EAAs are an effective protein synthesis driver in muscle, thus preventing skeletal muscle loss. It is a perfect low-calorie solution that provides all our critical amino acid needs without all the fat energy of animal protein sources. EAAs will not interfere in the formation of ketones, as insulin levels are not affected. We do not need much; even 1 – 3 teaspoons with each meal can make a huge difference to cells struggling to meet their protein needs. Remember, 15 grams (3 teaspoons) of EAAs provides maximum anabolic power for protein synthesis (Church, Hirsch et al. 2020).

We must remember that protein intakes were calculated in "***metabolically healthy***" older and younger adults to be 0.66 to 0.8 grams per kg of weight (Richter, Baerlocher et al. 2019) adjusted for lifestyle and illness. Who is metabolically healthy now?

EAAs are rapidly absorbed and distributed, ensuring struggling cells receive these critical amino acids to repair and restore cell function. It is a fantastic way to decrease meat consumption.

As stated in this book, meat will become a thing of the past. The writing is already on the wall for animal products. EAAs provide a way to meet (pun intended) all your needs. Suppose we supplement and have a whole food diet to ensure we get other nutrients, phytochemicals, non-essential amino acids, fibre, etc. In that case, we don't need to be concerned about a nutrient deficiency and certainly not an amino acid deficiency if we use EAAS in our diets.

Please think of the medical model as it now stands with drug-centric madness with no thought for nutrient adequacy. It has been shown that an evenly distributed protein (amino acid) intake resulted in a 25% increased muscle protein synthesis (MPS) (Weiler, Hertzler et al. 2023). In other words, spread this EAA dose out three times daily rather than getting all the EAAs in one hit. Remember, you can maximise protein synthesis with just three (3) teaspoons (~ 15 grams) 2 – 3 times a day and lessen whole protein intake, especially animal flesh that does you and the environment no favours. If you have some whole protein, then decrease the EAA intake to 2 teaspoons to ensure amino acid adequacy.

EAAs vs Plant-Based, Animal Proteins: Will you get enough protein your body needs? EAAs as a whole protein-sparing strategy

The only thing that matters in terms of protein sufficiency is getting enough amino acids, whether from a cow, a plant, a mealworm or crickets. The WHO and other expert bodies have documented animal flesh as dangerous. We are not Neanderthals that need these staples anymore. We need to get beyond this. As I have indicated, essential nutrients in animal products can be found in a wealth of other foods and supplements.

We are caught between a rock and a hard place regarding animal flesh versus plant-based protein and amino acid availability and digestibility issues. So what does one do? We are moving into a post-staples world, and animal protein is not exempt from this shift. With 3D printing of "meat" and plant-based proteins filling the shelves and fridges of supermarkets, you will witness a huge revolution in protein production and consumption, which has only just started. Insect-based proteins like mealworms or crickets and other insects will make up a large part of protein intake in future. This protein intake shift is a huge threat to farmers and meat and livestock boards. Be prepared for a barrage of gaslighting as protein intakes shift to new forms coming our way.

The problem is that if we continue to eat animal meat, we risk our health and the health of our planet. On the flip side, if we eat plant protein, we face issues with protein digestibility and amino acid availability (Day, Cakebread et al. 2022). EAAs are a huge benefit and a strategy to bypass these problems of adequacy and digestibility by boosting critical essential amino acids that our bodies and cells need with each meal. There are no digestibility issues here. EAAs are absorbed rapidly.

The days are numbered for all staples, including red meat. Staples such as meat, eggs, dairy, and grains have taken a massive toll on humanity, considering all the health damage caused by these foods. So the recommendation is to use plant-based foods packed with multicoloured veggies but ensure we have highly bioavailable Essential Amino Acids (EAAs) in all meals. We need to stop listening to corrupted dietetic advice and make sense of the dangers of food rather than listen to gaslighting. The fickle dietetic groups will gravitate to these new foods in future after destroying 100s of millions of lives. How much sooner could we have transitioned to new protein sources if dietetic groups said we were wrong and needed to move forward and away from staple foods?

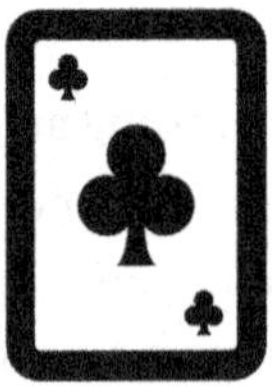 Whole protein portion size is used using a deck of cards as a guide, which is 3 ounces or 85 grams.	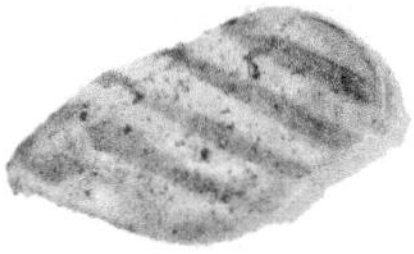 Chicken breast 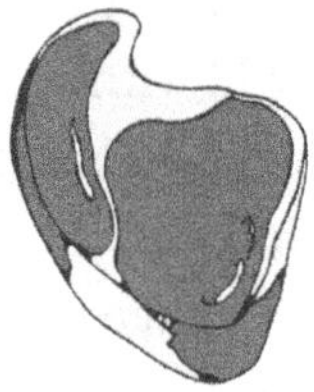 Meat	Equivalent to up to 30 grams of protein

It is truly surprising how little protein you need to consume to meet protein synthesis needs, and yet people think you need to eat a whole cow a day to satisfy protein needs. As a rough guide, a chicken breast slightly larger than a deck of cards is equivalent to 30 grams of protein. Thus, using a protein intake of 0.66 grams per kg of body weight, an individual weighing 70 grams needs only 46 grams daily. This amount could be slashed by using EAAs in the diet as well as animal flesh is energy-dense with all that fat, and a lump of animal flesh may not be digested well for various reasons such as proton pump inhibitors (PPIs) or age and diminishing stomach acid production.

We must remember the wealth of amino acids we get from nuts, seeds, vegetables, fruit, dairy or non-dairy foods, grain or grain-free foods, and egg or egg-free foods. We can easily overdo it in terms of protein intake. Dietitians often use the size of a palm to explain a protein portion size or a deck of cards.

One heaped teaspoon of EAA increases protein synthesis 3.5 times. Protein-sparing effect of EAAs cutting down on animal & plant protein

Even a very small dose of 6 grams (approx. one heaped teaspoon) of Essential Amino Acids (EAAs) can increase protein synthesis by 3.5x (Borsheim, Tipton et al. 2002). You won't need to consume a lot of animal or even plant-based protein if you use EAAs with that meal. All protein from plants or animals will have more calories than the negligible energy in EAAs. Cut animal or plant-based protein by half or 2/3s by having EAAs with that meal. Imagine the benefit to you and our environment. You will not suffer from micronutrients or protein deficiencies if you follow this supplement regimen. A nutrient is a nutrient, whether from food or a supplement. Don't be fooled by "gurus" who state otherwise.

Energy (calories) in EAAs are incredibly low, with no animal fat. EAAs can be a Godsend to struggling cells that need to repair damaged protein components. They are rapidly absorbed and distributed to cells with little to no digestive power required. EAAs may prevent a huge amount of cellular harm caused by Proton Pump Inhibitors (PPIs) that won't affect the digestion of free-form amino acids that don't require stomach acid for digestion. EAAs should be considered in anyone taking a PPI. Using EAAs during and after exercise can significantly improve protein synthesis after training, but you do not need carbohydrates or Non-Essential Amino Acids

(NEAAs) to drive this protein synthesis as all you need are EAAs (Borsheim, Tipton et al. 2002) (Volpi, Kobayashi et al. 2003).

> *There is a linear increase in muscle protein synthesis from 3 grams of EAAs to a maximum of 15 grams, beyond which extra EAAs won't benefit protein synthesis* (Church, Hirsch et al. 2020).

A flat teaspoon will contain around 3.7 grams of EAAs. There are three (3) teaspoons in 1 tablespoon in the USA, UK and NZ, but in Australia, there are four (4) teaspoons in 1 tablespoon. To keep things simple, use two (2) heaped teaspoons of EAAs with each meal if a whole protein is being consumed; otherwise, use three (3) teaspoons or 15 grams if no whole protein is consumed to ensure adequate protein synthesis will be adequate.

It would help if you avoided Protein Energy Malnutrition (PEM) at all costs. Insulin resistance weakens cells structurally and blocks amino acid entry into cells. So, we need a constant supply of EAAs to help cells repair and become functional. Most people, as discussed, will need around 0.66 grams of protein per kg of body weight (Richter, Baerlocher et al. 2019). As mentioned, the average protein intake intake for a 70 kg person is only 46 grams of protein per day. So, not the massive amounts people think they need. According to the WHO, this amount is the same for children and adults, as stated in the Richter et al. paper.

We forget that there is plenty of protein in fruit and vegetables, where 1 cup of spinach has 5 grams of protein, and 1 cup of cooked Edamame may have 17 grams of protein.

Food intake is hit-and-miss. Some may be scraping through with protein (amino acid) requirements, while others following a Paleo-type diet may eat huge amounts of animal protein.

The flawed research doctors and dietitians love to use to discredit nutrient management.

Please read on if you want to see how supplement use is undermined in medicine and dietetics. There are many biases against supplements from the medical and dietetic professions that keep quiet about Adverse Drug Reactions (ADRs), which are extremely common and far more deadly than any nutrient risk.

The following discredited studies have been constantly used to warn us about the dangers of supplements. It is as if doctors and dietitians have not bothered to look at the research flaws and counterarguments that don't just use soundbites and gaslighting.

1. The CARET Trial: Beta-Carotene and Retinol Efficacy Trial in 1996
2. The ATBC Trial: Alpha-Tocopherol Beta-Carotene Trial 1983 – 1993 by the National Cancer Institute (NCI)
3. The Homocysteine Trials

In both the ATBC and CARET trials using Beta-Carotene, those who took the beta-carotene saw an increase in lung cancer risk by 16% after six years in the ATBC trial and by 28% after four years in the CARET trial. However, it is important to point out that the age groups in these two trials were from 50 – 74 years, and these individuals were at a higher risk of cancer anyway. In the CARET trial, individuals who were heavy smokers and some with asbestos exposure were included in this study. Smokers and those exposed to asbestos are already at high risk for lung cancer, irrespective of beta carotene being taken. Naïve when you think that researchers would have expected a miracle in lung cancer protection by throwing one nutrient in the form of beta-carotene, a carotenoid, to individuals at high risk in the last few decades of their lives.

So, just one nutrient is used as monotherapy in beta-carotene against the horrendous exposures that predispose to lung cancer over a lifetime. These study subjects had lungs exposed to thousands of dangerous chemicals through smoking and other air-related toxicities, including deadly asbestos. Failure of this study seemed guaranteed with such a mix of high-risk individuals in the study.

Nutrient research is riddled with fantasy approaches like this, disregarding decades of damage over someone's lifetime but expecting miraculous reversal by one nutrient at high doses.

It is important to note that the carotenoid family has around 750 naturally occurring compounds. So, how can you cherry-pick any of them and use them in a potent pharmacological dose as the sole representative of that whole family of pigmented food compounds? These compounds don't work alone but synergistically to provide powerful phytochemical protection. Using one carotenoid in a high dose will block the effects of the others on cells. Also, phytochemical protection must occur throughout our lives in the form of a high vegetable and low fructose fruit intake, where we consume 100s of carotenoids on a regular basis. You can't just suddenly wipe away decades of neglect and cellular damage by throwing one or a handful of nutrients at this damage and expect it to work wonders. For this reason, I never suggest supplementation by itself; we need thousands of plant-based phytochemicals and fibre from whole food to help our cells recover.

Researchers say that a high intake of veggies and fruit protects against cancer. So, they thought, why not choose beta-carotene to represent all those vegetables, fruits and the 100s of carotenoids and 1000s of phytochemicals in plant-based foods? Amazing reasoning, right? One compound to represent 1000s of plant chemicals. Some research thinking is truly dumb. We don't cherry-pick nutrients but provide ALL micronutrients required by cells to be effective.

Surprisingly, a later study using Beta-Carotene was carried out in Linxian, China, with a younger cohort than the ATBC/CARET studies. This Chinese study used a broader mix of nutrients called 'Factor D'. This combination of 50 mcg of selenium, 30 mg of Vitamin-E, and 15 mg of Beta-Carotene was given to 29,584 adult participants. The research findings of this broader nutrient base:

> *"...led to decreased mortality from all causes, cancer over-all, and gastric cancer." (Qiao, Dawsey et al. 2009)*

Qiao et al. stated:

> *"The beneficial effects of selenium, vitamin E, and Beta-Carotene on mortality were still evident up to 10 years after the*

cessation of supplementation and were consistently greater in younger participants." (Qiao, Dawsey et al. 2009)

Imagine that! A broader set of nutrients used from a younger age had such an amazing, long-lasting effect on cancer protection, but it was still a cocktail of cherry-picked nutrients.

Instead of facts, doctors and dietitians tend to resort to catchy phrases when discussing studies on beta-carotene. It makes for a good fairytale story with no basis in reality. The gullible in medicine and dietetics listens intently and never challenges anything. All this does is create a bias towards what really matters in a nutritional sense and makes the "drugs are our only hope" sentiment or that whole food can provide all the nutrients we need that has seen chronic metabolic disease flourish and, in fact, rocket skyward.

Flawed research like this does chase people away from comprehensive supplementation and into the arms of drug-centric models of management. What a mess this model has created. What would the research results have been if ALL nutrients in upper RDAs were given along with the food-based ketosis approach that I discuss, drawing upon the enormous benefits of the Mediterranean Diet (MeDiet), the MIND Diet and the DASH diets, all of which are highly researched diets packed with phytochemicals and fibre? Instead, we love using meaningless piecemeal approaches.

The homocysteine story

Here is another story about flawed research regarding homocysteine affecting the lives of countless millions of people over the decades of mismanaging this compound. Homocysteine is a naturally occurring toxic amino acid normally produced by the body. It is highly damaging to our cardiovascular systems, our bones and brain. This harmful compound increases if we lack certain micronutrients like Vitamin-B6, B12 or Folic Acid or consume high methionine foods. Methionine is rich in animal protein sources.

Once again, we can see the huge benefit of micronutrient supplementation by having these vitamins daily to keep homocysteine levels in check. We can also help decrease homocysteine levels by reducing Methionine intake. Methionine is rich in animal meats, dairy, eggs, poultry and seafood. The problem with homocysteine research is that they throw a few nutrients to patients with high homocysteine levels that have been causing damage over a long period and then expect a lifetime of damage to be reversed rapidly by cherrypicked nutrients. The same happened in the CARET and ATBC trials.

Like glucose or LDL or any other biomarker we target, it will fail if we don't see all these biomarkers acting in a bigger picture sense and never in isolation from the many different impacts acting around them. Is it any wonder that throwing a cocktail of vitamins or just one micronutrient naively at someone with advanced damage to their cells, tissues, organs and vascular beds at a late stage of homocysteine-related damage? How can this approach reverse long-term damage? This story is similar to our microcirculation damage issue because when it occurs, this damage can't be reversed if left too long by trying to lower glucose – ***the metabolic memory***.

This homocysteine story is yet another one where intervention needs to start early in life and where micronutrients are vital in helping decrease a toxic compound throughout life and not at a late stage of life. Even mild to moderate elevations in Homocysteine can severely damage blood vessels in the heart, brain and other organs.

Homocysteine is underappreciated as a huge risk to our vascular systems (Koller, Szenasi et al. 2018). Homocysteine significantly increases the risk of microcirculation damage (our tissue and organ assassin). Just imagine this huge lifelong risk being controlled and fixed by what we put in our mouths by ensuring we have all the micronutrients needed for health and avoiding methionine-rich staples such as animal flesh and the use of supplementation known to keep homocysteine in check. A good multivitamin with activated B-group vitamins can do this.

Limited glycine intake

Glycine is a non-essential/conditionally essential amino acid. It can be a limiting amino acid for a wide range of critical compounds in the body:

> *"Glycine plays many important physiological roles, including collagen formation (glycine located at every third position in collagen), neurotransmitter function, glutathione production (glycine is one of the amino acids in the glutathione tripeptide), regulation of immune function, and synthesis of other biomolecules including DNA, RNA, creatine, serine, and heme." (Weiler, Hertzler et al. 2023)*

We can be significantly deficient in glycine, as discussed in the paper by Weiler et al. Glycine was found to be "considerably short" for healthy outcomes. For this reason, adding marine collagen to the intake of EAAs will be incredibly beneficial in ensuring you get a rich supply of glycine in your diet. Consider 1 – 2 teaspoonsful (5 to 10 grams) of Marine Collagen daily or a Glycine supplement. I often use essential amino acids (EAAs) with glycine added.

Getting enough amino acids, including Glycine, is vital to health. Adding HMB, an L-Leucine compound, can help decrease age-related muscle loss (sarcopenia). Let's not forget that creatine monohydrate can help increase muscle mass and cell energy levels, especially as we grow older. Also, ensuring your cells have all the necessary nutrients for energy (ATP) production will help drive anabolic processes to build muscle.

The RML Nutrient Resource Protocol

Thinking of diets is now an outdated idea, as we emphasise one macronutrient over another, such as carbs, protein, or fat. We now need to think about nutrition in terms of disease prevalence in populations, how we can bypass nutritional weaknesses to overcome factors that can lead to a bioenergetic decline in cells, and how best to support cellular repair and restoration of cell components. We must consider the after-eating (postprandial) harm caused by all foods as this one factor can drive metabolic disease toward organ failure faster due to the horrific impacts on our vascular endothelium and glycocalyx with every meal or snack.

Slapping foods on a plate based on taste and not nutritional sufficiency is a surefire way to end up chronically ill fast. The wonderful news is that it is not hard to understand and follow the golden rules. Our number one nemesis driving chronic metabolic disease is insulin resistance, followed by dietary patterns that come nowhere near supplying all the necessary nutrient resources needed by our cells to stay fully energized and functional.

1. We base this Nutritional Ketosis (NK) diet around a gentle nutritional ketosis strategy that is helped by episodic overnight fasting and C8:C10 MCT oil +/- Beta-Hydroxybutyrate (BHB) to boost ketone bodies as a fuel lifeline to insulin-resistant cells. Even episodic production of ketone bodies or low-grade ketosis will make a huge difference to starving cells by providing ketones as fuel for significant ATP production, which then triggers repair and restoration processes.
2. We draw upon the principles of highly researched diets mentioned in this book. So, this is not dietary guesswork but evidence-based wholefood-related principles. Researched diets need to be stripped of vested interest food recommendations, though.
3. We need to concentrate on veggies and more veggies. Use the Mayo Clinic 1-2-3 approach to understanding vegetable serving sizes. Keep in mind legumes are carb-heavy. Aim for 10 servings of vegetables and two servings of low-fructose fruit.

Food	One serve
Raw Vegetables	1 cup
Dark Green Leafy Veggies	3 cups
Legumes (Beans, Chickpeas) Legumes are high in starchy carbs, so keep these to a bare	½ cup

minimum or avoid them, as you do not need starchy anything in your diet unless you are an elite athlete or training for the Olympics.	

4. How you incorporate veggies will depend on your preferences. You can mash, blend, juice, pulverise, roast, eat raw, create veggie-rich dips, add veggies to stir-fries, and make a crudité plate with cut raw vegetables to dip into hummus, tahini, veggie dip (low carb, low calories), tomato paste or low-fat, coconut yoghurt dip. Sprinkle a few drops of black sesame oil to make the veggies delicious. An antioxidant plate is a great way to get a huge hit of phytochemicals and fibre - see point-6 below and Appendix-37. I like to say "***pump it up***" with veggies by ensuring you use a wide array of colourful and leafy vegetables in a bolognese sauce or curry. Just blend and add to the sauce. If you don't like vegetables and 95-99% of the population doesn't, as survey after survey has shown, find ways to include them as this is not negotiable for health. If you avoid them, then illness follows! Always add a vinaigrette to veggies, and use either olive, hemp or avocado oil plus vinegar or lemon juice to absorb fat-soluble nutrients. The vinegar can decrease the glycaemic effect (lower the GI) of food. The lemon juice provides a hit of Vitamin-C that can reduce LDL modification. Rotate the oils being used for diversity. Start your day not with pointless cereals out of a box but with a low-calorie, gluten-free, dairy-free soup pumped up with vegetables raw or frozen along with coriander or other herbs. A salad with fish, such as salmon, herring, or mackerel, is a great breakfast.

5. We need ten (x10) servings of mainly veggies daily. One serving of fruit and vegetables is 80 grams. Use the Mayo Clinic's serving sizes above to guide you. However, don't go

above the ½ cup of legumes as these are carb-rich, and in fact, you may only be allowed ¼ of a cup of legumes or lower to keep carbs and glucose levels low to trigger ketosis. Avoid legumes when you have diabetes or insulin resistance, irrespective of what dietetics teaches. Their high-carb recommendations are a sales pitch for grains, legumes and other starchy carbs. Think of the horrendous damage and deaths inflicted by high-carb recommendations. Remember the after-eating glucose-spiking effects of high-carb foods. We want ketosis and not glucose spikes where glucose can't get into cells in the first place. Forget about weighing anything, as this is usually disastrous when continuing with a diet. Being precise is not like NASA using calculations to land a rocket on Mars; thus, any dietary advice that says you have to be exact is misguided. So what is desired is 800 grams as a target for maximum benefit, according to the Imperial College London (Wighton 2017). The original study, which included 2 million people, was published in the *International Journal of Epidemiology* (Aune, Giovannucci et al. 2017). In summary, consuming this amount of mainly vegetables and a small amount of low fructose fruit has the following health impacts:
- It will save almost 8 million lives worldwide (probably a gross underestimate).
- Reduce heart disease by 24%
- Reduce stroke by 33%
- Reduce cardiovascular disease by 28%
- Reduce cancer by 13%
- Reduce the risk of dying prematurely by 31%

If only governments were smart enough to stop paying for incredibly expensive failed drug and surgical treatments and subsidize fresh food. Food advisory bodies don't push the ten servings, not that it is not extremely beneficial, but because if up to 99% are not even getting the recommended five (5) servings of veggies and 2 servings of fruit, then why bother to push ten (10) servings as you may scare people off? Find ways to "pump up the veggies" in food consumed.

6. Boost phytochemicals from whole veggies and low fructose fruit using smoothies and juicing. A well-structured smoothie that is not packed with high fructose fruits will beat anything coming out of a box by far for breakfast. Phytochemicals are critical compounds in the diet that can reduce oxidative stress and inflammation in the body and provide massive health benefits. There are 25,000 bioactive components in our diets, mostly from plants and collectively called phytochemicals. There are two broad categories of phytochemicals: 1) Carotenoids and 2) Polyphenols or just phenols. We have around 1000 carotenoids (the red, yellow, and orange pigments in veggies and fruit) and about 8000 polyphenols. These polyphenols include flavonoids, proanthocyanidins (anthocyanins), stilbenes (resveratrol), coumarins, lignans (soluble) and lignins (undigestible) (Blomhoff 2010). This huge family of polyphenols have antioxidant activity because of their ability to donate hydrogen (Blomhoff 2010).
We want to pack in these phytochemicals with our ten (10) servings of vegetables mainly and low-carb fruits, as shown in Appendix-8. We can also use low-fructose juicing to provide a huge "hit" of phytochemicals. Most dietetic practitioners would foolishly shoot this down and state with a knee-jerk reaction, saying, "But you are removing the fibre." This is a short-sighted negative statement when you consider the poor phytochemical intake in populations and the huge positive impact they have on health. We get a lot of fibre through the recommended whole food, veggie-rich diet anyway. Practitioners who denigrate juicing just because of being fibre-poor miss the point completely. Such negativity has no place as populations get sicker and sicker every year, especially when intakes of vegetables and fruit are woefully low. It is as if dietitians or nutritionists have to say something "clever" when asked about juicing. Avoid juices that include only fruit,

as this causes a big fructose hit.

You now know that fructose damages cellular ATP production. We need a broad vegetable hit in such a juice with some fruit, and berries are great. Do it at home or through a juicing outlet. I suggest 2 carrots, beetroot (make it blood red), ½ lemon, blueberries/mixed berries, cucumber, spinach or kale, and a small amount of watermelon (high GI but low in carbs). These are commonly available in juicing stations. My recommendation tastes great, with a huge phytochemical blast including beta carotene and a wealth of carotenoids, some of which can be converted to Vitamin-A. I normally get this phytochemical blend 2 – 3 times a week. Blending these as a smoothie will also give you all the fibre but will be thicker in consistency.

Interestingly, skin levels of carotenoids highly correlate with total blood carotenoids and vegetable intake. A higher carotenoid skin level is significantly associated with a lower risk for metabolic syndrome (MetS), lower insulin levels and decreased risk of cardiovascular disease (Matsumoto, Suganuma et al. 2020). Thus, a combination of wholefood vegetable and fruit intake and predominantly veggie juice consumption 2 – 3 times a week with the abovementioned ingredients will keep your tissues saturated with carotenoids and polyphenols, and this can help reduce skin cancer risk by a rich intake of the huge family of carotenoids. Lycopene has also been associated with less sun damage to the skin. Tomato paste is rich in Lycopene, a carotenoid that doesn't convert to Vitamin-A but is beneficial for health. This strategy will unsurprisingly result in a huge health benefit. Don't have too many carrots in the juice, though, as the carotenoid levels will be so high in your skin that you will look orange. Beetroot and dark green leafy veggies are rich in nitrate, which will help boost Nitric Oxide (NO) for vascular health. Low nitric oxide (NO) is an early hallmark of vascular disease, contributing to heart disease, strokes and microvascular deterioration. Add nitrate-rich beetroot powder to your smoothies and salads. Let's not forget the hit of magnesium and brain-protecting folate in this high vegetable and vegetable juice intake that will support the MIND diet recommendations for green vegetables to protect memory.

Some polyphenols may act as prebiotics for the gut microbiome. Still, phytochemicals can dampen down inflammatory processes within the bowel and alter the gut microbiome composition. Phytochemicals can be changed to form bioactive compounds such as enterolactone from lignans rich in flaxseed. Vitamin-A from carotenoids can protect the gut mucosa from pathogenic colonization, and phytochemicals can modify quorum sensing (bacterial signalling) (Dingeo, Brito et al. 2020). Boosting the intake of phytochemicals using an Activ8Health Antioxidant Plate designed by me, Dr Rodney Lopez, and discussed in Point-8 and Appendix-37, will ensure your cells get all the help they can to fight off oxidative stress and inflammation to help them recover lost energy levels and function.

7. The post-staple food era: Do you need animal products? Do you need dairy? Do you need eggs? Do you truly want to eat a Group-1 carcinogen in the form of bacon, listed in the same category as powerful cancer-forming agents such as Benzene or Asbestos? What about risky frankfurts, salami, or ham? Please revisit my BIG-10 list of drivers of disease and understand we have been conned by corporations and the dietetic groups embedded with these corporations into thinking staples are healthy. I have discussed the damaging effects of each staple food and that we are moving beyond these staples that have caused so much harm over humanity's history. In our primitive past, when we didn't have 3D food printers on the savannahs of Africa or insect protein-producing farms, it was understandable that primitive humankind needed to eat these foods to survive, although

eating insects was a part of early human history. In the 21st century, it is now very anachronistic that we continue to consume such damaging foods. Gaslighting from these industries will persist and try to muddy the water with paid and biased research, advertising, and marketing. Foods from the fourth agricultural revolution adopting AI technologies and huge data-driven innovations in farming and food manufacturing will hit our shelves in the not-too-distant future. For protein, consider fatty fish from sustainable fishing practices 2 – 3 times a week. Otherwise, explore the huge range of plant-based protein sources, from Quorn^{TM} to other proteins from plants that include "mince" or "steaks" to chunks you can use in kebabs. A walk down the aisles in any supermarket will show the vast change in food choices, even from 10 years ago.

Summary

I hope you have seen how easy it is to pull the plug from cellular energy production through a wealth of common 21st-century cell "shocks" throughout our lives. Our focus should be on bioenergetic decline, and preventing it is our challenge. Health through nutrient sufficiency through a food-based, nutrient-supplement-based approach is your only hope for a long health span. It is up to you to see if what the medical and dietetic profession is telling you is right or if what I am saying in this book resonates, but always keep in mind the absolute failure of medicine and dietetics to stop this carnage created by preventable chronic metabolic diseases after six (6) decades on their watch.

Please check my references in my Blog on my www.a8h.com.au website (see under bibliography) to see the wealth of ignored research that points to health and well-being rather than the explosion of disease prevalence we are seeing globally. My wish is for you and your family to enjoy healthy lifespans and to see through the dogma, gaslighting, blunders and downright lies of medicine and dietetics that are keeping this horrendous chronic disease pandemic in full swing.

In this book, I wanted to show how easy it is to turn off the lights in cells and to set the machine in motion towards lower and lower cellular energy levels, leading to higher and higher cell decay, disorder and deterioration (high entropy), ending up in an acquired chronic metabolic disease.

All diseases start in the womb or after birth. Common micronutrient insufficiencies, often referred to as 'hidden hunger', can lead to overt deficiencies. One of the most common is iron deficiency. Additionally, the simple act of overloading a plate with food can result in the consumption of excessive food energy, known as 'Nutri stress', to choke off cell energy production.

I wanted to inform you of the huge impact foods have in the after-eating phase of digestion and the distribution of digested nutrients that have powerful and damaging effects on our bodies. We seem to forget that the very nature of food itself can be the driver of this horrendous chronic metabolic disease pandemic despite decades of knowledge on after-eating (postprandial) impacts. It is not hard to see why vested interests have ensured this knowledge on food impacts is little known.

We discussed how after-eating (postprandial) effects make matters worse by piggybacking on all the damaging changes that occur along the metabolic dysfunction continuum to heighten the detrimental impacts of biomarkers and systemic inflammation meal-by-meal and snack-by-snack. The combined effect of the insulin resistance-metabolic dysfunction plus after-eating impacts lead to more and more microvascular damage that then drives biological rot, which is the ultimate vascular "hit men" that assassinate organ systems.

Fructose switches off cellular power rapidly and is found in virtually every food we eat. Avoid sugar and high fructose foods shown in Appendix-8. Women are at great risk for iron deficiency, and at perimenopause/menopause, a ***metabolic switch*** occurs to decrease the ability to use glucose in the brain. This change in brain glucose utilization puts a woman at great risk for Alzheimer's dementia and multiple sclerosis. The sad fact is that in these women and really in all of us, these damaging factors act simultaneously to drive cell energy down and entropy (cell disorder, decay and degeneration) up. Nutrition ketosis is a saviour for all these diseases and women undergoing menopausal change.

We must come to the realisation that all these diseases do not and cannot have a unique factor that causes a specific disease, as this is irrational thinking. It is far more logical to see one metabolic process caused by multiple factors that can lead to multiple organs failing simultaneously but at different rates and manifest at various times along this metabolic dysfunction timeline, as we have discussed.

I have singled out our microcirculation networks as the final and silent "assassin" of all our organs simultaneously. There are no single factors affecting specific organs. We have one process that results in organ damage. We can blame multiple organs being damaged simultaneously by our damaged microcirculation networks.

I have tried to outline that our vulnerable cells are biological entities that cannot run on air alone but need a wealth of nutritional resources to function and produce energy. We must keep our cellular 'batteries' topped up at all times to avoid entropy (chaos, decay) overwhelming us.

For the doubting Thomases sceptical of everything, even if it means they are risking their own health and medical destiny, I have taken a great deal of time and effort to show how easy it is for cells to be robbed of energy and then set on a path to organ failure.

We must embrace the Cell Starvation Model (CSM), which I have expanded upon in this book to provide a bigger picture of how and why our cells can become so damaged and lose energy so easily. Insulin Resistance robs our cells of their primary fuel (glucose) and so we must use alternative fuel (ketones) thus throwing cells a lifeline as an energy "spark" to get cells back to normal. Cellular energy is our key to overcoming cellular decay and organ degeneration.

I have discussed the use of Essential Amino Acids (EAAs) as a brilliant protein-sparing way to nourish our cells and provide all the amino acids needed for repair and balance that does not involve insulin spikes or high food energy.

You cannot roll back years and decades of nutritional neglect and cellular damage overnight. We discussed cells that are too weak and sick to utilize all the nutrients presented to them. After all, when you are severely ill, do you long to eat a huge meal? We coax cells back to health slowly but surely by just presenting nutrient resources to them at safe doses. Nutritional support is not an in-your-face drug strategy that wants immediate results, as this is not the reality of what needs to be done for cells limping along.

If we don't change soon, we will all be headed over a healthcare cliff in the not-too-distant future. This crisis is already in full motion, and crunch time is only around two decades away. Our medical and dietary professions need to brace themselves for an almighty backlash that is only around the corner. Public anger and more and more scrutiny will emerge as the media will start to dissect why a predictable medical crisis that could have easily been avoided was allowed to occur with the loss of 100s of millions of lives over six decades since the 1960s. Can this be justified in any way? There will be class actions galore in the near future, I predict, and perhaps the legal eagles will already be sharpening their knives to use against governments, the medical and dietetic professions and medical and dietary gurus who helped propel this healthcare disaster along to the nightmare it has now become.

Appendix-1: Fructose Metabolism

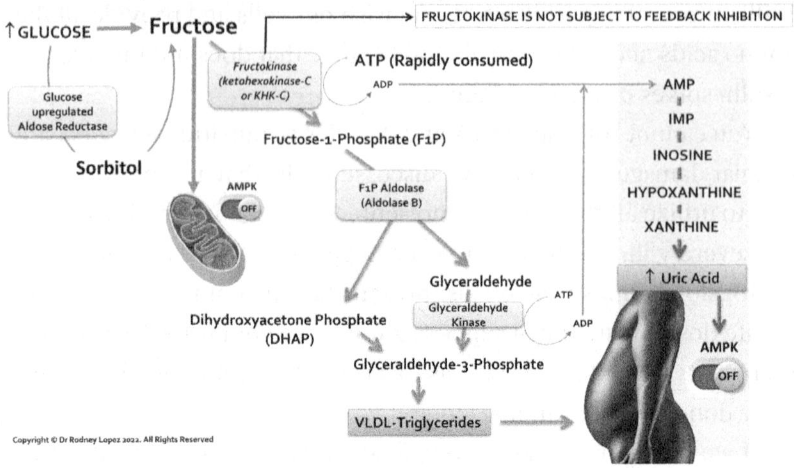

Expression of KHK-C is seen primarily in the liver, pancreas, kidney, and intestines. Expression of KHK-A is more ubiquitous and expressed at the highest levels in skeletal muscle[1] Aldolase-B is the most upregulated protein in pancreatic islets as a result of rising blood glucose levels[2].

The activity of KHK is different from that of other hexokinases because it induces transient ATP depletion in the cell. The mechanism is that KHK rapidly phosphorylates fructose to fructose-1-phosphate, resulting in marked ATP depletion. The activity of KHK (Fructokinase) is not subject to feedback inhibition, such as in the case of glucose metabolism; thus, the ATP depletion is profound. Since the majority of fructose metabolism occurs in the liver, the effects of this ATP depletion are exerted on numerous important hepatic metabolic processes. The depletion in ATP is also associated with intracellular phosphate depletion and dramatic increases in AMP generation. Both of the latter stimulate the activity of the purine nucleotide catabolic enzyme AMP deaminase, increasing degradation of AMP ultimately to uric Acid.[1.]"

References

1. http://themedicalbiochemistrypage.org/fructose.php#metabolism
2. Haythorne, E., Rohm, M., van de Bunt, M., Brereton, M.F., Tarasov, A.I., Blacker, T.S., Sachse, G., Silva dos Santos, M., Terron Exposito, R., Davis, S. and Baba, O., 2019. Diabetes causes marked inhibition of mitochondrial metabolism in pancreatic β -cells. Nature communications, 10(1), p.2474.

Appendix-2: AMPK Function

AMPK is an energy sensor within a cell. It is a protein kinase enzyme that will convert AMP to ATP in low cellular energy environments.

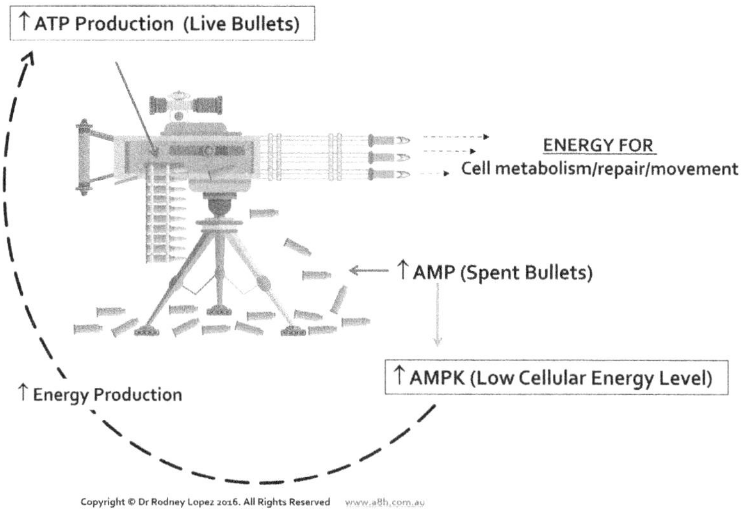

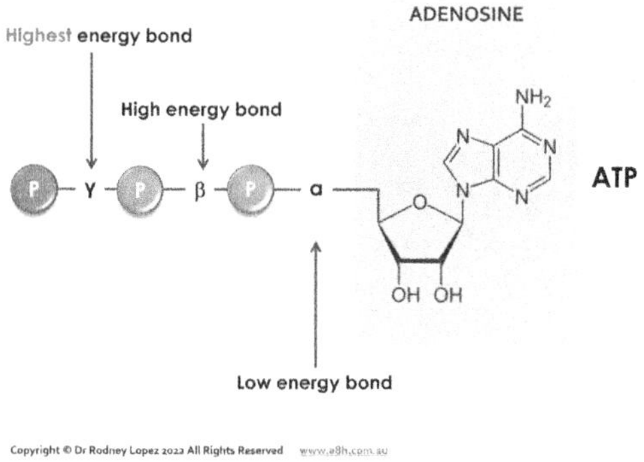

Adenosine Triphosphate (ATP) has three high-energy phosphate bonds, with the most distal (furthest) away from the adenosine anchor point having the most energy. Once that phosphate bond is cleaved to extract energy, you are left with Adenosine Diphosphate (ADP), which has two phosphate bonds left. When the second phosphate bond is cleaved for energy requirements, you are left with adenosine monophosphate (AMP), the lowest remaining energy molecule. The accumulation of AMP is a signal of low energy stores (empty bullet casings analogy) and that the cell needs more ammunition in the form of ATP. This is where AMPK, the cell's energy sensor, calls into action ATP production to re-establish intracellular energy levels.

Appendix-3: The Randle Cycle

The Randle Cycle is a way of understanding the competition between glucose and fatty acids. When we have insulin resistance and high glucose levels, the burning of fats (fatty acid oxidation) is blocked, and intracellular levels of fats can increase. These fats, in turn, can block the Insulin/PI3K-AKT pathway, preventing the translocation of GLUT4 receptors to cell membranes and thus blocking glucose entry to cells. Glucose levels will rise (hyperglycaemia) and be shunted off to other tissues and organs, such as the liver. Glucose can then also be converted to fructose through the Aldose Reductase pathway. This fructose further damages the energy reserve of cells through uric acid increasing intracellularly, consuming phosphate rapidly and dramatically decreasing intracellular ATP (energy)

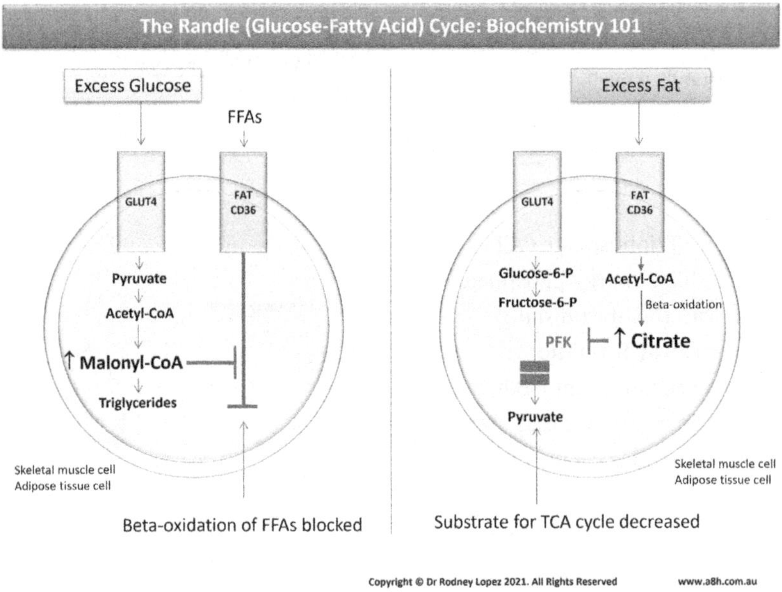

It is important to remember that cells cope at least initially. Increasing levels of glucose results in increased Malonyl-CoA blocking fat oxidation. In the case of excess fat in the bloodstream and tissues, as happens with insulin resistance, elevated Citrate blocks Phosphofructokinase (PFK) conversion to pyruvate. All of this greatly reduces energy supplies within cells.

Appendix-4: Excess Glucose & Intracellular Fat Cells

As insulin resistance worsens and insulin and blood glucose levels rise, we have an interplay that ensures excess glucose is shunted to triglyceride (fat) formation. This interplay ties in with the uricase gene silencing to maximise fat (energy) storage. These effects occur in skeletal muscle cells and adipocytes (fat cells), where the action of GLUT4 predominates. The skeletal muscle then accumulates fat, and insulin resistance worsens. The effect is to increase the supply of glucose throughout the body, particularly the liver, which is under siege due to fructose overload and ATP depletion in cells, causing a cellular energy crisis. This metabolic dysfunction happens when mitochondria are overwhelmed by unnecessary food intake in humans (nutrient overload and nutri-stress).

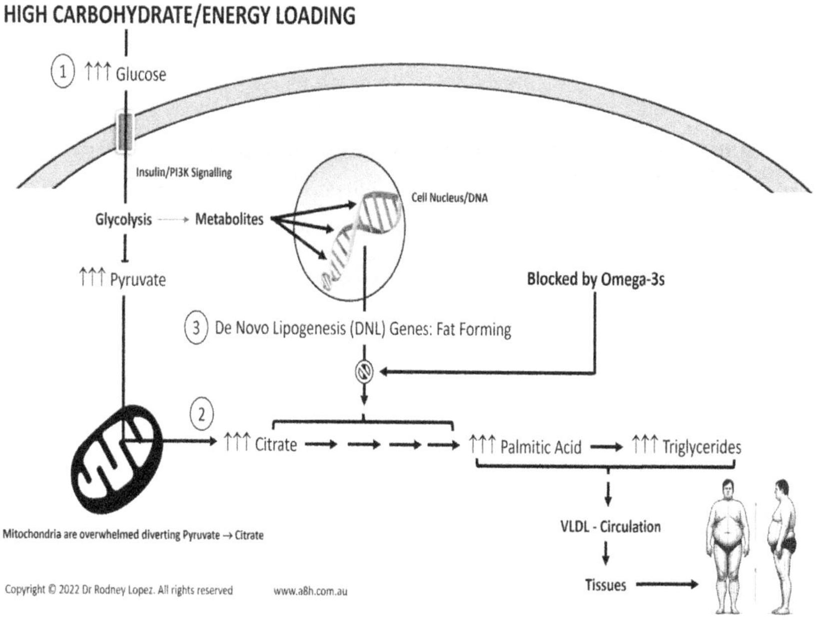

Appendix-5: Statins, Heme-A, CoQ10 Impacts

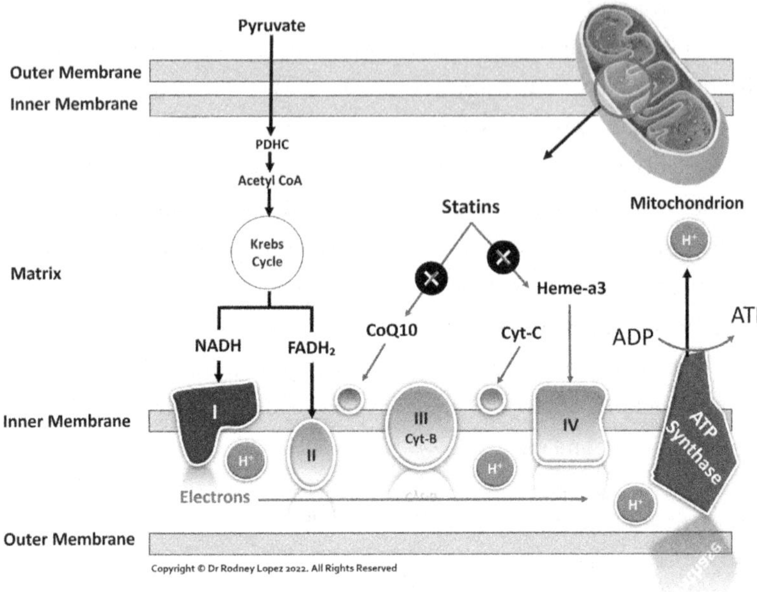

Statins are extremely common medications used in diseases with metabolic dysfunction in the heart of the disease process. Statins can benefit metabolic dysfunction, but perhaps for the wrong reasons used in medicine. Most doctors see statins as lipid-lowering agents, but this is a simplistic view of what these drugs do. They can be of help but also do great harm as well. They have pleiotropic effects (non-lipid lowering effects) that can benefit the starving cell concept, but they can also add to the starving cell process by having a high impact on the Electron Transport Chain (ETC) in two locations 1) CoQ10 and 2) Complex-IV where Heme-A is used to generate ATP. There is great complexity with the use of statins, and these conflicting benefits vs adverse effects need to be teased out in further research, but hopefully not by vested interests who only want to sell drugs.

Excellent diagrams on the Mevalonate Pathway can be found here (https://www.intechopen.com/chapters/48175)

Appendix-6: How Does Epigenetics Work?

The genetic material in chromosomes is incredibly long. Evolution has developed a way to compact the DNA around histones, analogous to a bobbin and sewing thread. The thread can be unwound through epigenetic markers at various points, allowing the unwrapping of the DNA to expose hidden (wrapped) genes. This graphic is a composite showing how this works. So, you can see that the genetic material of the DNA is not altered at all. Epigenetics only opens up that gene for expression. The Greek word 'epi' means on 'top' of, 'over' or 'around', so epigenetics works on top of the DNA, not within the coding. These epigenetic marks can linger for generations and are how dietary and metabolic factors can impact intergeneration. Epigenetics is Nature's way of passing information about the environment to future generations. A readily understood mechanism for survival was shown in the Dutch famine of 1944-1945, where babies born at this time were at high risk for adiposity after birth. This epigenetic communication was thus saying: "There is little food around, so store fat for survival after birth."

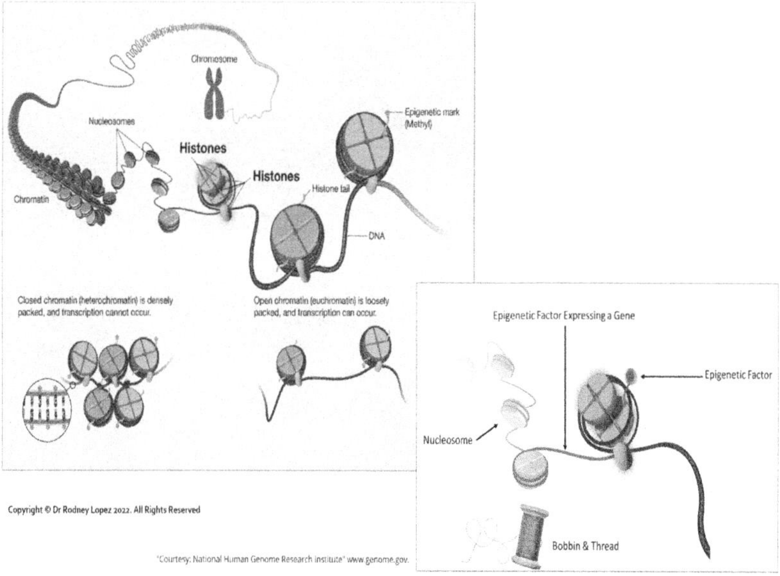

"Courtesy: National Human Genome Research Institute" www.genome.gov.

Appendix-7: The Krebs Citric Acid Cycle B-Group, Minerals and Other Vitamins

The Krebs Cycle requires pyruvate to be created from glucose predominantly in sufficient quantities to then feed into the Citric Acid Cycle (Krebs Cycle). Zinc is vital for pyruvate transport into the Krebs Cycle, and this cycle creates two critical compounds, NADH from Vitamin-B3 and $FADH_2$ from Vitamin-B2 (Riboflavin). These two compounds carry highly charged electrons that feed into the Electron Transport Chain (ETC) to begin the process of converting glucose to Adenosine Triphosphate (ATP), the currency of energy in cells. Vitamin-A controls the Pyruvate Dehydrogenase (PDH) enzyme and pyruvate utilization (Acin-Perez, Hoyos et al. 2010). Therefore, any enzyme defect in the Krebs Cycle due to a vitamin deficiency will severely restrict ATP formation in the ETC. The graphic below shows the steps in the Krebs Cycle with the corresponding B-Group vitamins needed at each step (Kennedy 2016).

Vitamin-B12 has a critical role in the Krebs Cycle in forming Succinyl CoA, where numerous intermediates enter and exit the Krebs Cycle, as shown below (Romain, Sviri et al. 2016).

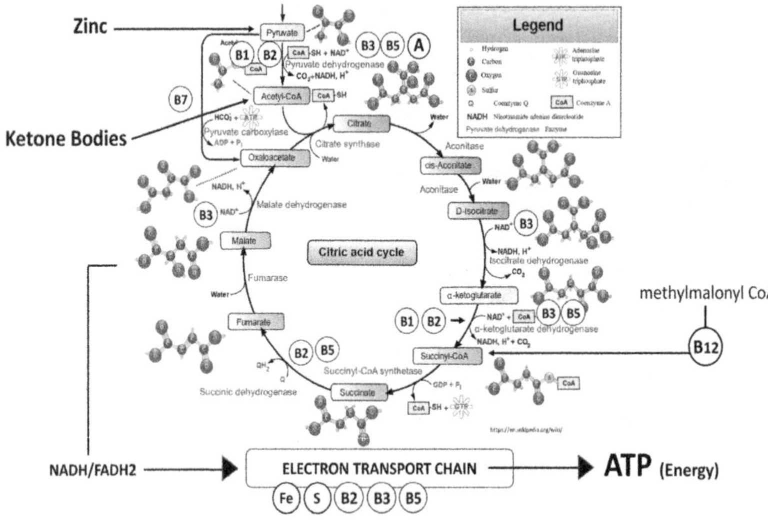

Graphic: https://en.wikipedia.org/wiki/Citric_acid_cycle

Appendix-8: High and Low Fructose Foods

Fructose effectively impairs cell ATP production and increases our level of body fat. Table sugar is 50% Glucose + 50% Fructose. Sugar is found in any pizza base; bread or burger buns will have sugar, including sauces or condiments. Think of kids.

Food	Low Fructose Foods	High Fructose Foods
Dairy	Unsweetened soy, almond, and oat milk. Cheese and yoghurt	Any sweetened milk, dairy or otherwise, includes yoghurts or kefirs. Choose unsweetened
Fruits	Mandarin, orange, strawberries (x3), fresh pineapple (1 slice), kiwifruit blueberries (x10), avocado (1/2), raspberries (x5) (Shepherd 2015)	Prunes, Dates, Raisins, Other Dried Fruit, Canned Fruit, Fruit Juice. A 200g Mangoes will have 30g carbs, of which 10 g will be fructose. Remember that just one glass of orange juice can significantly raise central arterial pressure (Pase, Grima et al. 2015). Jams are often loaded with sugar.
Grains	Gluten-Free, Buckwheat, Corn-Based, Quinoa, Rice, Rye. Remember, all grains are high-carb loads, so use minimal quantities (just 1/4 cup). With rice, it is better to use Basmati or Clever Rice.	Wheat-based are high in fructans (long chains of fructose), Pasta, Pizza Bases, Buns, Bread, Couscous, Wheat based Cereals (worse with sugar coatings like breakfast cereals), and fruit bread.
Protein	Meats that are not marinated in a sugar-based marinade. Tofu and Legumes but legumes need to be limited as per grains due to a high glycaemic load (high glucose effect)	Meats that are marinated in sugar or honey contain marinades. Consider stuffing as this may be wheat-based and hence rich in fructans.
Sweeteners	Artificial sweeteners (not recommended)	Honey (50% Glucose, 50% Fructose), Agave Syrup (70% - 97% Fructose) Table sugar (50% Glucose + 50% Fructose); High Fructose Corn Syrup e.g. HFCS-90 (90% Fructose), HFCS-55 (55% Fructose); Maple Syrup like cane or beet sugar is 50% Glucose + 50% Fructose
Vegetables	Bamboo shoots, beetroot, carrots, celery, chives, green pepper (note red peppers are high in fructose), parsnip, plum tomato, radish, rhubarb, sweet potato, greens such as Bok choy, kale, spinach and turnip greens, white potato, winter squash. Gas producing: Brussels sprouts, cabbage, cauliflower, lettuce	Broccoli (Stems), Onions, Okra, Leeks, Peas, Shallots, Mushrooms, Tomato Paste, Condiments, Sauces like Tomato Sauce, Red Peppers

Appendix-9: High Energy Triglycerides

Most of our dietary fat comprises triglycerides - ~95%. Triglycerides are made up of 3 fatty acids attached to a glycerol backbone. These three (3) fatty acids may contain a saturated, polyunsaturated, trans or monounsaturated fatty acid. Triglycerides are also known as triacylglycerols or TAGs. Triglycerides comprise the main form of energy storage as fat in the body and are produced when you consume more energy than you need.

The attached fatty acids can be removed to create free fatty acids (FFAs), which can be oxidized in the mitochondria to produce a wealth of ATPs.

A 16-carbon fatty acid can provide a net yield of 130 ATP compared to a glucose molecule, providing a net gain of 34-36 ATP. So, a fatty acid can deliver 3.6 times more ATP than glucose. (Cooper 2000).

If we view metabolic dysfunction from the perspective of an energy-starved cell, we can see why a cell would want fatty acids as an energy source to replace the energy deficit. Hence, the increased VLDL, LDL, and lowered HDL ensure cells are supplied with energy-rich fatty acids.

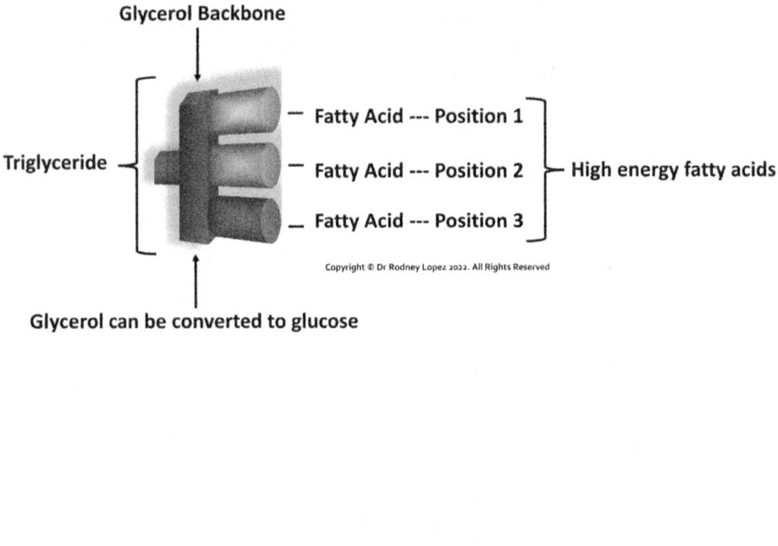

Appendix-10: Lipoproteins

Lipids are insoluble in an aqueous solution; they need a transport system to carry them in the bloodstream. This is achieved through apoproteins, which can be seen as cargo ships carrying lipid-rich cargo to cells. This enables the apoprotein to bind to phospholipids by hydrophobic forces to form spherical transport vehicles, the core of which are filled with triglycerides [triacylglycerols] and cholesterol esters. Lipoproteins share the same structure but differ in size, density, core lipid composition and the type of apoproteins present.

There are five major density classes of lipoproteins arranged in size, from the largest being the chylomicron to the smallest being HDL. There is only a small difference in diameter between IDL and LDL. [VLDL = Very Low Density Lipoprotein; IDL = Intermediate Density Lipoprotein; LDL = Low Density Lipoprotein; HDL = High Density Lipoprotein]

Around 80% of HDL is created by the liver. VLDL is the precursor molecule for IDL and LDL, which deliver lipids to cells.

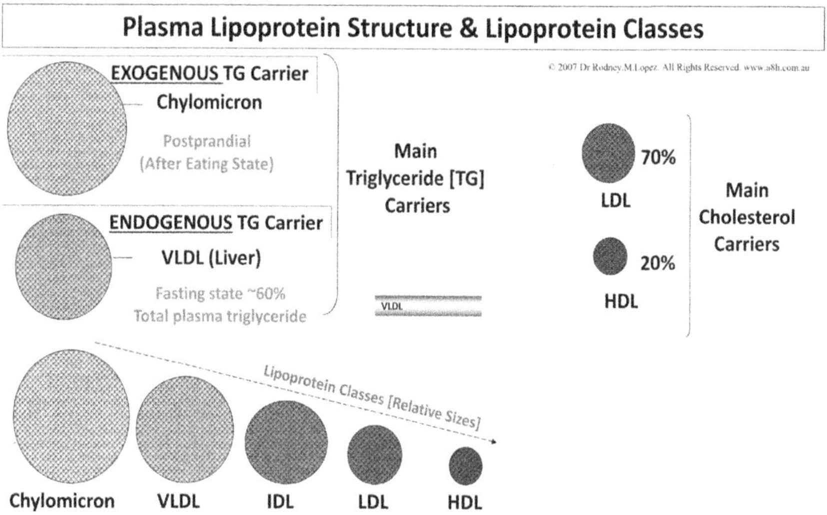

Reference:

Feher, M., Richmond, W, Lipids and Lipid Disorders: Pocket Picture Guide. 3rd Ed ed. 2001: Harcourt Health Communications [Mosby International]

Appendix-11: NAD^+

NAD^+ precursors such as Nicotinamide Riboside and Nicotinamide Mononucleotide are being hotly researched in the fields of ageing and longevity. Ageing decreases SIRT1, decreases mitochondrial biogenesis, causes damage to Complex-I of the mitochondrial Electron Transport Chain (ETC), and decreases cellular ATP (Imai and Guarente 2014). SIRT1 (located in the nucleus) is thought to play a critical role in ageing and cell longevity through its modulation of key transcription factors, such as p53. Both human and mouse SIRT1 are believed to promote cell survival by deacetylating and thus deactivating the p53 proapoptotic (cell death) gene. Adequate NAD+ levels maintain SIRT1 activity, which can delay apoptosis (cell death) and provide vulnerable cells additional time to repair, even after repeated oxidative stress insult[1]." An increase in NAD^+ has decreased the effects of Type-2 Diabetes Mellitus, MetS and NAFLD.

References:

1. Massudi, H., Grant, R., Braidy, N., Guest, J., Farnsworth, B. and Guillemin, G.J., 2012. Age-associated changes in oxidative stress and NAD+ metabolism in human tissue. PloS one, 7(7), p.e42357.

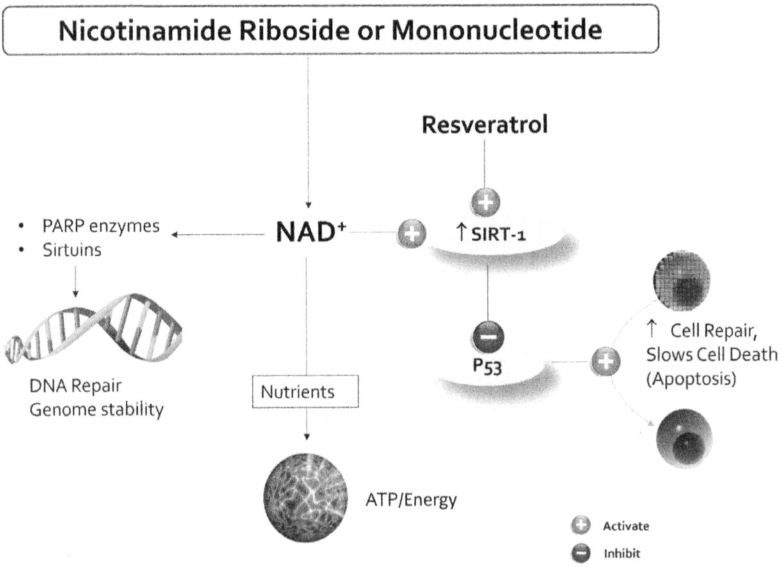

Appendix-12: Citrulline, Nitric Oxide & Erectile Dysfunction

L-Arginine can undergo extensive first-pass metabolism in the liver, leaving little for the body to use. L-Citrulline can bypass this first-pass metabolism by being converted in the kidney to L-Arginine and then into the bloodstream to cells and tissues needing to produce Nitric Oxide (NO) (Curis, Nicolis et al. 2005).

The little blue pill is used for Erectile Dysfunction (ED) when a man finds that he cannot get an erection strong enough to penetrate his partner. Erectile dysfunction is often the "canary in the mineshaft" and is an early warning sign that something is wrong medically. Often, ED is due to vascular injury, and Nitric Oxide is critical for an erection to occur. As shown below, soluble Guanylate Cyclase needs NO to activate it so cGMP can form. The PDE5 inhibitors given to individuals with ED do not form Nitric Oxide. This has to come from L-Arginine, which may be in short supply due to the added demands for nutritional resources in advanced conditions with vascular problems like MetS or Diabetes. L-Citrulline can be used successfully to help generate nitric oxide.

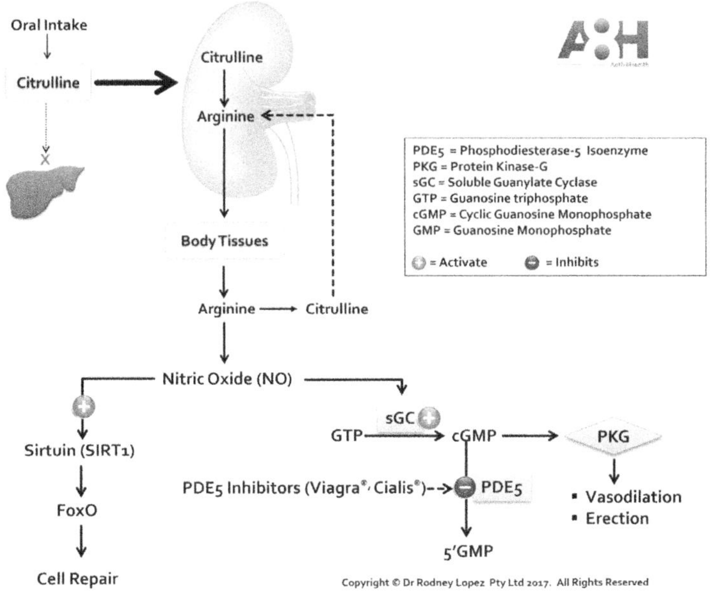

Appendix-13 Insulin Resistance

The mechanism of insulin resistance has been detailed in this book. Essentially, mitochondrial impacts and impacts on the Glycolytic, Krebs Cycle or Electron Transport Chain (ETC) will result in lowered cellular ATP energy production.

Cells low in energy can trigger insulin resistance and all the metabolic marker hallmarks that ultimately lead to a vast number of chronic illnesses. The insulin receptor does not respond to the insulin "key" in insulin resistance. The insulin key is vital to open the door (the GLUT4 receptor) to allow glucose to enter cells. A non-responsive door prevents glucose from entering cells, and then blood glucose rises. This sequence of events will set into play all the hallmarks of insulin-resistant diseases.

As insulin resistance worsens, insulin levels rise, and glucose levels rise. See Appendix-14

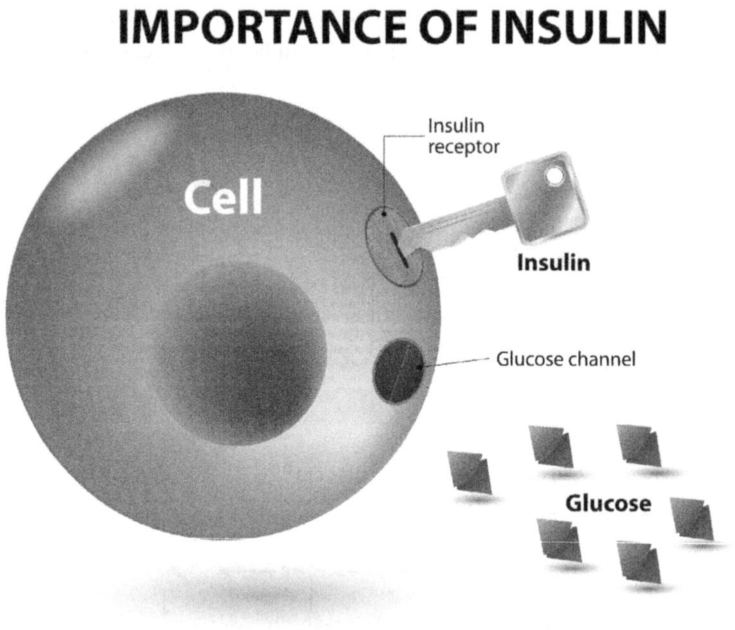

Appendix-14: Insulin Resistance & Diabetes

In Type-2 Diabetes Mellitus, we have insulin resistance, as described in Appendix-13. In the early stages, insulin gradually increases as the beta cells that produce insulin in the pancreas try to cope with the insulin-resistant receptors by sending in more "troops" – i.e. more insulin to overcome this resistance.

A Glucose Tolerance Test (GTT) with insulin levels at each stage can show this sequence of events as depicted in the diagram below. Blood glucose levels rise quite late in the process and can take a decade or two to show up in a fasting blood glucose level. If a doctor checks a blood glucose level as is commonly done in medical practice, they can miss this whole process by a mile. All tests or imaging must be put into clinical context and viewed with other results to conclude. It is an ominous sign when the insulin levels drop, as this indicates that beta cell burnout occurs when the beta cells are dying and struggling to cope. High-carb, protein, and fat diets will demand more and more insulin, putting beta-cells at high risk of failing.

Markers for the early mitochondrial decline may greatly benefit from picking up metabolic dysfunction early in the piece.

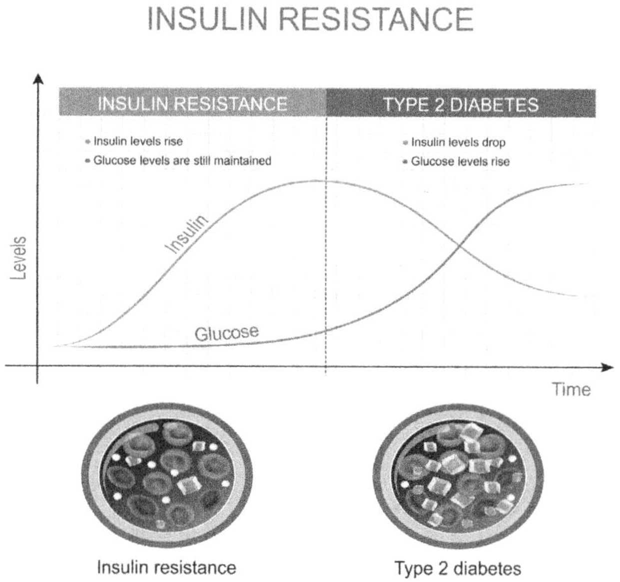

Appendix-15: The 3 Stages of ATP Production

The simple graphic below will give you an overview of the stages of glucose metabolism. Appendix-5 and Appendix-7 give you further information on metabolism. All these pathways have multiple-step enzymes or enzyme complexes as found in the Electron Transport Chain (ETC). None of these components work without a rich supply of vitamins and minerals acting as coenzymes or cofactors for enzyme systems. We must remember that all enzymes are proteins; all the Electron Transport Chain (ETC) complexes are protein-based; hence, we need the full complement of necessary amino acids to create them.

The numerous vitamins needed for the glycolytic pathway are shown in this paper (Tardy, Pouteau et al. 2020). Magnesium (Mg) is critical in the Glycolytic Pathway, Krebs Cycle and the Electron Transport Chain (ETC). Unfortunately, low magnesium levels exist in many populations. Thus, ATP production commonly will be greatly impaired in many individuals.

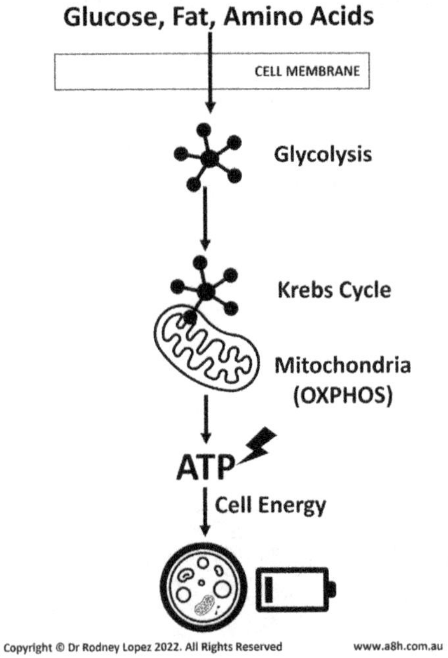

Appendix-16: OXPHOS

Oxidative Phosphorylation (OXPHOS) occurs in the mitochondria. Most of our ATP is generated through this process. Glucose is the main substrate for cellular energy pathways. One glucose molecule will undergo glycolysis (through the Glycolytic Pathway) to create x2 net ATPs and x2 Pyruvate molecules (Melkonian and Schury 2019). In aerobic conditions, pyruvate will enter the mitochondria to produce most of the ATP through the action of the Krebs Cycle and the Electron Transport Chain (ETC). Without oxygen, pyruvate will be converted to Lactate through anaerobic glycolysis. Anaerobic glycolysis is 100 times faster than OXPHOS through the ETC in mitochondria (Melkonian and Schury 2019). Anaerobic glycolysis in the absence of oxygen may be fast but less efficient, but it is called upon in short bursts of intense exercise. Glycolysis has an advantage in rapidly contracting skeletal muscle due to aerobic exercise or heavy weights lifted to exhaustion, thus depleting the oxygen supply. In this circumstance, the exercised muscle needs a lot of glucose and fast conversion to ATP. All these pathways depend on nutrient resources such as minerals or vitamins to act as cofactors or coenzymes. Amino acids are also needed in a constant supply to create the enzymes (proteins) and the components of the Electron Transport Chain. A lack of even one critical vitamin, mineral or amino acid will affect the whole energy-producing system. See Appendix-7 and Appendix-15

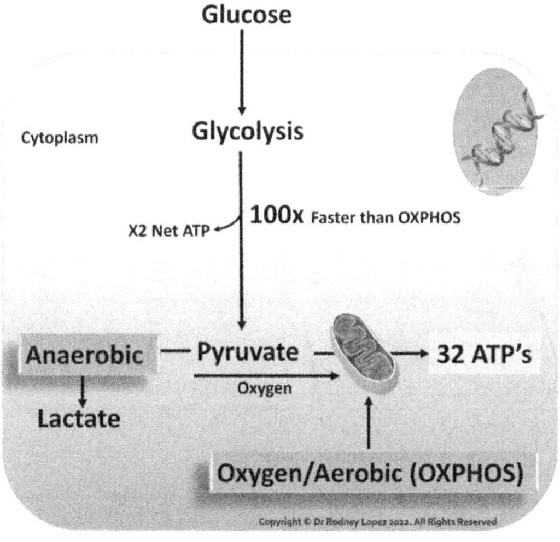

Appendix-17: Electron Transport Chain (ETC) Components

It is important to remember that the ETC is not some mechanical, non-biological energy-extracting machine. The components are highly complex proteins, and each complex has multiple protein subunits (Cooper 2000). In saying this, ATP Synthase is described as an ancient “nanomachine” as it creates ATP through a rotatory motor action (Kühlbrandt 2015). ATP Synthase is also described as “one of the most beautiful” enzymes in existence (Boyer 1997). ATP Synthase also does not function without magnesium. These ETC components are highly dependent upon amino acids to form protein complexes. Complex-I is the largest, with approximately 45 protein subunits. Most people get more than enough non-essential amino acids (NEAAs) but may be deficient in one or more essential amino acids (EAAs). Cytochrome B and C require iron to function. Iron deficiency affects the iron-sulphur-containing complexes I, II, and III but not IV and V (Hoes, Grote Beverborg et al. 2018). 30% of the world's population is iron deficient (Kumar, Sharma et al. 2022). In energy-deficient cells, making it as easy as possible to incorporate amino acids into cellular structures is important. Hence, supplementing early with easily absorbed free-form EAAs that are rapidly accessible to stressed cells can help provide amino acid resources for anabolic processes to fix structural cellular damage and to create new enzymes and ETC components.

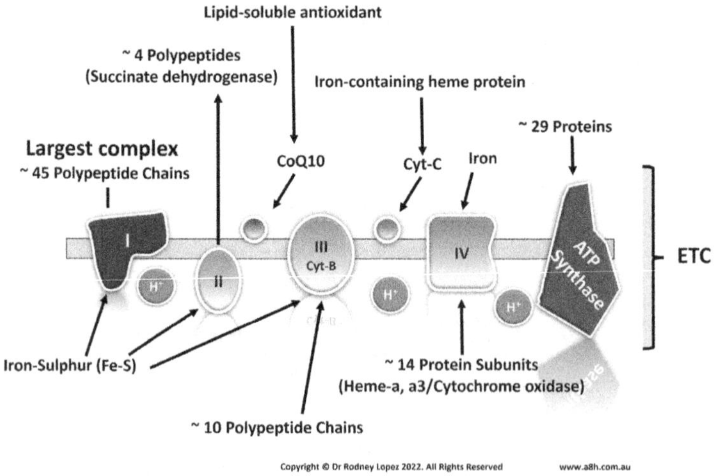

Appendix-18: Postprandial (After-Eating) Effects

We all need to see food in a different light—food damages all of us over time. After eating, impacts take us all out meal-by-meal and snack-by-snack. These incremental and cumulative effects spare no one. After eating, spikes in blood glucose and triglycerides (fats) can last 6 hours or more (Ceriello 2003). In those with insulin resistance, glucose and triglycerides may stay elevated 24/7 to damage proteins, tissues and organs constantly. Over this time, protein damage occurs from glycation (glucose damage) to oxidative stress and increased clotting factors after eating. Many people have a heart attack after a large meal. Our cells, organs and small blood vessels (microcirculation beds) are very vulnerable to these glucose and fat spikes after meals. Imagine all that damage overnight after a large meal eaten late at night. Yet, why is this effect of food not well known? Why do dietitians seem so unenlightened about these effects? These postprandial effects threaten our bodies (Margioris 2009).

We should listen to researchers like Professor Antonio Ceriello, who has published over 450 papers and knows what postprandial damage can do to the human body (Ceriello 2000). As shown in the graphic below, Professor Ceriello sees this postprandial effect as a wave or tsunami of destructive adaptations and defences against after-eating changes in the blood. These changes can eventually lead to ongoing and cumulative damage over our lifetimes. Processed and ultra-processed foods are highly damaging and ageing. Notice sympathetic system activation after eating is associated with abnormal heart rate variability (HRV), a heart attack risk. When do people stop eating in their waking hours? When do these spikes stop?

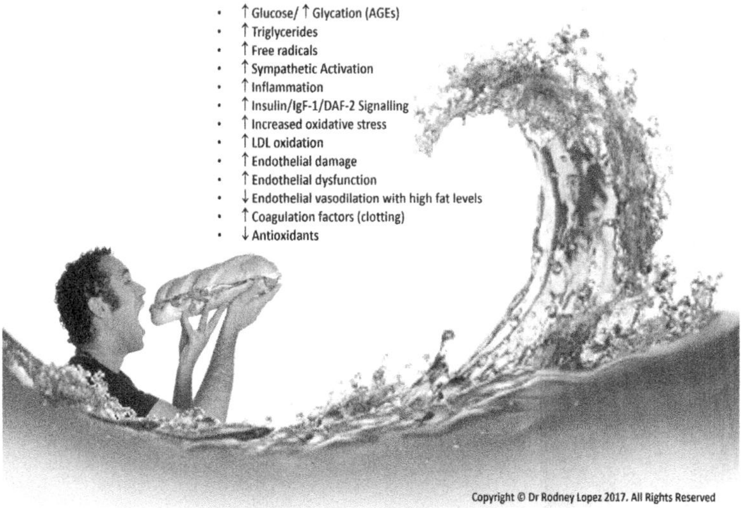

Appendix-19: Choline and the GABA Switch

Humans can produce small amounts of choline through phosphatidylcholine biosynthesis, which is insufficient for optimal health. The enzyme that is involved here in choline synthesis is oestrogen-dependent. For this reason, 80% of men and postmenopausal women (oestrogen-deficient individuals) will suffer from liver and muscle damage, but still, 43% of premenopausal women will have these adverse effects when choline-deficient (Fischer, da Costa et al. 2010). A co-authored paper by Professor Robert Freedman indicated that choline in the amniotic fluid activates ***alpha-7 nicotinic receptors*** in the fetus and facilitates cerebral inhibition. The neurotransmitter GABA switches from excitatory to inhibitory. Imagine GABA not being "switched" and kept in the excitatory state. Think ADD, ADHD, etc. This effect of cerebral inhibition implies a dampening down of certain neurological pathways, which may help prevent hardwired mental illness states from becoming established and all through micronutrient (choline) sufficiency. The authors noted that choline supplementation in pregnancy:

"...represents a paradigm-shifting approach to the prevention of psychiatric illness. It was a finding like this that led to the now routine regimen for pregnant women to take folic acid supplements." (Ross, Hunter et al. 2013). It's a pity that such a cheap (and essential) supplement is not commonly used in pregnancy. How could this impact mental health disorders like ADD, ADHD, anxiety and Schizophrenia prevalence? A huge missed opportunity.

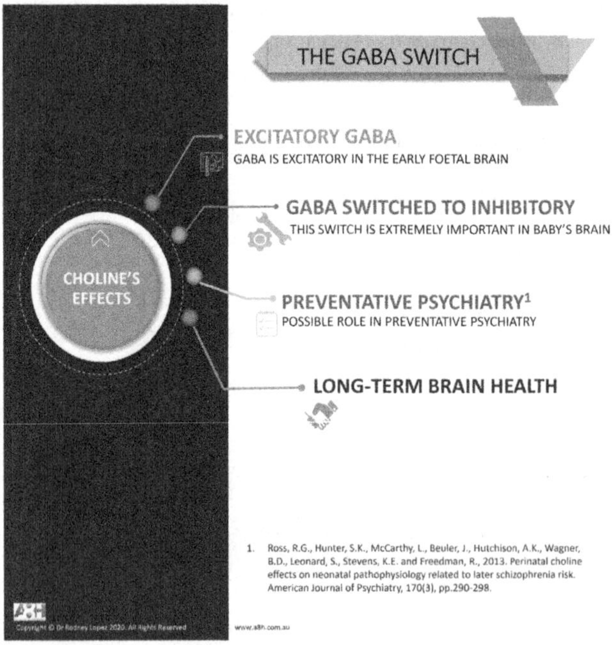

Appendix-20: The Critical Nature of Magnesium in Vitamin-D Activation

Magnesium is crucial in every step of Vitamin-D formation and activation (Dominguez, Veronese et al. 2021). Any research on Vitamin-D that does not measure red blood magnesium (RBC-Mg) sufficiency will have results that do not reflect the true benefits of Vitamin-D.

These are the intricacies of nutrients that few doctors or dietitians, for that matter, understand. One must wonder if researchers also know this information when designing a study on Vit-D. This lack of knowledge puts lives at risk as convincing data shows the immunomodulatory effect of Vitamin D, which has a vital impact on both the innate and adaptive immune system arms (Dominguez, Veronese et al. 2021).

Without magnesium, our inflammatory processes increase, keeping in mind that inflammation reflects an activated immune system, and this active immunity consumes vast amounts of energy, putting cells already energy-depleted at great risk.

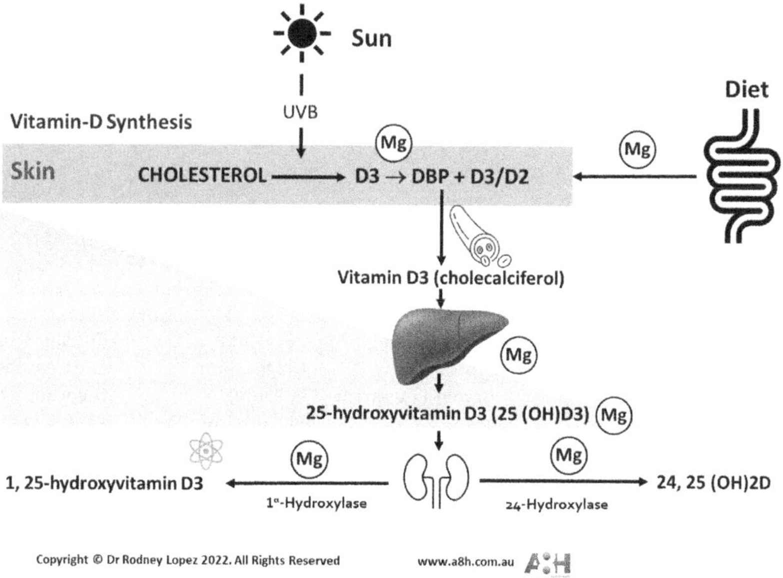

Appendix-21: Vegetable & Fruit Nutrients

The fact that 95% – 99 % of individuals in many Western populations do not get anywhere near the daily intake of vegetables and fruits for health is a huge indictment of the healthcare system as it currently exists. It is foolish that we spend vast amounts of money on drugs but couldn't care less about subsidizing fruits and vegetables for health outcomes. There is a wealth of nutrients from fresh fruit and vegetables or their juices but keeping fructose levels low (Płonka, Toczek et al. 2012). The soluble B-group vitamins are critical for energy-extracting systems (See Appendix-7). From adequate intakes of vegetables and fruit, we can derive numerous essential vitamins and minerals vital for 100s of biochemical reactions. Without these critical nutrients, our health simply diminishes, and our cells lose energy (ATP) and decline structurally.

Eating a gherkin in a hamburger doesn't count. It would help if you had a huge variety of multicoloured vegetables, either consumed whole or juiced, but keeping high fructose fruits out of the equation. We need ten (x10) servings of vegetables mainly and low-fructose fruit for optimal health.

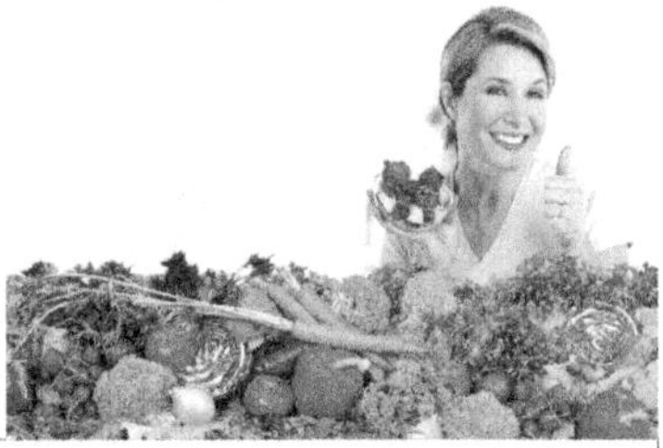

Water Soluble Vitamins	Fat Soluble Vitamins	Minerals	Other
C, B1,B2, B3, B5, B6, B9, and B12	Provitamin-A Carotenoids Vitamin-E, Vitamin-K1,	Potassium, Magnesium, Calcium, Phosphorus, Zinc, Iron, Copper, Manganese and Chromium	Choline + Lutein and Zeaxanthin (Avocado), Fibre, Phytochemicals

Appendix-22: Activ8Health Resources

As a medical practitioner, seeing the "holes" in the system, I have had to make my way in this area of interest concerning nutrition and nutrients. This critical area of knowledge is neglected in favour of drug-centric approaches. I work in Sydney and deal with medical and clinical nutrition problems, as many medical problems never improve but only worsen. I like joining the dots in medicine, which is often neglected as we focus on one failing organ and ignore the others failing simultaneously.

My website is Activ8Health, and the URL is: www.a8h.com.au

I can be contacted through email E: admin@a8h.com.au

This website has been designed to support precision nutrition assessments, which are difficult to find, or if you do find them, the expertise is lacking. Nothing is more satisfying when a client has a problem that is not improving or has been ignored when these problems can be halted and reversed by the right advice. I still see people working part-time at the Mosman 393 practice on Military Road, Sydney, as many want a different medical and dietary model presented to them to help drive back metabolic risk factors.

I look forward to meeting you one day if need be. Please send me feedback respectfully, as we can agree or disagree on aspects of this book, which is fine. Educated comments, insights, or disagreements can only make us stronger in our knowledge. Still, internet trolls are creatures I will totally avoid, as scientific arguments are based on intellect and backed by scientific data. Tone will never trump hard facts!

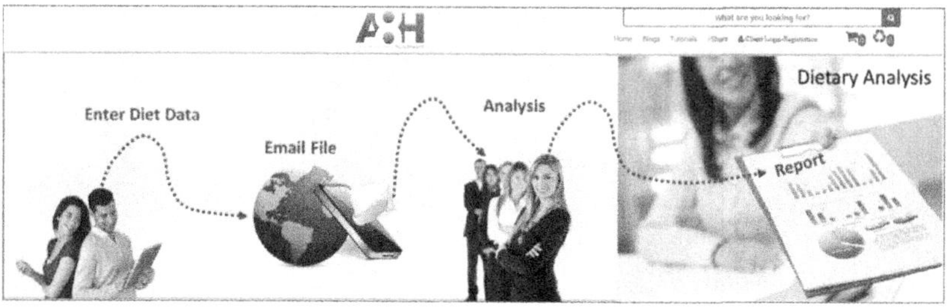

Appendix-23: Omega-3, Omega-6 Pathways

The Omega-6 essential fatty acids on the right of the graphic below go down a pathway that leads to Arachidonic Acid (AA). COX-1 and COX-2 enzymes then act on the AA to form the Series-2 and Series-4 eicosanoids, which are inflammatory. Aspirin, Ibuprofen, or COX inhibitors block AA from producing these inflammatory compounds. But this all started with a high intake of Omega-6s to make AA. If we look at the Omega-3 pathway on the left, you will see that we have Series-3 and Series-5 eicosanoids being produced from the long-chain Omega-3 EPA. These are anti-inflammatory. So, these anti-inflammatory series 3 & 5 eicosanoids counter the effects of the Omega-6 eicosanoids. Notice that both pathways use the same enzymes—notice also that the same enzymes produce a different subset of inflammatory or anti-inflammatory eicosanoids. So the trick here is to ensure Omega-6s don't flood cellular membranes and dominate as a substrate for the enzymes. This highly competitive system favours the most dominant type of essential fatty acid in cell membranes. If Omega-6s win the competitive battle, they profoundly affect background inflammation, which drives all diseases. So, the story's moral is to ensure an optimal Omega-3 intake and decrease Omega-6s found in vegetable oils, palm oil and richly processed and ultra-processed foods. Notice how DHA, a long-chain Omega-3 (bottom left), produces Specialised Proresolving Mediators (SPMs) that help switch off inflammation. These SPMs are the Resolvins, Maresins and Protectins.

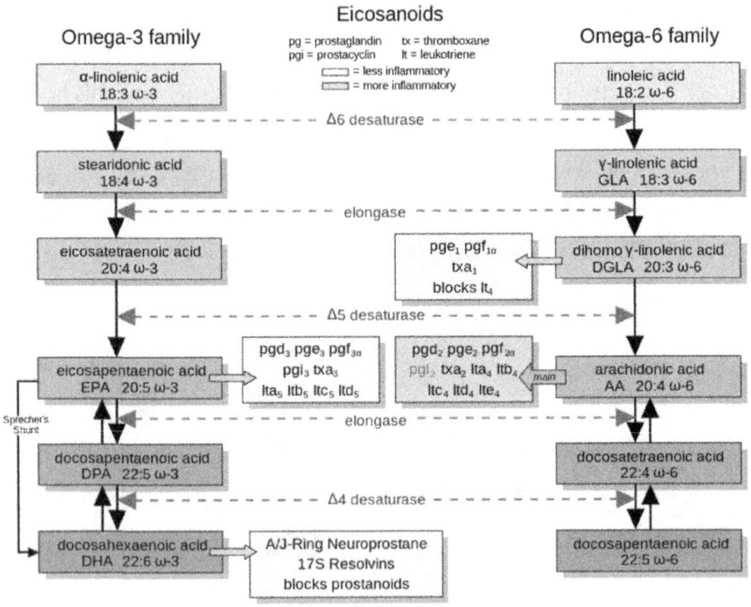

Appendix-24: Hidden Hunger. The Myth of an Optimal Diet

95-99% Low Vegetable & Fruit Intakes	This statistic, derived repeatedly in numerous surveys, shows how simplistic that throwaway line of "just eat an optimal diet" is (AIHW 2018). No green thing will ever touch my plate, which is a common sentiment among laypeople who deprive themselves of critical magnesium and various minerals and vitamins essential to drive ATP production in cells. Does anyone doubt that cell starvation is driving a pandemic of insulin resistance, diabetes and chronic diseases crippling healthcare?
Soils	Agricultural soils on the planet are deficient in numerous minerals, and we are running out of topsoil, with 40% of the world's soils classified as degraded or seriously degraded being lost at 10x to 40x the rate at which it can be naturally replenished (Time 2012).
Farming	Farming methods can strip the soil of carbon, making it weaker in soil nutrients.
Cultivars	Feeding billions of people means plant cultivars are selected for yield, not nutrient density.
Climate Change	With rising temperatures, we know that the cereals' carbohydrate component can change with altered gliadin to glutenin ratios and where zinc, iron and protein content can diminish by 5% to 10% (T.H. Chan School of Public Health 2022)
Paddock to Plate (P2P)	Nutrient loss occurs rapidly for many nutrients, from when they are picked to when they land on a plate.
Cooking	How one cooks meals can mean a significant loss of nutrients and even enzyme activity
UV Light and Heat	The UV light used as a treatment or high natural exposures can impact food composition in various ways to diminish nutrient composition.
Genetics	The eat an optimal diet statement becomes a real farcical saying when you delve into nutrigenomics and Single Nucleotide Polymorphisms (SNPs) that may demand more nutrients, specific nutrients or even lower nutrient intakes. Haptoglobin HP-2-2 is a case in point that can lead to Vitamin-C deficiency and scurvy.(Delanghe, Langlois et al. 2007)
Medications	These meds can truly distort nutrient needs. Powerful antacids called Proton Pump Inhibitors (PPIs) can dramatically decrease the absorption of many minerals and prevent protein absorption. Metformin can diminish Vitamin-B12, and alcohol can increase the need for Vitamin-B1. Books have been written about medication and nutrient interactions.
Individual Variations	Due to exercise, type of work, or medications, many individuals will need higher levels of micronutrients or macronutrients.
Acute & Chronic Illness	This factor is rarely considered by doctors or dietitians as there is a jump in the need for nutrient resources if someone is suffering a severe infection or recovering from trauma.
Ad Hoc Meals	It is also ludicrous to think that lay individuals who throw food components on their plates based on food preferences and rarely food nutrient composition will meet all their micronutrient requirements. Dietitians often fail miserably with meal plans that don't meet the targets for various critical nutrients (Dollahite, FRANKLINMS et al. 1995) .

Appendix-25: Drug vs Supplement Risk Bar Chart

Medical practitioners accept a perverted view that drugs are the only path to health once disease processes manifest. I am not saying that we don't need drugs because this is as much a right-wing view as stated about supplements and dietary management being hopeless. Nothing could be further from the truth.

The view that supplements are in any way dangerous is laughable when we compare the risk of a supplement to the risk of using a drug. The Alliance for Natural Health wants a natural revolution where we do not feed drug or food corporations. This graph from the ANH shows that in comparison to drugs, supplements are 62 thousand times (62,000 x) less likely to cause death than a drug reaction.

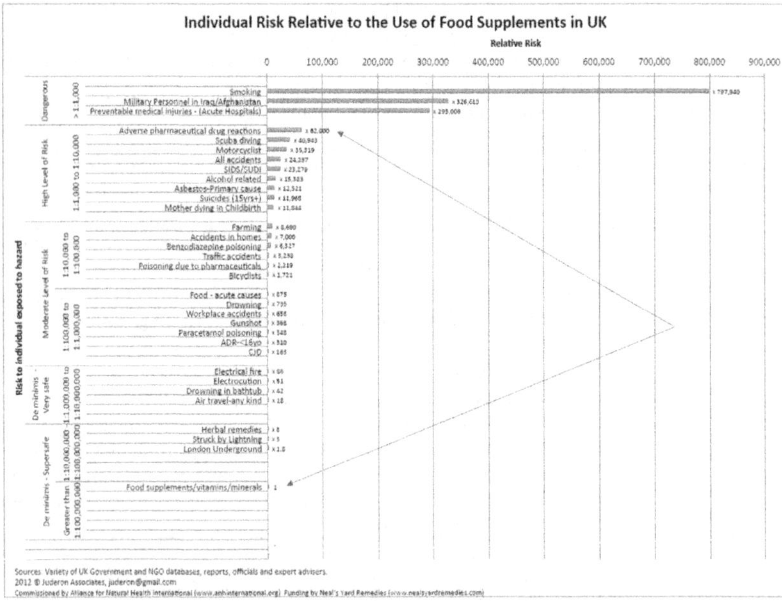

Source: Alliance for Natural Health International: ANH Website Link or search for ANH "Drugs as dangerous as war."

Appendix-26: Drugs vs Supplement Risk Bubble Chart

This graphical representation follows Appendix-25 and presents this vast difference in risk of death in a highly visual bubble chart format. Notice the incredibly low risk in the lower left area where you will find supplement risk, and then notice the whopping two bubbles in the top right for adverse drug reactions from pharmaceuticals and preventable medical injuries.

You can get a PDF of these charts on the ANH website: https://www.anhinternational.org/. This PDF will enable you to magnify areas of this chart that put the relative risk of death from supplements versus pharmaceutical drug reactions into sharp perspective. It is absurd and unbelievably sad that we have allowed distorted drug views to gain such prominence when they have failed to protect populations against the rise of chronic diseases caused by insulin resistance and diabetes.

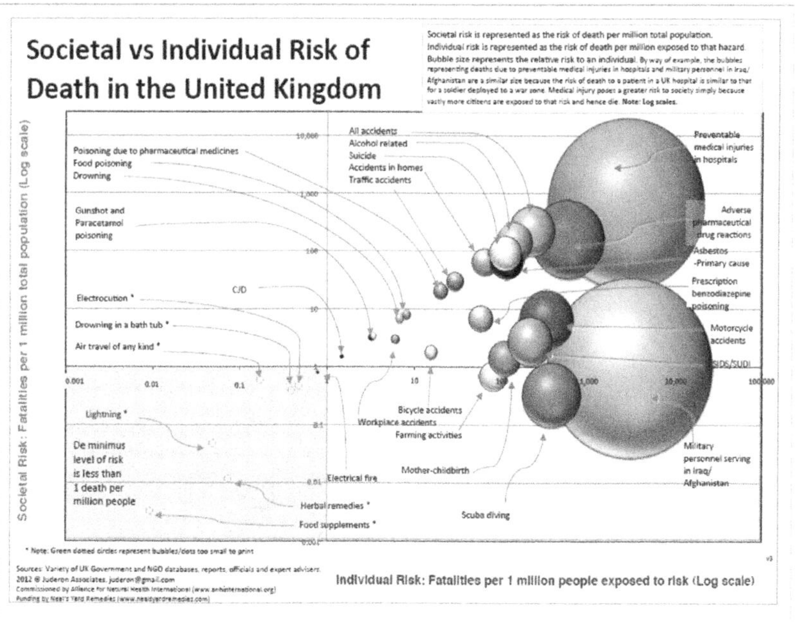

Appendix-27: NAD^+ Sirtuins and Protein Activation

Nutrient energy overload is a major problem in wealthy nations. Ultra-processed foods (UPFs) pack a huge punch with energy intake, and UPFs can make up 50% - 90% of energy intake for many individuals. High energy intakes can result in a marked drop in Nicotinamide adenine dinucleotide (NAD^+). NAD^+ is the electron donor to NADH, and it is NADH and FADH2 generated by the Krebs Cycle that carry high energy electrons to kick-start the ATP generation in the mitochondrial Electron Transport Chain (ETC) – this is shown diagrammatically in Appendix-29.

The problem with high food energy intake is the consumption of NAD+, a coenzyme critical to functioning a group of proteins called Sirtuins. Sirtuins are vital to activate a range of metabolic proteins through the deacetylation of proteins (post-translational protein modification). Without deacetylation, proteins will not be in an active form for the task they need to perform. Sirtuins and nicotinamide supplementation are highly researched topics. Optimal Sirtuin activity is linked to longevity. NAD^+ decreases as we age and with high food energy consumption, and thus, intermittent fasting works by preventing the decrease of NAD^+ by food restriction.

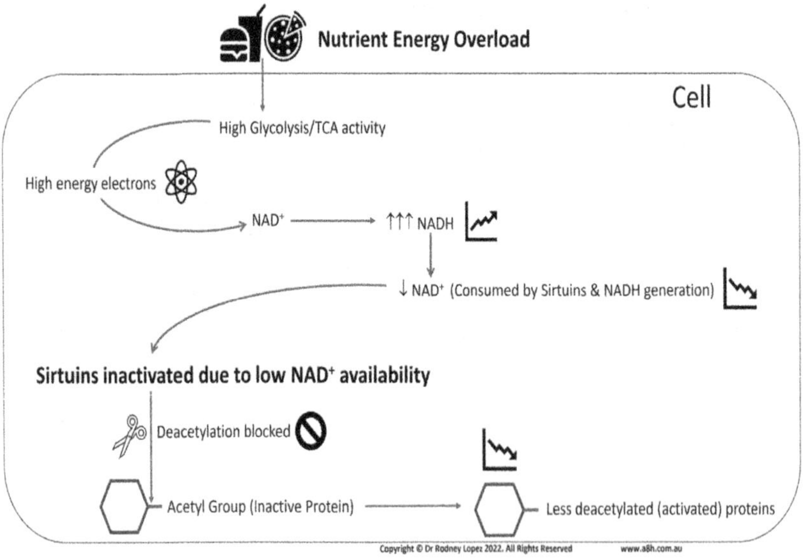

Appendix-28: NAD^+ vs NADH

NAD^+ and NADH are a redox couple, and the availability of these compounds can greatly impair cell metabolism and energy production if the balance is disturbed, as shown in Appendix-27. With high-energy food intake, this balance is disrupted, and this redox couple determines the metabolic destiny of cells' sirtuin, protein and metabolic activity.

The energy released from the breakdown of food components like glucose is captured by electron transfer to NAD+. These captured high-energy electrons are then transferred to NADH/FADH2, one of two compounds that generates the vast amount of ATP in mitochondria. An overview of this process is shown in Appendix-29.

Oxidation and reduction are the loss of electrons (oxidation) or the gain of electrons (reduction).

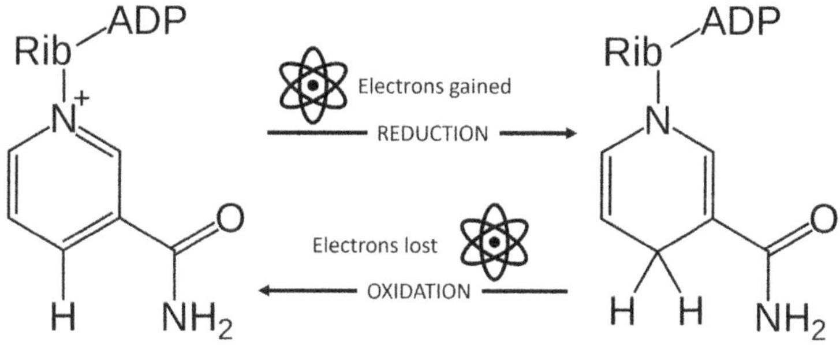

$NAD^+ + H^+ + 2e^-$

NADH
(Reduced form – gained electrons)

Appendix-29: Krebs Cycle NADH & FADH2

We looked at NAD^+ and NADH in Appendix-27 and 28, and the following graphic puts this into the framework of glycolysis (the Glycolytic Pathway), the Krebs Cycle and the mitochondrial Electron Transport Chain (ETC) to provide a complete picture of how these redox reactions work to generate vast amounts of cellular ATP energy. First, high-energy electrons from NADH and $FADH_2$ are fed through the Electron Transport Chain, as shown below, allowing this electron energy to drive Oxidative Phosphorylation (OXPHOS). Next, ATP is powered by this electron energy, creating a hydrogen gradient (chemiosmosis) across the inner mitochondrial membrane. This hydrogen gradient drives the ATP-Synthase rotatory nanomachine or "turbine" to produce ATP. ATP-Synthase. Described as one of the most beautiful molecules in the human body, ATP-Synthase is located at the end of the Electron Transport Chain, and the OXPHOS process requires oxygen to generate vast amounts of ATP energy (Boyer 1997).

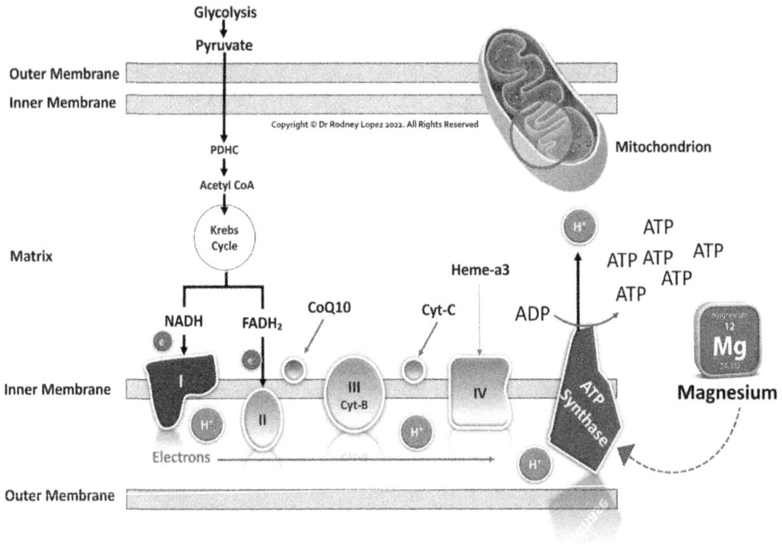

Appendix-30: Long-term trends in diabetes. CDC Graph

It is interesting to see a gradual increase in diabetes from the 1950s in an affluent country, but this increase was slow and gradual until the 70s and 80s. Then, a steep rise occurred from the late 80s and early 90s. This graph and the timing of the steep uptake in diabetes prevalence makes sense when considering that the Green and Farming revolutions happened in the late 60s and 70s. There was then a lag phase as the "geniuses" of the industrial machine turned their minds to food manufacturing and churned out irresistible, highly processed and ultra-processed foods devoid of nutrients but rich in energy using the glut of cheap grains produced in these food revolutions. The food farming revolutions also kick-started the fast-food revolution. And so, here we are in the 21st century, fighting diseases created by these food disasters. Yet, we cluelessly use drugs instead of food-based and nutrient-based management to offset the horrendous illnesses caused by horrendous foods in the first place.

Number and Percentage of U.S. Population with Diagnosed Diabetes, 1958-2015

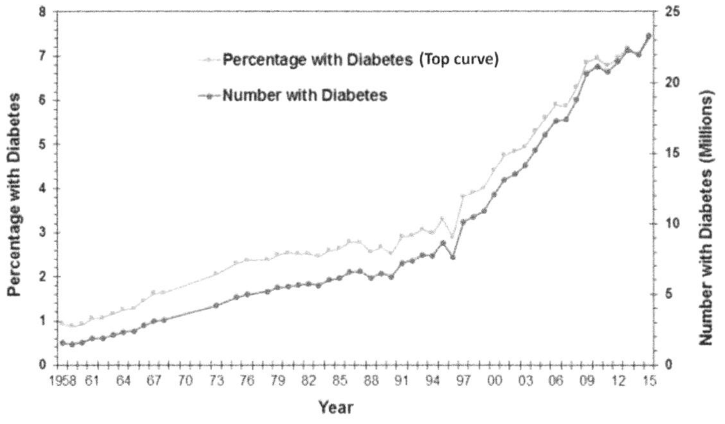

CDC's Division of Diabetes Translation. United States Diabetes Surveillance System available at http://www.cdc.gov/diabetes/data

Appendix-31: Early IR Markers

COMMONLY AVAILABLE BLOOD MARKERS	
Marker	**Comment**
ALT	Alanine Transaminase is a liver enzyme that is raised in Fatty Liver (NAFLD), now regarded as the liver manifestation of Metabolic Syndrome (MetS)
GLUCOSE	Look for a Quintile-Climb. A rise between the goalposts is needed for an early warning if the level is in the upper quintile.
GGT	Gamma-glutamyl transferase can increase due to POP exposures and is a marker for future NAFLD and Oxidative Stress and predicts CVD, heart failure and gestational diabetes. GGT in the highest quintiles predicts a 67% chance of cardiovascular risk (Lee, Evans et al. 2007).
Triglycerides	A high triglyceride level is a common IR signal. Look for a Quintile-Climb
VLDL	A high VLDL is a hallmark of insulin resistance (IR).
HDL	A low HDL may be a signal of IR.
Insulin	Look for a Quintile-Climb. A high fasting insulin level will predict future diabetes.
Uric Acid	A marker of ATP depletion
Other	α -Hydroxybutyrate, Adiponectin, RBP4, chemerin, A-FABP, FGF21, fetuin-A, myostatin, IL-6, and irisin, estimated glucose disposal rate (eGDR)[1], Cardiolipin[2] (Mitochondrial exclusive phospholipid), 8-OHdG[2] (oxidative stress in mitochondria)
PHYSICAL MARKERS	
Waist	Europeans $\geq$ 80 in women $\geq$ 90 in men and Asians 73.5 cm in women and 82.5 cm in men were optimal cut-off points to identify IR. Due to the higher visceral fat in Asians, the waist measurement is the better option.

References:

1. Park, S. E., Park, C.-Y., & Sweeney, G. (2015). Biomarkers of insulin sensitivity and insulin resistance: Past, present and future. Critical reviews in clinical laboratory sciences, 52(4), 180-190.
2. Reddam, A., McLarnan, S. and Kupsco, A., 2022. Environmental Chemical Exposures and Mitochondrial Dysfunction: a Review of Recent Literature. *Current environmental health reports*, 9(4), pp.631-649.

Appendix-32: AETT, Toxic Wounds, Perfume & Fragrance Toxicity

Smelling nice may cost you your health. Perfumes and fragrances as harmful is something that most users would never even consider. We spray on perfumes or deodorants as if there is no tomorrow, reeking of a scent that affects others around us and then mingling with others in their scented bubble with your 50 – 300 chemicals now colliding with another scented bubble that may have 50-300 other chemicals. As stated in the Guardian:

> *"About 4,000 chemicals are currently used to scent products, but you won't find any of them listed on a label. Fragrance formulations are considered a "trade secret" and, therefore, protected from disclosure – even to regulators or manufacturers. Instead, one word, fragrance, appears on ingredient lists for countless cosmetics, personal care and cleaning products. A single scent may contain anywhere from 50 to 300 distinct chemicals." (Guardian 2019)*

As I have mentioned, a 2020 inventory of industrial chemicals showed we have greatly underestimated the number of mainly untested chemicals out there. This inventory showed around 350,000 chemicals in the environment.

Let's look at one fragrance used for 20 years by millions of people until one day, they decide to test it. This fragrance is the cautionary tale of AETT, which was used to give clothes or sheets a fresh smell. Lab rats exposed to AETT became rapidly ill and developed a blue discolouration of internal organs, and their behaviour changed soon after dosing (Grenville 2018). These rats experienced muscular twitching and hyperirritability, and post-mortem, the nervous system on biopsy showed "Spectacular myelin bubbling" (Spencer, Sterman et al. 1979). AETT was said to have been withdrawn in 1978; however, it is interesting that there was a 30% increase in multiple sclerosis from 2013 (Walton, King et al. 2020).

A toxic impact can take years or decades to manifest as signs and symptoms. However, infinitesimally small amounts can have powerful effects like hormones. Fragrances are powerful hormone disrupters, so imagine the impact of disruption to estrogen or testosterone on a developing brain in the womb, causing sexual and behavioural changes in that individual.

Appendix-33: Lessons From The Laron Syndrome

Insulin and IgF-1 are like siblings and share 50% of their amino acid sequences (Friedrich, Thuesen et al. 2012). There is extensive overlap between downstream cell signalling after attaching to the receptor by both hormones. Insulin stimulates IgF-1 production in the liver (Friedrich, Thuesen et al. 2012). High insulin/IgF-1 levels are a cancer risk through cell mTORC1 (nutrient sensor) and cell proliferation. View the mechanisms in the graphic below.

Laron Syndrome describes a growth hormone (GH) gene mutation and IgF-1 deficiency. The insulin/insulin-like growth factor-1 (IGF-1) pathway regulates our lifespans. IgF-1, a potent anabolic hormone, stimulates cell proliferation. Interestingly, individuals with Laron Syndrome are short in stature but have a striking absence of Type-2 Diabetes Mellitus (T2DM) and an almost complete absence of cancer (Melnik, John et al. 2011).

C. elegans is a small worm. Prof Cinthya Kenyon, in 1993, discovered a mutation in the DAF-2 gene in c.elegans that blunted IgF-1 signalling. These worms lived twice as long as other worms without the mutation. Those who practice intermittent fasting (IF) have significantly lower IgF-1 signalling, an important part of extending lifespans and healthspans and decreasing cancer risk. Many common staple foods can cause tremendous elevations in IgF-1 signalling, increasing the risk of cancer and metabolic diseases. Many aspects of ageing can be attributed to Insulin/IgF-1 action.

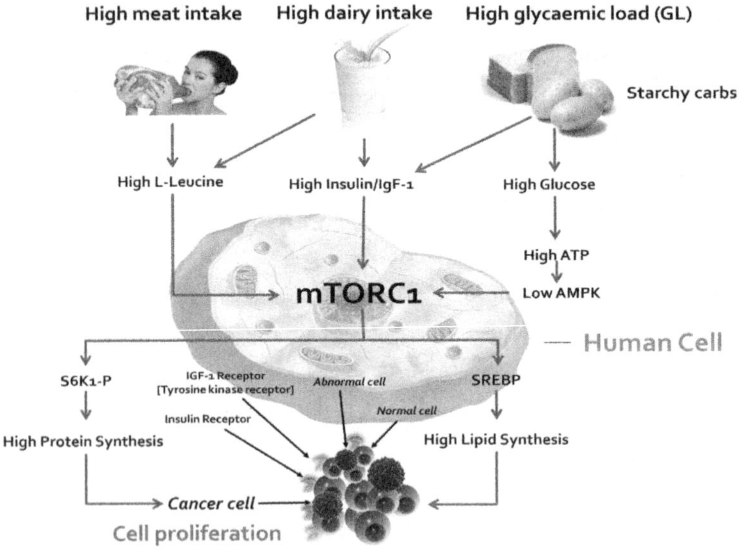

Appendix-34: Brain Impacts

The graphic below shows the various inputs leading to neurodegeneration and mental health disorders. Brain atrophy can occur due to ageing and is associated with mental health disorders and neurodegeneration. All we need to do is think about cell loss due to diminishing blood supply (microcirculation damage) and bioenergetic decline. Microstructural damage occurs over time as a result of diminished energy and nutrient supply. Appendix-19, discussing the GABA "Switch", explains how you can be programmed for a range of mental health disorders in your mother's womb.

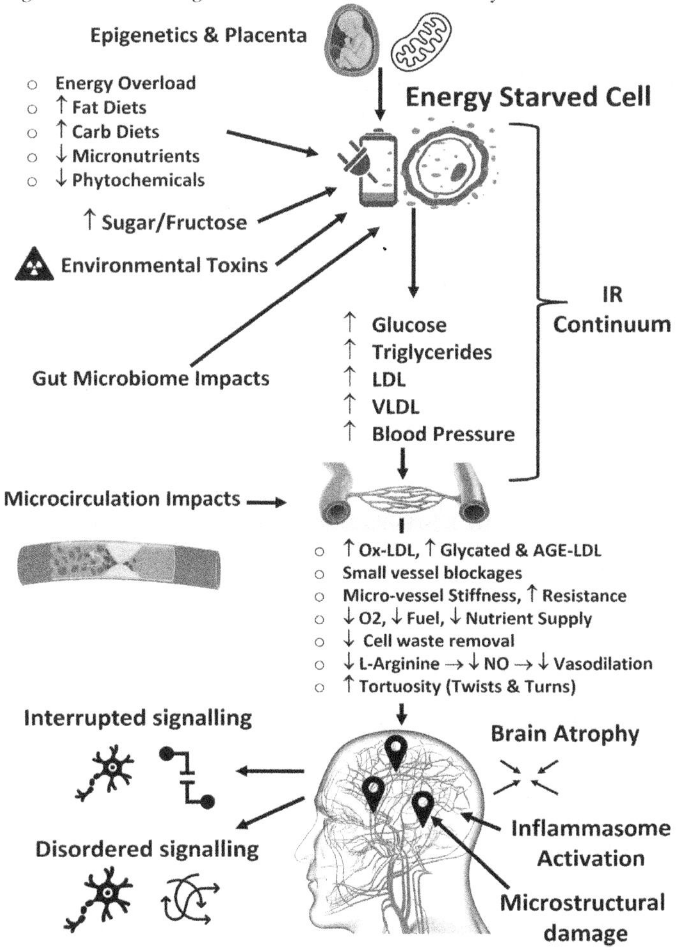

 www.a8h.com.au

Appendix-35: Adverse Drug Reactions (ADRs)

The following has been taken from my book *Slow Kill*. A study published in the prestigious Journal of the American Medical Association (JAMA) indicated that around 100,000 deaths in the United States of America every year are due to lethal Adverse Drug Reactions (ADRs) (Lazarou, Pomeranz et al. 1998). This astonishing figure was disbelieved by many "experts" who criticised the data, and this was understandable as the figure was so high and frightening. The figure reflected a 0.13% incidence of fatal ADRs. This figure was vindicated when a British study published in the equally prestigious British Medical Journal (BMJ) looked at 18,820 hospital admissions in the United Kingdom (Pirmohamed, James et al. 2004). This UK research group found a higher 0.15% incidence of fatal ADRs when adjusted for population number differences between the UK and the USA. The study produced a similar or even greater number of deaths due to lethal adverse pharmaceutical drug reactions.

The USA ADR mortality figure is equivalent to two Vietnam wars every year and to the number of US military casualties of WWII every four years due to pharmaceutical-related deaths! Justifiable? The authors estimated ADRs ranked from the fourth to the sixth leading cause of death depending on whether the lower or higher mortality rate was considered. And medical gurus worry about the safety of nutrients provided in recommended daily allowances (RDAs) – how absurd when we look at the massive number of drug reactions and deaths occurring year by year.

A study from Sweden, one of the richest countries in the world, was published in the British Journal of Clinical Pharmacology in 2007; it found that fatal adverse drug reactions accounted for 3% of all deaths in the general population but 5% of deaths in hospitalised patients. Fatal adverse drug reactions were estimated to be Sweden's seventh most common cause of death (Wester, Jönsson et al. 2008). The numbers are simply staggering! Moreover, just one supplement associated with an adverse event will make headlines in a medical newspaper, magazine, and even the mainstream press. How ridiculous! Who benefits from this misinformation or fake news?

Appendix-36: Multivitamin Components

For twice-a-day dosing: Ingredients as a guide only. Taken under practitioner guidance only and to be taken with a recommended diet and never as a substitute for a wholefood diet, as discussed in this book.

	Per Capsule or Tablet
Ascorbic Acid (Vitamin-C)	100 mg
Beta Carotene	4 mg
Biotin	100 mcg
Boron as Borax	1.5 mg
Choline Bitartrate	25mg
Chromium Picolinate	25 mcg
Citrus Bioflavonoids (Mixed) & Mixed Flavonoids	12.5 mg
Copper as Gluconate	13 mcg
Inositol (Myo-Inositol)	12.5 mg
Manganese oxide	500 mcg
Molybdenum trioxide	50 mcg
Selenium	25mcg
Taurine	25 mg
Vitamin-A (Retinyl Acetate) Not suitable for pregnancy)	170 mcg
Vitamin-B1 (Thiamine Hydrochloride)	25 mg
Vitamin-B2 (Riboflavin)	15 mg
Vitamin-B3 (Nicotinamide Riboside or NMN)	100 mg
Vitamin-B5 (Calcium Pantothenate)	75 mg
Vitamin-B6 (Pyridoxal-5-Phosphate (P5P))	50 mg
Vitamin-B9 (Folic Acid)	200 mcg
Vitamin-B12 (Methylcobalamin or Mecobalamin)	200 mcg
Vitamin-D3	100 IU
Vitamin-E (Mixed 8 isomers, 4 Tocotrienols, 4 Tocopherols)	150 mg
Vitamin-K1 (Phytomenadione)	50 mcg
Vitamin-K2 (Menaquinone or MK7)	75 mcg
Zinc Bisglycinate	15 mg

Notes:

- No calcium is included as a food-based diet rich in vegetables and fruit needs no added calcium as a supplement
- No Magnesium, as you need a full dose of multiple forms of magnesium, which would be more than can be provided in a multivitamin formulation
- Boron is a protein serine protease inhibitor, and Prostate Specific Antigen (PSA) is a serine protease enzyme (LeBeau, Kostova et al. 2010).
- Selenium and Myo-Inositol in early Hashimoto's Thyroiditis have an advantage by improving TSH sensitivity. Perhaps very important in early Hashimoto's Disease (Nordio and Pajalich 2013).
- The formulation should have mixed carotenoids + mixed flavonoids such as Lutein Zeaxanthin, Lycopene, and Anthocyanins.

Appendix-37: The Activ8Health Antioxidant Plate (One variation)

The key to good health is an absolute diversity of plant-based foods, hence the term “eat the rainbow”. Doing this provides a huge variety of phytochemicals – carotenoids and polyphenols. So, if you follow the Nutritional Ketosis (NK) diet, you will have the healthiest of diets you can. A daily antioxidant plate complements this diet. You can use lycopene-rich organic tomato paste as a dip for raw or frozen veggies. Have one square of polyphenol-rich 95% dark chocolate. Kelp sheets provide many trace elements, including iodine from kelp. In the graphic below, in the middle, you can use a low-fat probiotic-rich coconut yoghurt dip for the crudites or make your dip from tamarind paste + prune (or date) paste or prune juice: some fructose, yes, but a huge benefit. Tamarind is rich in antioxidants, fibre, mucilage, gums, and many minerals. Mucilage is sadly lacking in Western diets. It is all about making food count to add to the health of individuals and not a fleeting taste sensation that will take years off your life if healthy dietary inputs are forgotten. Nutrient density and fibre diversity are key to healthy outcomes.

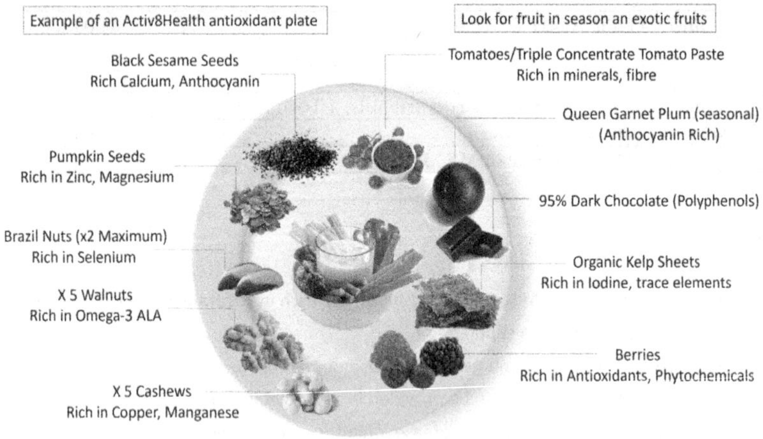

Appendix-38: The Food Pyramid 1992 – 2005

With a flood of cheap cereal grains from the Green and Farming Revolutions of the 60s and 70s, food pyramids were devised to meet "basic nutrition needs". The United States Department of Agriculture (USDA) produced a food pyramid to inform people about "healthy" eating patterns. Notice the 6 – 11 servings of starchy carbs that comprise the pyramid base. Then imagine the huge postprandial (after-eating) surges in blood glucose after eating this vast carb load, and the massive food energy "hits" with plates full of pasta, bread, biscuits, crackers, breakfast cereals in a box, buns, pizza bases and so on. As you know, food energy hits can incapacitate cellular ATP production, as we have discussed. Is this a clever recommendation when vast numbers of populations globally have insulin resistance, obesity, and diabetes? These individuals cannot tolerate glucose, and blood glucose spikes from all these carbs become highly toxic to them. Starchy carbs = glucose spikes in the blood = insulin demand. High insulin levels = high IgF-1 levels and all the problems caused by this hormonal duo. See Appendix-33 *Lessons Learnt from the Laron Syndrome*. Remember, persistent high insulin levels will result in cells becoming "deaf" to this insulin prodding, thus ultimately leading to persistent insulin resistance (Del Prato, Leonetti et al. 1994). It is interesting how agriculture and food boards have such a huge impact on politics and then public "health" policy on food consumption, resulting in a deterioration in health. Dietetics needs to wake up, stop being influenced by corporations, and only concern themselves with population health.

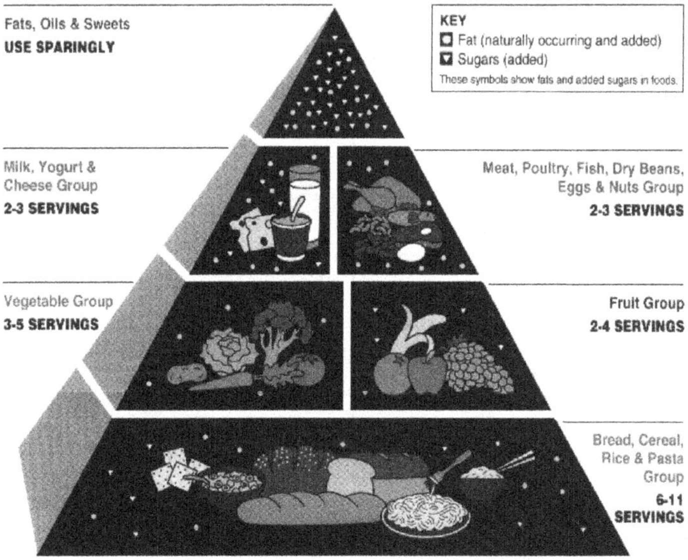

Appendix-39: The DASH Diet: Recommendations & Flaws

A US government body created the DASH Diet. Hence, they have to be mindful of farming or food boards. Notice the emphasis on grains, meat, vegetable oils, sugar products and dairy. We want to go beyond these staples that have caused so much harm. None of them are essential. Only nutrients matter!

Source NHLBI – US NIH For a 2000 Calorie diet	
DASH Components	Improvements
Grains: 6 – 8 servings **Vegetables**: 4 – 5 servings **Fruits**: 4 – 5 servings **Low-Fat Dairy**: 2 – 3 servings **Lean meats, Poultry, Fish**: 6 or less **Nuts, Seeds, Legumes:** 4 – 5 servings **Fats & Oils:** – 2-3 servings– soft margarine, vegetable oils, mayonnaise, safflower oil **Sweets and added sugars**: – 5 or less	• Notice the number of grains. High glycaemic loads (high-GL) • Not enough vegetables 7 – 10 ideal • Too many serves of fruits – high fructose loads in already energy-lowered cells • Why meat when forests are being cleared for cattle? The risk of meat and colorectal cancer. Plant-based sources of protein are far healthier for us and the planet. • Legumes need to be limited due to a high glycaemic load (lots of starch and glucose elevation after eating, causing insulin levels to rise and increasing insulin demand on beta cells) • High Omega-6 intakes in vegetable oils are not recommended. • Notice the sweets allowed. Sugar is 50:50 glucose + fructose, so not a good idea with energy-starved cells.

Appendix-40: Exercise

Aim for a mix of aerobic fitness and, importantly, muscle strength. Concentrating on aerobic exercise will allow muscle loss (sarcopenia) to progress throughout our lives. It needs to be a combination. Please check with your doctor before beginning any exercise program. If you are new to resistance training, seeing an Exercise Physiologist is your bet to get you doing this safely.

Always warm up with a treadmill first, and when using weights, "pyramid-up". In other words, slowly increase the weight to the muscle exhaustion point where you cannot do another rep. Aim for 12 reps to exhaustion if you can. I suggest doing a total body workout at least once a week, or if you like gyms, then doing the lower half one day and the other half another – a split routine. A total body workout that is done just once a week is fine. The Big-5 works for all the major muscle groups, and you can add more targeted exercises for your biceps, triceps, Quad, shoulders, hamstrings, etc.

Along with this gym component (home or commercial), do some brisk walking and, if possible, intersperse this walking with brief yet fast runs a few times a week. Use Essential Amino Acids (EAAs) during and after a workout. Muscles can't grow without amino acids. Discuss exercise with your doctor and get help from an Exercise Physiologist. Check out the prediabetes chapter.

The Big-5	Exercise	Muscles worked
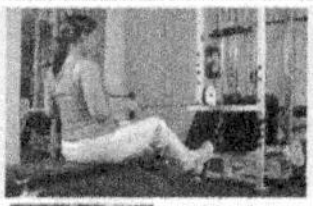	Seated row	Forearms, biceps, triceps, lattisimus dorsi, the rhomboids, paravertebral muscles, core muscles
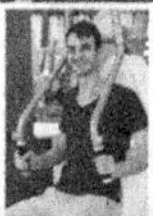	Chest press	Pectoral muscles, deltoids (shoulder), forearms, biceps, triceps
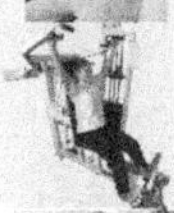	Overhead press	Shoulders, with strong involvement by the triceps and pectoral (chest) muscles, core muscles (stabilization)
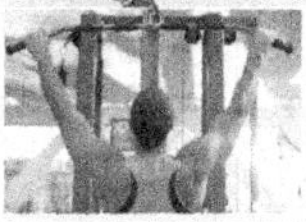	Pulldown	Upper back, pectoral, forearms, biceps, triceps, shoulders , core muscles (stabilization)
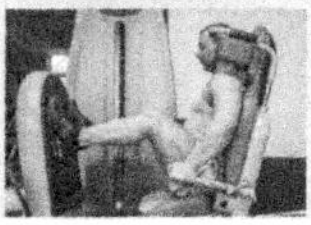	Leg Press	The lower body from waist and lower back to ankles, strong activation of buttocks, quadriceps, hamstrings, calves, core

Appendix-41: Vitamin-C, Scurvy and the Haptogobin (HP-2-2) Genetic Variant

In humans, a weaker form of the haptoglobin gene exists, producing the HP 2-2 version with less binding capacity for free haemoglobin after haemolysis (rupture) of red blood cells. Red blood cells have a half-life of around 120 days and are recycled, releasing free haemoglobin. Doctors and dietitians need to be aware that a huge 35% of the white population and over 50% of South and East Asians have this weaker HP 2-2 version that can predispose them to have subclinical or clinical scurvy in times of oxidative stress (Delanghe, Langlois et al. 2007). Insulin resistance is associated with significant oxidative stress in the background. Suppose an effective haptoglobin molecule does not mop up free haemoglobin, preferably HP 1-1; heme iron will be exposed after RBC rupture and subject to oxidation, just like iron rusts if exposed to the elements. The iron will then undergo reduction (gains an electron) by Vitamin-C from Fe3+ to Fe2+, leading to the creation of highly reactive hydroxyl radicals, which, in turn, leads to a rapid decrease of Vitamin-C in the body, as Vitamin-C is consumed in its antioxidant role. With HP 2-2, more free haemoglobin will be present, exposing more iron to oxidation. With chronic leg ulcers needing Vitamin-C to heal, we must consider this mutation. Vitamin-C and other vitamins and minerals are critical for tissue repair and collagen production. Scurvy is not uncommon in the 21st Century, contrary to popular belief.

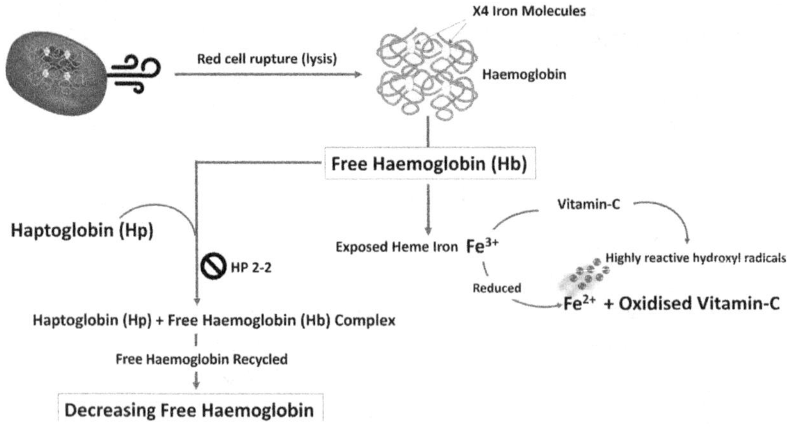

Bibliography

The bibliography for Cell Shock is very extensive and will increase the word count considerably, thus increasing the cost of the book. For this reason, I have added the bibliography to my website's blog area. The advantage is that hyperlinks make it easy to jump to a website reference or, if desired, copy and paste the article into a search engine to find and look up the original article.

To access this bibliography online, please follow these steps:

1. Go to www.a8h.com.au
2. Look for "Blogs" on this website and click on it
3. In the Blog's search box, type in "Cell Shock Bibliography."

For constructive comments or respectful feedback, please don't hesitate to get in touch with Dr Rodney Lopez through this email: admin@a8h.com.au

Index

"

"Normal" Ranges · 126
"Tap" and "Sponge" analogy · 114

3

3M factory · 105

4

40 kg of ATP · 251

8

80% of ATP consumption in the brain · 226

A

ACCORD study · 201
Aconitase · 277
AETT · 108
Agave syrup · 315
Aldous Huxley · 9
allostatic loads · 407
Alzheimer's Disease (AD) · 205
Amara Strande · 105
amyloid · 207
Anaerobic glycolysis · 218
Animal Flesh · 172
antioxidants · 175
apoE4 · 206
Arkansas Diet Manual · 276
Astrocyte-Neuron Lactate Shuttle · 218
Astrocytes · 218
ATP Synthase · 269

B

back pain · 227
balloon and conveyor belt analogy · 189
Barker Hypothesis · 145
Benjamin Franklin · 9
Beta-amyloid · 211
BIG-10 Womb-to-Tomb List · 154
Bioenergetics · 254
Bowel cancer · 172
brain microbiome · 211

C

Carb cheating · 418
CARMA study · 131
Cartesian Divide · *See* Dualism
Cell Starvation Model (CSM) · 233
Choline · 316
choline and betaine 81% lower visceral fat · 317
Chrononutrition · 415
chrononutrition effect · 156
citrate synthase · 277
Cogito ergo sum · *See* Dualism

continuing professional development (CPD/CME) · 397
COVID-19 · 290
COX-2 inhibitors · 204
crisis signalling · 292
CTEP inhibitor · 364
Cytokines, pro and anti-inflammatory · 374

D

Dairy · 169
Dark Waters · 106
DASH diet · 378
Dietitians Association of Australia (DAA) · 390
Dr. Mark Hyman · 101
Dualism · 76

E

EAAs 15 grams maximum · 460
Eat Like the Animals · 456
Eggs · 168
Electron Transport Chain (ETC) · 266
Endocalyx™ · 210
endometriosis · 429
endothelium · 198
Environmental toxic impacts · 176
Epigenetic mitochondrial programming · 176
essential amino acids (EAAs) · 458
Every Patient Tells a Story" Lisa Sanders · 242

F

$FADH_2$ · 266
Fasting insulin · 132
fatty liver · 184
ferritin · 278
Finding early risk · 91
Forward-looking infrared (FLIR) · 92
fragrances · 108
Framingham Study · 347
fructose 50% to 80% lower ATP in hepatocytes · 296
fructose 7 – 10 times more glycating · 313
fructose 80% of ATP depletion in 5 minutes · 297
fructose 90% lower liver protein synthesis · 296
fructose, 200% increase ROS · 303
fructose, a weapon of mass destruction · 297

G

GDM developing diabetes · 289
gene silencing · 303
Genome-wide association studies (GWAS) · 103
gestational diabetes mellitus · 145
Glial cells · 218
Glucose Hypothesis · 137
Glucose to Fructose in the brain · 152
glycated LDL (gLDL) · 355
glycocalyx · 210
Glycocalyx · 92
GORD/GERD · 280
Gordian's Knot · 81

grand unified theory · 209
Guardian Angels, Ketones · 424

H

haemoglobin · 279
HbA1c · 215
heme iron · 172
Hidden Hunger · 248
Hippocrasy
How Doctors Are Betraying Their Oath · 182
hormone disrupters · 105
hydrotrope · *See* ATP
hyperinsulinaemia · 216
Hypertension · 197

I

ILLUMINATE CTEP trial · 365
Index · 522
Inflammation · 202
insulin · 259
Iron deficiency · 273
iron-sulphur (Fe-S) complexes · 277
isocitric dehydrogenase · 277

K

ketogenic diet · See Mental Health
ketone bodies · 422
Krebs Cycle, · 277

L

lactate · 218
Laron Syndrome · 270
L-Citrulline · 205
LDL Paradox · 353
Lipid Hypothesis · 137
lipoproteins · 346
low carbohydrate diet (LCD) · 214
Lyon Diet Heart Study · 229

M

magnesium deficiency · 252
magnesium-ATP (Mg-ATP) · 252
Magnetic Resonance Spectroscopy · 243
Mark Ruffalo · 106
menopausal transition · 425
Metabolic Dysfunction-Associated Steatotic Liver Disease (MASLD) · 308
Metabolic memory · 142
Metabolic Psychiatry · 219
Metabolic Singularity · 82
metabolic switch, menopause · 426
Metabolomics · 89
MetS · 85
Microcirculation Armageddon · 223
Microcirculation, 60% - 70% of oxygen supply · 275
micronutrient insufficiencies and deficiencies · 173
microplastics · 105
microvascular density · 195
Microvascular disease (MVD) · 190
MIND diet · 219, 379

mitochondria transplants · 89
mitochondrial DNA (mtDNA) · 255
Mitochondrial handicaps · 241
mitochondrial overheating · 257
mitochondrial transplants · 89
Molecular Velcro · 142
Multiple continuums · 87
multivitamin · 269

N

NAD$^+$/NADH redox couple · 159
NAD+/NADH Redox Pair · 257
NADH · 266
neurodegeneration · 209
Nitric Oxide (NO) · 205
nonalcoholic steatohepatitis (NASH) · 308
Non-Essential Amino Acids (NEAAs) · 458
Nutrient overload (nutri-stress) · 159
Nutrient-Rescue · 414
Nutritional Ketosis · 414

O

Obesity Continuum · 97
one teaspoon EAAs 3.5x protein synthesis · 463
Oral Glucose Tolerance Test (OGTT) · 147
overfat · 297
oxidised LDL (ox-LDL) · 357
OXPHOS · 254

P

Pain Hustlers · 393
PCOS · 429
PFAS · 106
phosphate · 323
phosphoglycerate kinase 1 (PGK1) · 210
phytochemicals · 175
Planck's Principle · 242
PM2.5 micron particles · 104
Poiseuille's Law · 196
polymath specialists · 384
polyol pathway · 312
Postprandial (after-eating) effects · 155
Prediabetes · 178
PREDIMED study · 371
pre-disease continuum · 185
Pre-disease continuum · 182
Prions · 211
Professor Anthony Linnane · 254
Professor Ed Bullmore · 77
Professor Edwin Gale · 136
Professor John Yudkin · 299
Professor Lisa Sanders · 242
Professor Marion Nestle · 120
Professor Robert Lustig · 300
Professor S Sethi · 219
protein decoys · 456
Protein Leverage · 456
Protein-Energy Malnutrition (PEM) · 249
Proton Pump Inhibitors (PPI) · 279
pseudogene · 303
Pure, White and Deadly · 298

Q

Quintile-Climb · 128

R

Reactive Nitrogen Species (RNS). · 256
Reactive Oxygen Species (ROS) · 256
relative risk reduction (RRR) · 368
René Descartes · *See* Dualism
Rosetta Stone · 233

S

Scandinavian Simvastatin Survival Study (4S) · *See* Lyon Diet Heart Study
scientific reductionism · 82
Second Law of Thermodynamics · 72
Selenium · 451
selfish super-systems · 286
Serotonin Hypothesis · 453
small dense LDL (sdLDL) · 356
soluble transferrin receptor (sTfR) · 279
speaker programs · 394
succinate dehydrogenase · 277
Sugar taxes · 247
supplements · 436

T

Terazosin · 210
The exploding worldwide cancer burden · 109
Thomas Kuhn · 111
Thrifty Gene · 304
Tik-Tock · 196
Toxic breakfasts · 315
Toxic wounds · 103
Type-B LDL pattern · 356

U

Uric acid · 228
uricase gene · 301

V

vascular steal syndrome · 225
VCAM-1 · 198
visceral fat · 309
Vitamin-A · 450
Vitamin-B6 (Pyroxidine) · 447
Vitamin-C · 306
Vitamin-D · 290
Vitamins A, D, E, and K · 449
Vit-C HP-2-2 genetic variant · 361
VLDLs · 316

W

Warburg effect · 305

Α

α-Hydroxybutyrate · 404

ABOUT THE AUTHOR

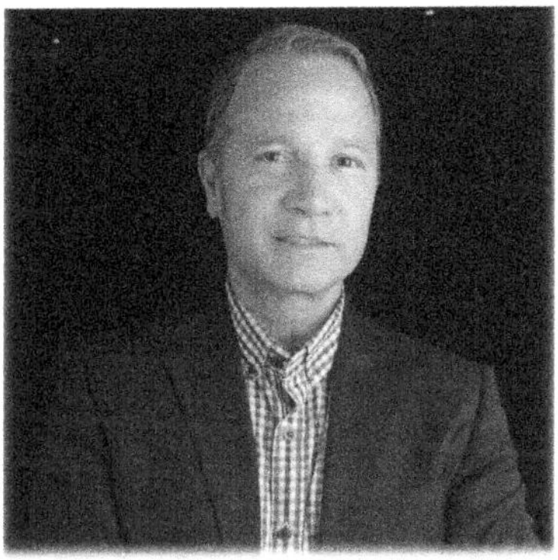

Dr Rodney Lopez is a Sydney University medical graduate. Prior to undergraduate medical studies, he was a fully qualified laboratory technician working at the ICPMR and then for Westmead Hospital, performing laboratory tests for the Accident & Emergency Department and the wards. As dux (Cum Laude) of his HSC year, he was accepted into the Faculty of Medicine at Sydney University while still working in the labs. Disillusioned by the fact that patients were never cured of metabolic diseases that dominated medicine, he went on to postgraduate study in clinical nutrition through RMIT University (Melbourne) and recently became a Fellow of the Australasian Society of Lifestyle Medicine (FASLM) after finishing exams at the American College of Lifestyle Medicine (ACLM). He had to build his clinical nutrition framework through meticulous study and then find a way to incorporate that understanding into a drug-centric medical world where both doctors and patients seemed oblivious to the critical role of powerful nutritional impacts on disease causation, prevention, or aggravation.

Dr Lopez works part-time in Mosman, a harbourside suburb of Sydney, and his passion is to use his in-depth knowledge of medicine and clinical nutrition to connect the dots for individuals struggling with metabolic disease or mental health problems that are never cured by conventional means and where these problems only seem to get worse with traditional models of management. Contact me through E: **admin@a8h.com.au**.

Made in the USA
Monee, IL
05 November 2026

67806918R00292